ANTICANCER LIVING

Lorenzo Cohen, PhD, is the Richard E. Haynes Distinguished Professor in Clinical Prevention and director of the Integrative Medicine Program at the University of Texas MD Anderson Cancer Center in Houston. He is the former vice chair of the Academic Consortium for Integrative Medicine and Health and is a founding member and past president of the Society for Integrative Oncology. Dr. Cohen has published more than 125 scientific articles in top medical journals and has edited two books on integrative medicine for cancer care.

Alison Jeffries, MEd, has worked extensively as an educator. She is a former president of the MD Anderson Cancer Center Faculty and Family Organization and works closely with Lorenzo Cohen to foster health and wellness in individuals and their communities.

Cohen and Jeffries live in Houston with their three children.

●　●　●

Praise for *Anticancer Living*

"The health care revolution continues with a great new book. . . . A valuable resource that presents an accessible, science-based approach to wellness."
—Andrew Weil, MD

"An invaluable guide for both professionals in the health field and the general public . . . Written by authors with impeccable credentials."
—Deepak Chopra, MD

"*Anticancer Living* will empower millions of people with information they can use to reduce their risk of getting cancer and improve their chances of surviving a cancer diagnosis. Highly recommended!"
—Dean Ornish, MD, author of *The Spectrum*

"*Anticancer Living* . . . blends expert insight, practical experience, deep compassion, and clear writing to produce a formula that can change lives—and save them. This is an important, empowering book."
—David L. Katz, MD, author of *Disease-Proof*

"*Anticancer Living* is an excellent resource that outlines the types of health behaviors that can reduce cancer risk and also improve the quality of life of those undergoing cancer therapy."
—David S. Rosenthal, MD, former president of the American Cancer Society

"It should be required reading—not only for laypeople, but for physicians too."
—Neal D. Barnard, MD, author of *Dr. Neal Barnard's Program for Reversing Diabetes*

"Adults and children, men and women can benefit by applying the sound advice and easy to follow guidelines presented by Cohen and Jefferies."
—Margaret I. Cuomo, MD, author of *A World Without Cancer*

"*Anticancer Living* presents scientific evidence that changing the way we live can reduce deaths from cancer and other major diseases. It shows us how to go about altering our lifestyles in order to achieve this goal and feel better every day. This much-needed book provides a prescription for better health, from experienced professionals who want passionately to help you improve your life."
—John Mendelsohn, MD, former president of the MD Anderson Cancer Center

"Lorenzo Cohen and Alison Jefferies are picking up the mantle from the late David Servan-Schreiber, and not a moment too soon! This book promises to be an important guide to reducing the risk of recurrence of cancer and the risk of getting it in the first place."
—Susan M. Love, MD, MBA, author of *Dr. Susan Love's Breast Book*

"The cheapest, most effective form of health care is not getting sick in the first place. For cancer patients and anyone seeking to avoid a future cancer diagnosis, this book will be a bible providing a practical, achievable path toward an anticancer lifestyle." —Gary Hirshberg, chairman and cofounder of Stonyfield Farm

"I thoroughly believe in the Cohen/Jefferies approach to prevention and healing and I think this is an important book for all people to read."
—Yogrishi Swami Ramdev

"My brother's book, *Anticancer*, has already helped millions of patients around the world. *Anticancer Living* discusses the latest research, shares inspirational stories, and gives us practical advice. This is an indispensable book for all of us."
—Franklin Servan-Schreiber

"It is not hyperbole to state that there is a desperate need for this book. An astonishing number of Americans will be diagnosed with cancer during their lifetimes. Dollars spent on cancer research are devoted primarily to treatment and cure—or, to use an image from this book, 'mopping up' once a cancer diagnosis has been made. *Anticancer Living* provides a concrete, evidence-based guide to 'turning off the tap'—lowering inflammation in order to prevent cancer in the first place."
—Meg Cadoux Hirshberg, founder of the Anticancer Lifestyle Foundation

"A must-read for those caring for cancer patients as well as patients themselves who will find it informative and inspirational." —*Houston Medical Journal*

"[Cohen and Jefferies] offer some fresh perspectives and evidence . . . These are basic, sustainable, synergistic lifestyle adjustments that can reframe how we deal with cancer at any stage, including prevention. . . . It may save your life."
—*Galveston County Daily News*

Anti
cancer
Living

Transform Your Life and Health
with the Mix of Six

LORENZO COHEN, PhD
ALISON JEFFERIES, MEd

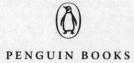

PENGUIN BOOKS

PENGUIN BOOKS
An imprint of Penguin Random House LLC
penguinrandomhouse.com

First published in the United States of America by Viking,
an imprint of Penguin Random House LLC, 2018
Published in Penguin Books 2019

ISBN 9780735220430 (paperback)

THE LIBRARY OF CONGRESS HAS CATALOGED THE
HARDCOVER EDITION AS FOLLOWS:
Names: Cohen, Lorenzo, author. | Jefferies, Alison, author.
Title: Anticancer living : transform your life and health with
the mix of six / Lorenzo Cohen PhD, Alison Jefferies.
Description: New York, New York : Viking, [2018] |
Identifiers: LCCN 2018013075 (print) | LCCN 2018013436 (ebook) |
ISBN 9780735220423 (ebook) | ISBN 9780735220416 (hardback)
Subjects: LCSH: Cancer—Prevention—Popular works. |
Self-care, Health—Popular works. | BISAC: HEALTH & FITNESS /
Diseases / Cancer. | HEALTH & FITNESS / Healthy Living. |
HEALTH & FITNESS / Healing.
Classification: LCC RC268 (ebook) | LCC RC268 .C62 2018 (print) |
DDC 616.99/4052—dc23
LC record available at https://lccn.loc.gov/2018013075

Printed in the United States of America
1   3   5   7   9   10   8   6   4   2

Set in Warnock Pro
Designed by Daniel Lagin

*To all cancer patients and survivors and to those who care for them.
You inspire us to live in the moment and lead purposeful lives.*

*With love and gratitude to our parents—Paola, Jon, Susan, and Robert—
who set us on our course; and to our children—Alessandro, Luca,
and Chiara—who keep us focused on the priorities of life.*

CONTENTS

Preface   ix

Introduction   xii

PART ONE
The Anticancer Age   1

CHAPTER ONE
The Anticancer Revolution   3

CHAPTER TWO
Our Healing Powers   17

CHAPTER THREE
What Causes Cancer, Anyway?   38

CHAPTER FOUR
A Cell's Quest for Immortality   46

CHAPTER FIVE
The Epigenetics of Prevention   59

CHAPTER SIX
Synergy and the Mix of Six   69

PART TWO
The Mix of Six   81

CHAPTER SEVEN
The Foundation Is Love and Social Support   83

CHAPTER EIGHT
Stress and Resilience   122

CHAPTER NINE
The Need for Rest and Recovery   162

CHAPTER TEN
Moving for Wellness   196

CHAPTER ELEVEN
Food as Medicine   221

CHAPTER TWELVE
The Environment and the Quest for Health   263

Concluding Thoughts   291

Appendix   301

Acknowledgments   329

Notes   335

Index   405

PREFACE

March 8, 2018 was the day Alison and I signed off on the final version of this book. It was ready for the printers. The next time we saw the book, it would be in its finished, printed form. It felt like the culmination of years of work—but we didn't get the chance to celebrate.

That same day, I went to the doctor's office to get a biopsy. Two weeks earlier, I had noticed a slight tingling pain in my left armpit during a morning yoga session. Over a short period of time, I found a swollen lymph node. As the node started to grow, I suspected something was not right. Moments after the biopsy was taken, an empathetic pathologist entered the room. I was still lying on the biopsy table, Alison sitting beside me. The pathologist told us she saw malignant cells in the sample. She could not determine what kind of malignant cells they were, but it was unmistakably clear—I had cancer.

It would take another five days to conduct a thorough pathology work-up to determine the source of the cells. The malignant cells, I was told, were melanoma. In that moment, I joined the one in two men and one in three women in the United States who will be diagnosed with cancer in their lifetime; and the legions of people being diagnosed with melanoma, one of the cancers on the rise.

The irony of getting cancer after studying and coauthoring a book on anticancer living is not lost on me. As the primary risk factor for melanoma is excess sun exposure in childhood, there is not much I could have done recently about the initiation of the disease due to my multiple sunburns as a child. Yet my subsequent lifestyle choices likely influenced the establishment of the disease.

I have tried to follow the tenets of anticancer living for the past ten years, but this has not always been the case. Also, effectively managing stress in my life and fostering calm has been a challenge. I am passionately devoted to my career in cancer research, and I have often driven myself far beyond what was healthy for my body. We now know that while diet and exercise are important, managing stress and healthy sleep habits are also crucial. I'm sure that my stress levels were far from optimum for my immune system.

After the initial shock of the news, Alison and I quickly sought to incorporate this new reality into our lives. Having a life-threatening illness can certainly be a wake-up call. After discussing all the conventional options with medical and surgical oncologists, as well as several medical colleagues, I started combination neoadjuvant immunotherapy. The collateral damage from the cancer treatment has been significant. From excruciating mouth sores to chronic dry mouth to hypothyroidism, these side effects have had a hugely detrimental effect on my day-to-day well-being. What has helped to alleviate the side effects from the conventional cancer treatment has been incorporating an integrative approach, such as specific foods and spices, acupuncture, energy work, exercise, various mind-body practices, and physical therapy.

After three courses of combination immunotherapy, my tumor had shrunk. In mid-June, I underwent an axillary lymph node dissection. The post-surgical pathological report showed that I was now classified as having no evidence of disease. As I responded well to the presurgical immunotherapy, I will continue the immunotherapy for one year.

Alison and I realize that having no evidence of disease does not mean it is okay to go back to my life as it was before. Melanoma is a cancer that is controlled through the immune system. In fact, it is one of the most immunogenic of all cancers. That is why the best way to control melanoma is through treatments that boost the immune system. This means that lifestyle factors such as stress, exercise, diet, social support, and sleep are all critically important, as each independently and synergistically influence immune function.

Cancer diagnosis and treatment can take us off the nicely paved highway and onto a more circuitous, bumpy road. How we navigate the trip down the bumpy road is where the journey's gifts are found. However, it also means making difficult choices on where we spend our limited time and energy. Having cancer has given me the permission to take care of myself in a way that I had never done before.

I now prioritize exercise and my mind-body practice on a daily basis, something that I did not consistently do before. In fact, I have now started a 200-hour yoga teacher certification course. I can honestly say that I have never felt healthier: physically, mentally, or spiritually. Although some might read this and feel sorry for me or see my diagnosis as a tragedy, I do not view it in this way. I feel fortunate to be in this good place. With that said, we welcome all your good thoughts, positive energy, and prayers. Love and support, after all, is the foundational pillar of anticancer living.

Although I knew that following the tenets we laid out in *Anticancer Living* were important to my health and well-being, having cancer puts the necessity of following the prescription in a different light. As we say in the book, "Anticancer living is built on a belief that self-care is health care and that greater wellness is available to us all." No matter where we are on the spectrum of anticancer living, we should always be striving to improve ourselves. It should not take a life-threatening illness for us to take care of ourselves and engage in our true purpose—we must remember that we always have the permission to take care of ourselves. As integrative medicine has helped me so much in the short time I have been dealing with cancer, I feel more dedicated than ever to continue the important work documenting how an integrative approach in cancer care is the key to controlling side effects and improving clinical outcomes. I look forward to continuing my research in integrative medicine and anticancer living and to have this approach become the standard of care for all.

My close colleague David Servan-Schreiber, author of *Anticancer: A New Way of Life*, shared his deeply personal cancer experience with the world. We saw how his relationship with cancer transformed his life and became his guide and teacher. Now I too have my own cancer experience that is unfolding. As so little time has passed between my diagnosis and the publication of the paperback version of *Anticancer Living: Transform Your Life and Health with the Mix of Six*, the content of the book has not changed and remains as it was before my diagnosis. But let's just say that the message is now more important to Alison and me than ever before.

INTRODUCTION

What if we could make basic, sustainable lifestyle adjustments that might push back the onset of cancer or even prevent us from ever getting it? What if those with cancer could change the way they live to reduce their risk of recurrence and improve their chances of living long, vibrant lives? What if the missing link to cancer prevention and treatment is not the next pill or the latest scientific breakthrough but the choices we make every day that influence our body's natural ability to maintain and restore balance and health? What if we could make changes in the way we live now, today, that would help us beat the odds, survive a diagnosis, or possibly remain cancer-free for life? I've devoted my career to trying to answer these questions.

We have reached a critical moment in terms of cancer research, treatment, and prevention. It is now clear from scientific research that how we live in our bodies, in our communities and the broader world—how we eat, sleep, work and play, manage stress and face life's challenges, create our support networks and make choices about our environments—has a profound effect on our health and wellness; and on cancer in particular.[1–9]

The work that forms the basis for this book was inspired in part by David Servan-Schreiber, author of *Anticancer: A New Way of Life* and a true pioneer in the quest to demonstrate the links between lifestyle and cancer.[10] Together, David and I designed and launched a pioneering study at MD Anderson Cancer Center in Houston, Texas, to better understand these deep connections and, most important, to develop research-based recommendations both for patients and for the ever-growing community of those concerned with prevention.[11]

My own work and David's had been running on parallel tracks for decades, but there was a significant difference between us: David was living with a brain tumor, diagnosed at the age of thirty-one. David's original cancer had been treated "successfully" with surgery, but it had returned five years later, and the prognosis was not good. The average survival time for this kind of recurrence is typically twelve to eighteen months, with five years considered to be the maximum. David had no choice but to undergo another risky surgery, followed by a year of chemotherapy and radiation.

This marked the start of his journey to the work that emerged in book form as *Anticancer: A New Way of Life*. As the title suggests, for David this became a new way of living—with cancer. David made a deeply felt and very personal decision to listen to his body, to learn to tune in to its signals with a different kind of attention, and to trust its guidance. He amassed all the scientific evidence available at the time and used this to help guide his life style choices. He became curious to the point of obsession about how our daily actions and choices affect what he called the cancer "terrain"—our genetic, cellular, and regulatory systems. He became interested in how he might influence his own biology in ways that would enhance his immunity, decrease inflammation, and suppress the tendency of cancer cells to proliferate, while simultaneously improving his quality of life. He quickly discovered that with each lifestyle improvement he made, he felt better, healthier, and more present—not just in body, but also in mind and spirit.

David set out to answer this question: Does how we live—the quality of our relationships, what we eat, how we care for ourselves—determine cancer's progress? He dedicated the rest of his life to understanding how our finely engineered bodies can sustain health, even in the presence of cancer. He wanted to find out if we could modify how we behave in our daily lives to prevent cancer, prolong remission, or simply improve and extend a cancer patient's life. In fact, after making some of these adjustments himself, he led a rich and productive life for another nineteen years, outliving his statistical prognosis by a factor of four.

In 2009, following the publication of his book *Anticancer*, David and I hatched a plan to raise money for a clinical trial to examine the effects of comprehensive lifestyle change on survival and quality of life for cancer patients. David was instrumental in helping us design the early phase of our Comprehensive Lifestyle Study, a study of women with stage II and III breast cancer, which is now fully under way and ongoing here in Houston. Formal data will be available once the study is completed, but we are already seeing profound transformations in the lives of the study participants. They are truly the inspiration for this book. I also find inspiration in the broader community of patients, doctors, care providers, researchers, and scientists, all of whom are adding to the literature on how lifestyle heals.

The publication of *Anticancer Living* coincides with the tenth anniversary of *Anticancer*'s initial publication—and is in part a celebration of David's achievement and clear evidence of how far we've come. A decade later, it's undeniable that lifestyle should be as vital a component of comprehensive cancer treatment as traditional frontline medical treatments such as surgery, chemotherapy, radiation, immunotherapy, and new targeted therapies. In fact, the pace at which new scientific evidence is connecting the dots between lifestyle factors and cancer progression and recovery is accelerating. It is, we are discovering, the synergy of both specialized medical treatment and lifestyle changes that offers cancer patients the best outcomes. But what the anticancer community has been wanting is a complete and simple plan for living the "anticancer life." This book is intended as a road map toward the journey ahead, how we as individuals can work in tandem with the scientific community and doctors to support our own health even as new discoveries are being made. Mounting research suggests a clear link between lifestyle and wellness, and we will share the scientific evidence alongside the stories of cancer survivors to help bring that science to life. While each person's journey is unique, we believe the cumulative impact points to a clear path forward.

Part 1 of this book outlines the cancer landscape and sets the stage for the role each of us can have in our own health, whether or not we have cancer. Each chapter in part 2 presents the latest research, inspiring stories and testimonials, and ends with evidence-based recommendations for adopting the six pillars of anticancer living. The key takeaway is this: Our daily choices in life have a direct, measurable impact on cancer and other chronic diseases. If that seems daunting or discouraging at first, we hope you will come to embrace your role in this discovery and understand it as truly empowering. Each of us can reduce our cancer risk and increase our chances of surviving a diagnosis. This book is our effort to share and spread this message and to provide you and the ones you love with a step-by-step plan to maintain and foster your health.

Cancer does not grow in isolation. It develops within an environment we help create by the things we eat day after day, by our stress levels, our physical activity, our support network, the quality of our sleep, and our exposure to environmental toxins. We have chosen to focus on what we have identified as the six most crucial areas and how they work together synergistically. Taken together, these lifestyle factors, which we call the "Mix of Six," have the capacity to impact our risk of disease and our chances of survival after a diagnosis.

With Alison Jefferies, my wife, coauthor, and full partner in devising a forward-looking plan for *Anticancer Living*, I aim to present a comprehensive plan based on scientific evidence, for lifestyle changes that improve health, reduce cancer risk, and help to control disease. Alison has the remarkable energy and drive to implement in the daily life of our family many of the changes I've been studying for years. After a long career as an educator, she is uniquely adept at trying new ways to foster anticancer living, both in our home, in our community, and as a co-presenter of this material at talks we give across the United States. If I can make a convincing case that lifestyle choices really do have a biological impact on cancer risk and our chances of surviving a diagnosis, Alison can show us how to make changes in our own lives that will improve our own health and the health and outlook of our loved ones.

Together, we have created a supportive system that will help you put into effect the message that David Servan-Schreiber gave us so compellingly in *Anticancer*. The purpose of this book is to educate all of those currently dealing with a cancer diagnosis as well as those who have, so far, been fortunate enough to avoid cancer, to show how changing daily habits can bring enormous health benefits, and to demonstrate that increasing the odds of disease prevention is available to all of us if we begin to view our lifestyle choices as health choices.[12,13] Anticancer living is a low-cost option that has the potential to dramatically impact health without any harmful side effects. Yet, its benefits may be priceless.

It is my wish that this book embolden and inspire, if for no other reason than we might spend our days feeling healthier and happier, stronger, more resilient, and better supported in an ever-more-challenging world. Anticancer living is built on a belief that *self-care is health care* and that greater wellness is available to us all. Those who have shared their stories in this book and countless others are real-life examples of this. Actively engaging in the protection and promotion of our own health is potent medicine that can and will bring immeasurable joy, as well as the empowering feeling that we are taking some measure of control over our health and well-being.

I thought of David often as Alison and I worked on this book. He was a remarkable friend and colleague who lived the anticancer life eloquently and powerfully. His work and his example have inspired so many of us not just to survive but to thrive. And it's been extremely gratifying to share the ever-increasing body of scientific evidence that validates and reinforces David's central message—that it is within our power to reduce our risk of cancer or improve our chances of surviving a cancer diagnosis by changing the way we live. Now, more than ever, it is vital that we all take this message to heart.

PART ONE

• • • • • •

The Anticancer Age

CHAPTER ONE

The Anticancer Revolution

As director of the Integrative Medicine Program at MD Anderson Cancer Center in Houston, I have spent much of my career working to incorporate evidence-based, unconventional treatment modalities and lifestyle changes into the medical community's thinking and alongside conventional practices. As more research has emerged showing a clear link between our mental and physical state and lifestyle factors and our ability to avoid and survive cancer and other diseases, even the more skeptical within the medical community have begun to take notice. Over the years, more times than I can count, cancer doctors across all disciplines have confided in me that they have long suspected that their patients' mental state and lifestyle plays an important role in their ability to survive a cancer diagnosis and restore themselves to wellness. What is becoming increasingly evident based on solid science and our improved ability to measure and document the biological effects of lifestyle changes is this: comprehensive lifestyle change, combined with conventional cancer care, is powerful medicine that can help control, and potentially prevent, cancer.[1–3]

Living with Cancer

Once, a cancer diagnosis was basically a death sentence. Although it could, with a lot of medical might, be beaten back, it would rarely be defeated. Over the past couple of decades, however, this has begun to change. Cancer is now, for many, considered a serious, chronic disease. What this means in practical terms is that more people are living longer with cancer.[4] And this is very good news. But survival raises new questions: Are these people who are living longer with cancer feeling better—healthy and well—even if they are not cured?

Some oncologists might wonder why, if the patient is surviving, this question is relevant at all. In my area of expertise, the world of integrative medicine, this question is everything. I spend my workdays helping cancer patients make choices so that they will feel healthy—even as they undergo difficult, sometimes debilitating, treatments—because it's precisely these lifestyle changes that will also increase their odds of survival. And while I focus on their quality of life, my colleagues continue to better understand how cancer cells work, guiding the move from a one-size-fits-all approach to more nuanced, personal treatment. Much of this shift from a "hit it hard and fast" mind-set to more of what is being called "precision medicine" is due to the relatively recent breakthroughs we've made in understanding how our genes and cells work.[5] We're also developing and harnessing technologies that allow us to detect many cancers earlier—and the earlier a cancer is found, the better the prognosis and treatment outcome.[4]

These innovations are incredibly important, and alongside these ad-vancements are exciting discoveries being made not by scientists in labs or surgeons in operating room suites but by regular people in their kitchens and homes; on jogging trails; and in grocery stores, yoga studios, gyms, and wellness centers. Everyday lifestyle choices give us a surprising amount of control and influence over the trajectory of a cancer diagnosis and of our cancer risk. By making simple changes to the way we live, we can diminish the side effects of conventional cancer treatments, extend (and sometimes shatter) expected survival rates, decrease the chance for recurrence of dis-ease, and potentially prevent the onset of cancer diseases in the first place.[1,6–9] It's an exciting time to be in the realm of integrative care, but it took us a very long time to reach this point, and it's taking even longer to get the word out that lifestyle change is legitimate, effective medicine to help prevent and control cancer.

Are the Odds Really Stacked Against Us?

During the last fifty years, tremendous advances have been made in front-line treatments such as surgery, chemotherapy, and radiation therapy. These treatments, along with the innovative developments in targeted therapies (aimed at the abnormal proteins controlling cancer growth) and immunotherapy, have saved or prolonged the lives of millions of people.[4] In fact, our success rate at keeping people alive after a cancer diagnosis is better than ever.[4]

Yet despite these medical advances, nearly 1.7 million Americans are projected to receive a cancer diagnosis in 2017.[4] During that same twelve-month period, cancer will claim the lives of more than six hundred thousand people in the United States.[4] Around the world, cancer remains a leading cause of death, and new cases are expected to increase by 70 percent in the next two decades.[10] In 2015, the disease took the lives of 8.8 million people globally.[10]

Based on current models, one-third of all American women and half of all American men will receive a cancer diagnosis in their lifetimes.[4] Worldwide, nearly one out of every six deaths is due to cancer.[10] This means that the odds are extremely high that both you and I will one day join the more than 15.5 million Americans who are currently living with cancer and the tens of millions of cancer survivors around the world.[11]

Given these staggering numbers, it's unlikely that we'll eliminate cancer anytime soon, though this will not stop us from trying. Also unlikely is the discovery of one drug or treatment—a magic bullet—that will eradicate this increasingly complex range of diseases. What is more likely—as we are beginning to see now—is that we'll continue to understand how cancer cells respond to various stimuli and learn to slow or "turn off" their progression. Similarly, we hope to better understand the processes that trigger cancer's growth and target them with effective treatment. We're already seeing compelling evidence that lifestyle factors may be the missing ingredient of the existing cancer treatment model.

Cancer, first and foremost, is a disease of aging: Our odds of getting most cancers rises significantly each decade we live past the age of fifty.[12] This puts us in a bit of quandary, since we are—thanks in no small part to modern medicine—living longer and longer lives. The onset of diseases such as cancer adds a terrible burden to the already great challenges of aging, as our cells become more vulnerable to damage and corruption.

Although most cancers strike when we're older, there are some types (including colorectal and breast cancers) that are striking people at increasingly younger ages, and these cancers are often quite aggressive and fiercely resistant to treatment. In fact, recent data suggest that younger people are not only being diagnosed with colon cancer more than ever before but also dying of the disease in higher and higher numbers.[13] Some childhood cancers are also on the rise.[11]

So far, the medical establishment's response to the uptick appearing in the young has been to call for earlier screening, which is, of course, a prudent place to start. But early detection, we've found, isn't always the best or only answer. There are instances of early detection with some cancers, such as early-stage, low-grade prostate cancer and very-early-stage breast cancer, that lead to overtreatment with no demonstrable survival benefits.[14,15] In fact, the current recommendations have changed from "all men over fifty need to be screened to prostate cancer" to "all men over fifty should have a conversation with their physician about prostate screening." Could there, then, be a better way to prevent or delay the onset of cancers, including the aggressive types that seem to strike people so young? I believe the answer is yes.

Current cancer statistics can be sobering, even frightening, but the larger picture offers good news. There has been a positive, almost radical shift in cancer survival rates. Fifty years ago, only one in four Americans survived cancer for more than a decade; today that ratio is one in two—a doubling in overall survival rates. Is this because treatments and technologies have improved? In part, yes. Absolutely. But now we're beginning to understand that medical advances are not the only reason for improved outcomes.

Still, it is the unpredictable nature of cancer that often makes us feel powerless. Despite all we know of the disease and all the money that has gone into research and treatment, cancer has a way of defying our expectations and striking those who seem least likely candidates for a diagnosis. There is the singer who never smoked a day in her life who is diagnosed with lung cancer. Or the vegan runner who has been lean and fit his whole life and prides himself on his "clean" diet, only to be diagnosed young with stage IV colon cancer. And, most cruelly, there is the very young child who must battle an aggressive form of leukemia before she even has the words to describe what it all feels like. Why is it, we can't help but wonder, that my body, anybody's body, would let this happen? What could trigger such an awful disease within us?

It is perfectly normal to run the gauntlet of these thoughts and feelings and ask ourselves all these questions, but it is even more important that we don't beat ourselves up or blame or shame ourselves into resignation or passivity. Meg Hirshberg is a friend, breast cancer survivor, and the founder of the Anticancer Lifestyle Program, a nonprofit, evidence-based lifestyle program for people diagnosed with cancer. She recently spoke to me about why it's so important to resist blaming yourself if you get cancer: "Our message is always, 'Begin now. Don't look back. We have no idea what caused your cancer and we never will. But we do know that there are things you can do differently that will make a radical difference in how you feel. There is also scientific evidence that shows how these lifestyle changes will positively influence the results of your treatment.'" For Meg and the people who go through her program, this forward focus is accompanied by active education about the healing power of making lifestyle changes and the healing benefits of a loving community. As she continues, "Knowledge is power and, where cancer is concerned, knowledge has the power to enable survivors to lower the odds of cancer recurrence. There is data to back this up and we want to share that science with our community in ways that make people feel more hopeful, more powerful, more inspired, and more alive."

Where Cancer Is Concerned, Daily Choices Count

At least 50 percent of cancer deaths could be prevented by making healthy lifestyle changes, and the percentage could be even higher.[1,9] Dr. David Katz, one of the leading authorities on lifestyle change and founder of True Health Initiative, believes that as much as 80 percent of chronic disease and premature death could be prevented by healthy living.[16–18] A 2016 study by Harvard researchers who reviewed data from more than 135,000 people they have been following for more than forty years found that not smoking, drinking in moderation, maintaining a healthy weight, and exercising regularly could prevent 41 percent of cancer cases and 59 percent of cancer deaths in women and two-thirds of cases and deaths in men.[19] The exact percentages may vary from study to study, but the consistent message is that we can prevent at least half of cancers and cancer deaths. Graham Colditz, a professor of epidemiology and the coauthor of an editorial that accompanied the Harvard study, summed up the findings like this: "As a society, we need to avoid procrastination induced by thoughts that chance drives all cancer risk or that new medical discoveries are needed to make major gains against cancer, and instead we must embrace the opportunity to reduce our collective cancer toll by implementing effective prevention strategies and changing the way we live."[20]

While we continue to work toward increasing public awareness about the health dangers from behaviors and practices that have become so ingrained in Western culture, it is important to note that anticancer living is in no way at odds with standard medical care. David Servan-Schreiber understood that aggressive medical treatment was the "bull's-eye" of effective cancer treatment: He never considered forgoing surgery, chemotherapy, or radiation. In fact, with his first diagnosis, he dismissed any suggestions that he try "alternative" treatments at all. What mattered most to him was that the medical professionals he chose to work with related to him first and foremost as a human being, not simply as a host for cancer. He needed to trust that his doctors truly had his best interests at heart. As it turned out, this instinct was right on target. A commitment to living wholly as a human being rather than allowing himself to be limited by his diagnosis was foundational to his approach.

The Tobacco Lesson

Anyone who doubts the impact of lifestyle choices on our collective risk need only look back to what we learned in our not so distant past about the connections between lung cancer and smoking. In the early 1960s, a coalition of agencies, including the American Lung Association, the American Heart Association, the American Tuberculosis Association, and the American Public Health Association, pressed President John F. Kennedy to address the public health crisis being brought on by cigarette smoking. In 1962, Kennedy followed through and pulled together a broad alliance of experts who then spent two years combing through more than seven thousand scientific studies and articles.[21] In 1964, Surgeon General Luther L. Terry released the group's findings. The conclusion: Cigarette smoking was responsible for a 70 percent increase in mortality rates for smokers relative to nonsmokers. Since then, the tireless work by subsequent surgeons general, public health advocacy groups, and the activists behind successful, highly publicized lawsuits against tobacco companies has kept up public awareness of the causal link between tobacco (whether chewed or smoked) and cancer.[22] Yet it remains alarming that 15 percent of the U.S. population still smokes and that rates remain exceedingly high in many Asian, African, European, and

Middle Eastern countries.[23] Australia, which has smoking rates comparable to the United States, in an effort to reduce rates to zero will continually increase taxes on cigarettes through 2025, when they will cost up to forty dollars a pack.[24,25] The rule of thumb in the United States is that a 10 percent price increase on a pack of cigarettes results in anywhere from a 2.5 percent to a 5.0 percent overall decline in smoking, with most studies showing an average 4.0 percent drop.[25] In Russia, where cigarettes are much cheaper, 60 percent of men and almost 40 percent of the general population smoke.[26]

What's more, we have allowed the tobacco industry to reinvent itself with the advent of vaporized nicotine (vaping), bringing with it a slew of other chemicals that have not been adequately tested, including chemical compounds that have been linked with cancer.[27] So, although the rates of youth starting to smoke cigarettes have declined, teenagers are now turning to vaping (purportedly invented to help people quit smoking) as a new method of nicotine consumption.[28]

It also is worth noting that although the rates of lung cancer among American men have declined, the rates of lung cancer among American women—who began smoking publicly and freely much later than men—continued to rise through 2000 and have just recently started to decline slightly. Again, this is likely because lung, throat, esophageal, and other tobacco-related cancers are most common among the elderly, and so women who began smoking, say, during the 1960s and '70s, may just now be facing the cancer-related consequences. Unfortunately, tobacco is not the cause of just lung cancer but is now linked with fourteen different cancers.[29]

This recognition, that tobacco consumption—an avoidable (though addictive) behavior—is a direct cause of cancer, revolutionized the public's understanding of the links between behavior and disease. There was no longer any denying that our actions do matter, where cancer is concerned. This awareness launched the new field of cancer prevention, the search for other lifestyle or environmental factors connected to the onset of cancer.

Additionally, funding for cancer research began to increase, and it continues to pour in today. Yet—somewhat puzzlingly, if you think about it—the majority of these resources are invested in seeking cures. Funding for prevention research is dwarfed ten to one by the dollars invested in developing treatments and testing new drugs to thwart cancer.[30] I battle this discrepancy on a near-daily basis, despite how black-and-white the causal links between lifestyle factors and cancers may be. But the example of tobacco and lung cancer shows what can be accomplished when we put our minds and dollars toward the cause. What if we had the same level of public outcry against processed red meat (like bacon and hot dogs), which has been labeled as a carcinogen by the International Agency for Research on Cancer?[31] What if we had higher taxes on junk food and sugar-sweetened beverages? What if we had public service announcements warning against the excess consumption of sugar and processed foods, which have been tied to the obesity epidemic and a host of chronic diseases, including cancer?[32-34] We'd be living in a very different world.

We Are More Than Just Statistics

When diagnosed with a life-threatening illness, statistics and probabilities are a challenge not only to understand but also to know if and when they apply. David's work led him to challenge the statistical models of survival that most oncologists rely on to predict outcomes for their patients. How could columns of numbers account for all the very human variables that make up the unique and complex details of an individual's life? How could all the forces, the choices, of what we think of as "lifestyle," the gestures of our lives, *not* come into play when dealing with a cancer diagnosis? Never mind the intangibles, such as grit, the will to live, or faith in a higher power. What about diet and exercise? What about psychological aspects of wellness, such as hopefulness and gratitude? What about exposure to known carcinogens such as coal dust, asbestos, tobacco, or even the rays of the sun? David wanted to better understand all these factors. He craved a full, three-dimensional understanding of how lifestyle might affect cancer's ability to develop and grow.

This approach was, and still is, revolutionary. David embraced the fact that he had no choice but to learn to live well with cancer present in his body. What he modeled for us was a radical form of *acceptance*. He knew that cancer had become an integral part of him, and this acceptance empowered him to live with the illness powerfully and purposefully.

I don't know whether David lived his life with the goal of defying the odds and outliving his cancer the way he did, but I do know that he was instrumental in helping us understand how fluid these numbers can become when we decide to actively change the way we live with cancer.

In a chapter in *Anticancer* called "Escaping Statistics," David writes about the cancer experience of legendary scientist and writer Stephen Jay Gould, who was diagnosed at age forty with abdominal mesothelioma, a rare cancer that is linked to asbestos exposure. Gould immediately underwent surgery, but afterward, when he couldn't get a straight answer from the oncologist about his prognosis, he did what great scientists have always done: research. He learned that his type of cancer was considered "incurable" and that the median survival time was eight months from diagnosis.[35] He was stunned. He was also, fortunately, versed in how to read a bell curve. Gould noted that there wasn't much time for half of those who were diagnosed with mesothelioma (zero to eight months of life), so he focused his attention on the other side of that statistical bump. He saw that those who lived beyond the median (the middle figure in a set of numbers), the people to the right side of the curve, enjoyed a significant amount of breathing room, in terms of projected mortality. At the far end of the survival "tail," a person with mesothelioma could live three to four years. That was far better than eight months, and it would give him the time he needed to figure out how to improve those odds further. He was determined to become an outlier among outliers.[36]

Although naturally optimistic and curious, Gould acknowledged the dangers that statistics might pose for a cancer patient's state of mind. Impersonal data sets had the potential to seriously dampen a patient's attitude and outlook. In his essay, "The Median Isn't the Message," Gould wrote: "Attitude clearly matters in fighting cancer. We don't know why . . . but most people with the same cancer for age, class, health, socioeconomic status, and, in general, those with positive attitudes, with a strong will and purpose for living, a commitment to struggle, with an active response to aiding their own treatment and not just a passive acceptance of anything doctors say, tend to live longer."[36]

Gould exemplified this by living twenty years beyond his diagnosis. Both he and David Servan-Schreiber significantly exceeded the expected survival times for their (very different) types of cancer, and I feel certain that this was not just a stroke of luck or some random "miraculous" occurrence. Both studied the science and came to the same conclusion that I have reached: healthy lifestyle change is the key to preventing cancer and to extending the survival curve for every type of cancer.

Proactive Healing: Molly M.'s Anticancer Journey

Every summer, Alison and I take our family on an annual pilgrimage to a rustic cabin on an island in Georgian Bay, north of Toronto. The location, near the town of Perry Sound, is one of those magical summer places where we can connect with nature, escape our hectic lives, and leave all our troubles and cares behind—including our cell phones and our computers. The silent evenings are periodically interrupted by the call of loons on the glass-still water, and the whole area is perfumed by the scent of white pine and cedar. Over the years, we've become close friends with Molly M., a clear-eyed woman in her late fifties whose family has been spending their summers on the bay since the early 1900s. Molly is an avid outdoorswoman with an epic backstory. In her youth, after spending almost a year by herself on an island in the bay, she taught in the High Arctic and was the first woman to complete a 100-mile ski race. She knows the landscape like the back of her hand. For the past eighteen summers, we have shared meals, raced canoes, and watched sunsets on the reefs together.

Molly has survived for eighteen and a half years with glioblastoma multiforme, the most aggressive form of brain cancer—defined as terminal and incurable—the same kind of cancer that eventually took David Servan-Schreiber's life. In May 1999, when she was a forty-year-old high school science teacher, she began suffering from exhaustion, debilitating migraine headaches, vision issues, and other symptoms that she later found out were due to the brain tumor. One afternoon, after driving an hour to get home, she had a major seizure. When she went to the local hospital, they diagnosed her with a stroke and epilepsy but refused to provide the MRI she told them she needed. A month and several more seizures later, she saw a specialist in a large city hospital, had an MRI, and was diagnosed with a brain tumor that doctors wanted to remove immediately. She assumed her debilitating migraines would end, and she spent the night writing exam answers for a course she knew she wouldn't be there to mark. The resident sitting with her wept.

She didn't use the C-word for three months, but instead she set about finding the best facility to get radiotherapy. She hoped to return to teaching—a job she loved—but one after another doctor gently increased the recommended time off work from six months to a year to permanently. She was, after all, given a prognosis of six to eighteen months. Three brutal chemotherapy drugs followed the radiation, along with steroids.

When told she had six months to live, Molly told the nurses in the chemo clinic that she didn't know what she had been put on the earth to do. Their response: "You can be a miracle; miracles happen every day." Molly took that to heart and decided not to be a statistic. But then, almost exactly six months later, the cancer came back. Molly underwent a second surgery. She virtually walked out of this second surgery, unlike the first, and began a newly approved chemotherapy. She insisted on receiving the drug until "either I die or the cancer dies." At the same time, she started researching complementary treatments and worked with an herbalist who is an expert in cancer care. When I spoke to Molly recently, she reminded me that being forced out of teaching had not been easy. "I'd already had so much loss, having had several miscarriages. Never being able to have children, the kids at the school became my life. I hated leaving them, forced out by the seizures and cancer, especially when I felt like I was really hitting my stride as an educator."

Molly realized that she would have to focus all her attention and time on getting well. As she put it, "You have to accept the reality of your situation, even if it sucks—and believe me, cancer sucks. I had to have four different kinds of chemotherapy and they really knocked the stuffing out of me. I was forced to slow down and really learn to listen to my body and I began to change the way I lived one day at a time." Molly had heard the statistics that made her survival seem unlikely. Although she was told she had between six and eighteen months to live, she decided not to trust that prognosis. As she explains, "I'm not a number on some doctor's chart—I'm a person. I decided that I would educate myself and do everything within my power to defy the odds and to live as well as I possibly could for as long as I possibly could."

To make that happen, Molly has changed virtually every aspect of her life, from the way she eats to the way she thinks (reframing negative thoughts) to the company she keeps. The news can be toxic and addictive, so when alone she rarely turns on the radio. She starts every day with a mind-body practice that involves meditation and visual imagery, and she has learned to listen to her body in a way that is both gratifying and astounding. She is a living, breathing example of how anticancer living can not only extend our lives but also sustain and nurture our spirits so we can better enjoy the time we have.

Here's how Molly explains her new mind-set: "You have to decide you are going to live differently. This kind of acceptance is the opposite of resignation. It's about deciding you really want to live." Molly has survived more than eighteen years and counting with an aggressive brain cancer. I'm looking forward to seeing her up at the bay again this summer.

Molly's example is especially poignant in our current age, when so many of us (and our loved ones) are facing life with cancer. In 2016, the number of Americans living with cancer was more than 15.5 million.[37] That number is expected to exceed twenty million by 2026.[37] The World Health Organization predicts that the number of new cancers diagnosed worldwide will rise to twenty-two million within the next twenty years, a 70 percent surge.[10] Most of these cancers (60 percent) will be identified in Africa, Asia, and Central and South America, where 70 percent of all cancer deaths now occur.[10] In the United States the rate of breast cancer is expected to increase more than 50 percent between 2015 and 2030.[38] These projections make clear that we need to start educating people across the globe about the prevention and healing effects of adopting a healthy lifestyle. If we adopt and promote an anticancer living plan, I believe that we can see cancer rates decline in my lifetime. This, to me, would be the greatest indicator that we are moving toward a real cure for cancer and other deadly chronic diseases.

Imagining a New Bell Curve

As more oncologists, surgeons, and other treatment providers begin to understand that lifestyle can enhance the efficacy of conventional cancer treatments and encourage their patients to make lifestyle changes, the right side of the prognostic graph, which charts mortality, keeps extending for many types of cancers, while the smaller tail on the left side, which identifies the date of initial diagnosis to the date of death for some patients, has remained static.

Let's stop and imagine a new kind of bell curve: a different kind of statistical graph, one that will completely change our idea that a cancer diagnosis is an inevitability for almost half of us at some point in our lifetime. What if we found a way to track and quantify our ability to prevent the onset of cancer in the first place?

I've thought a lot about what this kind of graph might look like. In this new graph, the pinnacle of the "bump" is now the date of onset—or, more accurately, the date of initial diagnosis, since cancer usually grows quite slowly and can take years, even decades, to become large enough to be detected. Our new graph encompasses the ideas supporting the improvements in the survival graphs from the time of diagnosis, showing the lengthening tail of survival to the right, but in a *prevention graph* we now we have a

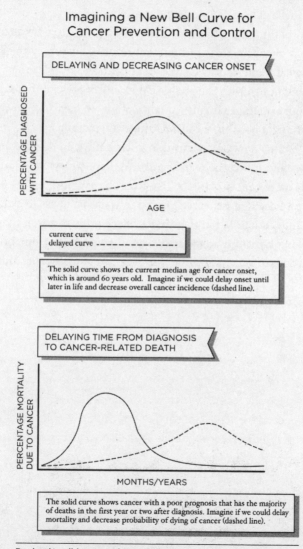

Imagining a New Bell Curve for Cancer Prevention and Control

DELAYING AND DECREASING CANCER ONSET

PERCENTAGE DIAGNOSED WITH CANCER

AGE

current curve ————————
delayed curve - - - - - - - - - - - -

The solid curve shows the current median age for cancer onset, which is around 60 years old. Imagine if we could delay onset until later in life and decrease overall cancer incidence (dashed line).

DELAYING TIME FROM DIAGNOSIS TO CANCER-RELATED DEATH

PERCENTAGE MORTALITY DUE TO CANCER

MONTHS/YEARS

The solid curve shows cancer with a poor prognosis that has the majority of deaths in the first year or two after diagnosis. Imagine if we could delay mortality and decrease probability of dying of cancer (dashed line).

Developed in collaboration with Laura Beckman.

growing tail of *prevention* to the left. If we think about our health, our bodies, and our control over both, and we decide to focus on prevention (whether initial diagnosis, recurrence, or progression), the graph becomes dynamic in new and exciting ways.

There's not just the possibility to live better and longer with cancer; now we open up the possibility that we might be able to "push off" a diagnosis further into the future, or perhaps if we dream big enough—and I am all about dreaming big where cancer prevention is concerned—we are able to push off getting a cancer diagnosis indefinitely.

This way of thinking is a dramatic shift—I would go so far as to call it a "revolutionary change"—from our current reactive posture with cancer detection and treatment. At the heart of an anticancer lifestyle is a new way of thinking about health with the purpose not only of preventing or overcoming disease but also improving the quality of life we have left, however long or short that might be. This is the anticancer revolution.

Backed by this new way of thinking, what if we all decided to modify our lifestyles now, much the way David and Stephen Jay Gould and Molly and so many other cancer patients I have met have done after their diagnoses? What if we decided we weren't going to wait for illness to strike before we stepped into action? What if we had the scientific research that showed us that making healthful adjustments now would fortify our bodies and increase the odds of our aging while free of cancer and other life-threatening diseases?

Imagine the possibilities.

CHAPTER TWO

Our Healing Powers

*C*ancer. It's the word none of us ever want to hear, and yet, most of us will at some point in our lives. It has certainly touched my own life in multiple family members. Ten years ago, my father was diagnosed with prostate cancer. Like most patients with early-stage prostate cancer, he was told by his doctor to pursue his normal routine and received no advice about lifestyle changes. "No need to do anything special," he was told. "We'll just re-biopsy you in a year."

Even in 2008, Alison and I knew all too well that this was not in keeping with the latest research. A year earlier, Dean Ornish, the renowned doctor and nutritionist, had shown in a randomized controlled trial that patients with early-stage prostate cancer who changed their diet and lifestyle for a year could slow the progression of their disease and greatly reduce the need for surgery.[1] Solid scientific research was thus increasingly pointing to the power of modification in lifestyle to alter the course of cancer's progression, especially when it was caught early. I urged my father to embrace these changes, to start meditating, to increase his physical activity, to cut back on meat and dairy consumption, and to start drinking green tea. I recommended, in addition, two teaspoons of tomato paste and one Brazil nut a day. (Brazil nuts have high levels of selenium, a trace mineral that has been shown in several studies to reduce prostate cancer risk. The lycopene in tomato paste has been shown in laboratory and animal studies to slow cancer cell growth.) My father took some of my advice. Eventually, he elected to have surgery. He does, however, continue to eat a healthy diet, one high in vegetables and fiber, low in meat and dairy products, to exercise daily, and to practice qigong. These routines help keep his body fit and outlook positive.

Coming to Terms with Cancer

My father took his cancer diagnosis in stride, but his cancer was caught early and his prognosis was good. For others, the psychological impact of a diagnosis can be devastating, not only to the patient but also to the family and friends. As a psychologist, I worry that our deep fears about cancer make us feel powerlessness when confronted with the news that we have this disease. The truth is we are anything but powerless. As we continue to lift the veil on the mysteries of cancer, thanks in no small part to our new understanding about how genes work, we are learning that our bodies are, by their very nature, robust disease-fighting machines, and our task is to ensure our everyday lifestyle choices and habits help our bodies do what they are programmed to—heal themselves.

Before we can step into action, however, it's important to stop and acknowledge the tough questions that will arise when we or those we love are diagnosed. Many cancer patients can't help but wonder: Why did my own body allow the creation of something so destructive? How do I reconcile myself to this kind of biological betrayal? Did I do something wrong? The paradoxes presented when cancer appears work cunningly to separate us in body, mind, and spirit at the precise moment when we need to be our most whole and integrated selves so we can make well-informed choices.

With this disease, we tend to lose trust in ourselves, in our bodies, and this can make it difficult to take daily actions that will support our natural defenses and promote our ability to heal. It's important for us to try to accept a diagnosis with a certain amount of curiosity, if for no reason other than that we are, inevitably, going to have to make some important treatment decisions. What if we decided that rather than convincing ourselves that we had no ability to participate in our care, we followed the examples of David Servan-Schreiber, Stephen Jay Gould, and our friend Molly M. and decided that we would listen to our bodies and make a commitment to give them what they need to heal? Taking it a step further, what if we took such a course of action while we are still healthy?

Envisioning a New Standard of Care

With all the innate potential of our bodies to help in the prevention or overcoming of cancer, why is it that some doctors—even if they try to educate themselves beyond the current "standard of care"—still do not recommend healthy eating, regular physical activity, and stress management to all cancer patients? The truth is that, despite the growing evidence that lifestyle plays a role in cancer risk, recurrence, and survival, many doctors remain reluctant to suggest lifestyle change as part of prevention or treatment, to some extent because it is not included in their training.[2-8] For many top surgeons, radiation oncologists, and medical oncologists, lifestyle remains an afterthought, a "complementary" treatment—helpful, but perhaps not necessary. Their focus is on their role in the process, how to shrink the tumor before cutting it out and then radiating the area to get anything they missed. The idea that the patient could have a measurable impact on this high-tech, specialized medical process has been vastly underestimated in conventional practice.

To help illustrate the extent of this disconnect, let me tell you the story of a woman I encountered not long ago who was getting her radiation treatment for breast cancer at MD Anderson after having her chemotherapy in her hometown. Elaine W., a thirty-seven-year-old mother of two, had been diagnosed with an aggressive stage II breast cancer. She was in good shape, ate what she considered a healthy diet, and stayed active. Like most Louisianans, Elaine grilled ribs once a week and, like most Americans, regularly ate pizza and cheeseburgers. But she also mixed in vegetables or a salad with almost every dinner and tried hard to limit her intake of sweets (if you don't count daiquiris). In terms of physical activity, Elaine wasn't the type to sit around watching TV or playing video games. Before they had young children to keep them busy, she and her husband, Henry, competed in CrossFit Games, running obstacle courses, flipping tires, and climbing ropes.

During her first visit with her medical oncologist after she was diagnosed with breast cancer, Elaine asked about the importance of diet. "Doc, tell me. I read articles online. I'm aware of things I have been hearing for several years that cancer feeds on sugar. Tell me right now and I will not eat any more refined sugars," she told him. "I will cut out whatever you tell me right now."

"You know what, Elaine," her oncologist responded, "cancer feeds on everything. Eat what you want. You're going through a hard time right now and you just need to be comfortable. Chemo sucks, so you eat what you want." His attitude was not uncommon; in fact, it's been the standard of care in the United States for cancer: a complete disconnect between treatment and lifestyle choices.

Elaine took her doctor's words to heart—happily. After her appointment, she went straight to a fast-food restaurant and ordered a large soda. That night, understandably too tired to cook, she ordered pizzas for the family—everyone's favorite comfort-and-convenience treat. The next morning, feeling a little bleary, still tired, and sorry for herself, she ate a donut someone offered her at work, *and* indulged in a midmorning chocolate cupcake.

A self-reinforcing "binge" pattern had begun, and it continued through her six months of chemotherapy. Sweets and junk foods felt like a reward for what she was going through. "It was a six-month pity party," she told me later, shaking her head.

Despite intensive chemotherapy meant to shrink her tumor, her team of doctors found, at the end of her six-month treatment, Elaine's tumor had almost doubled in size. After she was done with chemo, Elaine had a double mastectomy. Despite the surgery, her oncologist told her that the type of breast cancer she had, triple negative, had a 33 percent chance of recurrence. With triple-negative breast cancer, survivors don't have the option of taking a daily pill to block estrogen to prevent recurrence. Elaine was told (by the same oncologist who said, "Eat what you want") that there was not much she could do.

"Nothing I can do?" she asked in disbelief. Elaine had spent her life as a proactive person who took charge of situations. The prospect of helplessness did not sit well with her.

"Well, there is something . . ." Her oncologist glanced around the room as if he were about to tell her a secret he didn't want anyone to overhear. "But I'm saying this off the record." He told her to look up *Anticancer* by David Servan-Schreiber. "I'm telling you to look into this book not as your doctor but as a friend," he said. "It's not what they teach in medical school, but more and more, I'm becoming convinced there's something to it."

This is a graphic example about what I mean when I talk about a "disconnect" between what doctors "know" and the advice they feel comfortable giving their patients. The oncologist himself had become a vegan based in part on his belief that diet influenced his risk of chronic disease. But he was reluctant to share that belief "on the record" because he did not feel the connection between nutrition and cancer stood up to a medical standard of proof. I hear stories like this all the time. What makes it so frustrating to me is that we do have the proof. The cumulative evidence is overwhelming.

Oncologists who remain reluctant to share the connection between lifestyle and disease with their patients are doing them a disservice and possibly reducing their chances of survival.

That night, Elaine's husband, Henry, ordered five copies of *Anticancer*, one for himself, one for Elaine, one for her parents, one for his parents, and a final copy for a close family friend. When the books arrived, Henry immediately started reading, highlighting, and inserting Post-it Notes. Forty-eight hours later he declared, "We're changing the way we live." Soon after, Elaine and Henry celebrated their seventh wedding anniversary by going out for a fancy three-course dinner, complete with a bottle of wine and dessert. They also celebrated with an intimate conversation about their hopes, dreams, and goals for themselves and their children, and for their lives together.

The next morning, Henry cleaned out the pantry and refrigerator of every box, jar, and can of processed food. "We're done," he said. "You now need to drink three cups of green tea a day." He held up a small spice bottle. "This is called turmeric. It's our new favorite spice."

Elaine described that moment as the most romantic thing anyone had ever done for her. She realized just how deeply Henry cared about her. He wanted to live alongside and support her making changes that could help her survive cancer, at the same time they adopted healthy habits that could reduce the chances that he or their young children would ever face such a daunting diagnosis.

Still undergoing radiation therapy, Elaine now eats a mostly plant-based diet and is training with Henry for another CrossFit challenge. She starts each day with ten minutes of meditative silence, during which she concentrates on her breath. "That way, I spend the rest of my day free of that heaviness that comes along with cancer," she told me. She's less tired in the mornings, and she's also working to improve her sleep, without pills. These changes have led to her losing sixteen pounds. They also helped to clear up her skin. More important, she feels the power of her own choices in controlling and maintaining her health.

"I am at a completely different, more peaceful place than I was six months ago when I was just relying on chemo and doctors to fix me," she explains. "I'm not waiting for someone to just write me a prescription or to pump something into a port that's in my chest. I can make decisions every day that are going to help."

While Elaine's turnaround is inspiring, her initial encounter with her oncologist and his response to her concerns about how lifestyle affects cancer are all too common.

David Servan-Schreiber defined the paralyzing anxiety he felt in relation to his own brain cancer as a "false hopelessness," which the medical community tends unintentionally to reinforce when cancer is being addressed. Most oncologists and surgeons are so focused on the "cure" that they fail to enlist their patients' help in getting there. Like Elaine, David experienced this firsthand when he found that his doctors had no advice or encouragement to give him regarding what he could do to help save his own life when the recurrence of his brain cancer shook him to his core. As Elaine's story illustrates, many well-meaning cancer physicians inadvertently do the same thing to this day. They come up with a medical treatment plan and then send their patients off with the message, "We'll do everything we can. You just go back to your life and do what you've always done." But the unintentional discouragement that is expressed in this message could make the difference between life and death.

In terms of our own lives, Alison and I are not waiting for the medical community to catch up to the science. We have adopted an anticancer lifestyle in our home and promote it actively with our friends and in our community. The road has been challenging, for sure. I have given up pasta (which for an Italian borders on sacrilege), but that was not as difficult as giving up smoking (which I did after college). We have gradually moved to a more vegetable-based diet (a path that began for me when my father received his diagnosis), and we have striven to raise our children without processed sugar and on regular bedtimes to assure they maintain healthy sleep patterns.

We are certainly not perfect, but we are always trying our best. Why? The simple and obvious reason is this: I have seen so many people suffer and die from this disease that I want to do everything I can to help my children adopt habits now that will help them avoid or survive it, if it ever comes to that. I know what it is like for patients, and I know how difficult the process can be for survivors and their families. Cancer is life changing and all consuming. It is challenging on every level and in every imaginable way. If Alison or I could avoid a cancer diagnosis by changing the way we live, why wouldn't we do everything in our power to make those changes? If our lifestyle could influence our children's cancer risk, how could we not put every effort into being healthy role models and leading them down the anticancer path? Beyond preventing cancer, and perhaps even more important, this way of life simply feels better.

Unlearning Helplessness

Although much of the medical community is still not tuned in to this message of living a healthier life, I am fortunate to work at an institution where incorporating lifestyle in treatment plans is gaining traction. It has been a long, slow learning curve, even at MD Anderson, but I think we're approaching a tipping point. It's all about gathering strong research and data and making sure this information is available to both the medical and lay communities. But first, we must get past the "learned helplessness" that seems to be everywhere—especially when it comes to lifestyle and health care.

Treating ourselves well, unfortunately, isn't a quality that we value very highly in our society. We think that we have to overwork to be successful (despite that studies show the opposite); that going to bed early or sleeping in somehow means we're weak (yet sleep is one of the most healing and immune-balancing activities we can engage in); and that if we take time out to learn something like dancing or singing or improv, we're just being silly when, in fact, all of these actions are really good for our bodies and our health and they also, as an added bonus, strengthen our relationships.[9,10]

It's time we understand that there is a sweet spot where wellness and disease intersect, and it's where so many important breakthroughs in understanding how lifestyle disrupts the power and progression of cancer are occurring. This is the complex and fascinating space in which I live and work.

My days at the hospital are spent working with my team to teach simple, low-cost, nonmedical lifestyle techniques to cancer patients, even while they undergo chemo or radiation, stem cell transplants, or other rigorous treatments, which are often physically, psychologically, and emotionally taxing yet absolutely necessary. We help people with cancer make key lifestyle adjustments that will augment their treatment in ways that are vital to the success of those treatments and will also safeguard their health from other diseases and illnesses.

For instance, we encourage patients to engage in regular physical activity in order to strengthen their immune system and combat fatigue and to help their bodies become less hospitable to cancer growth and better able to sustain the rigors of treatment.[11-15] We help patients feel fitter, more rested, and free of anxiety or depression so they can experience and maximize their overall sense of "well-being," even when facing an often terrifying and challenging diagnosis. Most important, we help patients reconnect with their own bodies in a grounded and meaningful way, so that they can begin to identify the lifestyle areas they need to make changes in themselves. What we teach them, and continually remind ourselves, is that we can all take steps to improve our overall health dramatically by making our daily lifestyle choices healthy ones.

The goal is synergy, a phenomenon in which the whole is more than the sum of its parts. In terms of cancer risk reduction, this means that changing your lifestyle in a number of areas—as I mentioned, we have focused on six of them—makes each change more effective than it is on its own.[16-18] Even though many oncologists still treat lifestyle as an afterthought, the mounting research on the power of lifestyle change is getting through, and some major cancer organizations are taking note. The American Cancer Society and the American Institute for Cancer Research have clear guidelines for cancer prevention and cancer survivors in the areas of body weight, diet, and physical activity.[19,20] A number of large studies published in the last five years show that the more cancer prevention guidelines someone follows, the greater the reduction in cancer risk and cancer-related death.[21,22] For example, compared to people who follow only zero to two of the guidelines, people who followed seven to eight of the recommendations had a 12 percent reduction in the risk of developing any cancer and a 20 percent reduction in cancer mortality.[5] The risk reduction for certain cancers was especially high, with a 50 percent reduction in incidence of colorectal cancer for those following seven to eight of the guidelines.[5] For head and neck cancer the rate is higher, 63 percent; for endometrial cancer, 59 percent; and for breast cancer, 22 percent. The same holds true for cancer mortality. The more guidelines for cancer prevention and control people follow, the greater the reduction in deaths from cancer. For some cancers, the impact is modest (10 percent for ovarian cancer in one study) and for other cancers much larger (breast cancer, 33 percent; colorectal cancer, 61 percent).

All six lifestyle areas of the Mix of Six—social support, stress, sleep, diet, exercise, and environment—are interlinked. Emerging evidence demonstrates that success in one of the areas of lifestyle will influence

The More Lifestyle Guidelines You Follow, the Lower Your Risk of Cancer and Cancer-Related Mortality

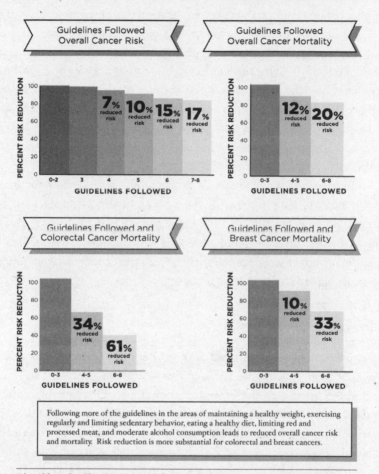

Following more of the guidelines in the areas of maintaining a healthy weight, exercising regularly and limiting sedentary behavior, eating a healthy diet, limiting red and processed meat, and moderate alcohol consumption leads to reduced overall cancer risk and mortality. Risk reduction is more substantial for colorectal and breast cancers.

Adapted from: C. A. Thomson, M. L. McCullough, B. C. Wertheim, et al., "Nutrition and physical activity cancer prevention guidelines, cancer risk, and mortality in the women's health initiative," *Cancer Prevention Research* 7, no. 1 (January 2014): 42–53.
    Adapted in collaboration with Laura Beckman.

success in the other areas.[23] Multiple studies show that stress can sabotage all good healthy intentions.[24–26] Programs that combine mindfulness meditation with a dietary intervention are more effective than dietary changes alone.[27] At this point, the science is clear: it is critical to move forward in multiple areas to improve your chances of sustaining lifestyle change and reducing risk of disease or disease recurrence.[22,28,29]

Cancer patients tend to recognize the synergistic benefits of anticancer living in themselves. I see it time and time again: Cancer patients make the connection between living well and feeling good because they see the positive effect healthy lifestyle adjustments have on their treatment and prognosis. For example, a breast cancer patient who distances herself from the toxic relationships in her life and aligns her core values with her actions and behaviors shares with me that she now feels "free and truly alive" for the first time in her life. The patient who starts eating a more plant-based diet, exercising regularly, and managing her stress sees that she is now sleeping better, has more energy, and describes her life as "infinitely better" than before her cancer diagnosis despite having undergone surgery, six months of chemotherapy, and six weeks of radiotherapy.

To understand why lifestyle factors can have such a dramatic impact, it's necessary to have a better understanding of cancer, in its most basic terms. It's also helpful to see how we've approached treating cancer over time so that we can understand more fully why the bulk of our medical and scientific resources were used to study how to treat cancer in isolation from the whole person and with little focus on prevention.

A Prescription for Hope

In my more than twenty years working in integrative oncology, I've watched as patient after patient goes through this brutal but necessary regimen of medical treatment only to be told that they are, for the moment, "cured" of the disease and their medical care, as it were, ends there. I watch these people leave this medically intensive initial phase of their cancer experience in a state of deeply compromised health and well-being, lacking the information or tools they need to go home and begin the important work of healing. They may be physically disfigured, in chronic pain, suffering from treatment-induced illnesses or secondary diseases, be depressed, depleted, and feeling anything but healthy. And yet it is at this moment, for many, that the real work of healing begins.

This moment, when they are post-treatment but not yet well, is when most people come to a crucial crossroad: they either grasp that their true healing and long-term health is really in their own hands or surrender to the crushing blow dealt them by the cancer and the aftermath of treatment.

Our bodies aren't designed to be cut into, doused with chemicals, or exposed to radiation without there being serious consequences. On the contrary, our bodies are designed to stay balanced, stay regulated, and to biologically resist disease—as long as we make choices that promote and support this natural imperative.

The inherent design of the body to heal itself is what anticancer living is all about. It's about shifting our focus and becoming conscious of the fact that how we live either promotes healing or does not, and that this is true whether or not we have cancer.

Medicine Is Everywhere: Diana Lindsay's Remarkable Healing Path

To see a living illustration of the healing powers of lifestyle change, we need look no further than health-care activist Diana Lindsay, who has lived with cancer for twenty-five years, including almost a dozen years with stage IV lung cancer.

Diana was first diagnosed with cancer when she was forty-one years old. The year was 1993 and her diagnosis was stage I rectal cancer. This prompted a lot of surgeries, and ultimately what was categorized as a "cure."

Then, in 2006, at the age of fifty-four, Diana was diagnosed with stage IV lung cancer. This time, the cancer was advanced, spreading from both lungs to her lymph nodes, her brain, and possibly to the lining around her heart. She was told she was not eligible for surgery and there was no cure, then placed in palliative care. However, her doctor had a hunch, broke with standard protocol, and put her on Tarceva, a targeted agent that is now used to treat advanced or metastatic non-small-cell lung cancer but which, at that time, was being tested in clinical trials. She also had Gamma Knife brain radiation. Diana had an extraordinary response to both treatments until eighteen months later, when a CT scan showed that the cancer was growing again. She then tried experimental stereotactic radiation (also now part of standard therapy options), which gave her nine more months without progressing. She then also incorporated qigong and Reiki for another nine months, until, ultimately, she was eligible for a groundbreaking lung surgery.

From the moment of diagnosis, Diana began to make profound changes in the way she lived. First and foremost, she took a leave of absence from the company she and her husband owned, a marketing communications business that supported multinational companies like Microsoft. This allowed her to focus on her health and maintain her health insurance (this was at a time when having a preexisting condition made it impossible to get health insurance). She eventually sold the company, providing her a sense of freedom and access to resources that are not available to most people in her situation, but as we will later show, Diana put this gain to wonderful use in terms of her own learning, and later on behalf of her community.

Before giving up the business, Diana often worked a stressful twenty-hour day, cutting back on sleep, overworking, traveling a great deal, and de-prioritizing much else—such as eating well and exercising enough. She prided herself on her ability to "do it all"—run a company, engage with her new granddaughter, and contribute to her community. Then, nearly overnight, she went to not working at all. After some soul-searching, and freed of the mental strain of planning, executing, and managing, she found herself able to more closely listen to her dreams, her body, and her intuition about what she needed to do to heal. As she recently told me, "I made a complete commitment to healing, gave everything up, and just completely dedicated myself to it. I learned to listen to my body and discern what it needed, and what it thought I should do to get better. And what I learned, pretty quickly, is this: medicine is everywhere."

From the perspective of Diana's doctors, her medical options were limited. Diana had been brought up to believe that healing began and ended with conventional Western medicine. She trusted doctors and respected their authority over human health. But as soon as she realized they didn't have enough answers for her, she began to look beyond that framework. "I began to realize, 'Hey! Food is medicine, and laughing with my family and friends is medicine, and long walks are medicine, clean air is medicine, too, and so is feeling relaxed and stress-free.' The list of things that I began to identify as medicine grew the more I allowed myself to explore the unknown. I knew I had to add things alongside what they could come up with as the best in medicine."

Diana began to make daily lifestyle choices based on a simple, straightforward criterion: "Does this make me feel better?" She found that, over time, she was able to listen to what her body was telling her and to provide it with what it needed to be healthy and strong.

When she was diagnosed with stage IV cancer, her odds of surviving to five years were 1 percent. Her doctor thought she would die within three months. Diana realized that if she was going to defy the odds and be the one in one hundred cases, the 1 percent who survived stage IV lung cancer, she had to learn everything she could about how to heal herself. As she explains, "I had to seize the moment and make the most of what I had."

That was twelve years ago. Diana has found a healthier path to live a fuller life and to extend her newfound sense of well-being to others. Today, Diana can say with confidence that every day since her awful diagnosis, her life has been an adventure into a great, vast, and very healing unknown. She felt called to invent a way, where few paths had been laid.

Diana was unusual in her ability to make this kind of life change relevant to her job, which of course for most of us is bound up with our and our families' access to conventional health care, as well as any resources with which to explore alternatives. Her open-mindedness, willingness to learn, and ability to be flexible and creative served her as well in her healing process as it had in her business career. Her path is not available to all, but she used her position, as well as the reward for the hard work she'd put in to build her company, to pioneer real and healthy change in her entire community.

One thing that makes Diana so exceptional is how wholeheartedly she trusted her body to guide her toward healing. She didn't let the reality that a "cure" was not available to her dim her hope or keep her from trying to make changes that would support her body to heal itself. She made a commitment to side with hope, and then she acted. She educated herself and used what she learned to craft her own unique anticancer living plan.

If Diana Lindsay was able to turn a dire diagnosis of stage IV lung cancer into a decade-plus adventure in anticancer living, just think what adopting these lifestyle principles will do for those of us who have not yet had cancer or another chronic or life-threatening disease?

The Difference between Healing and Curing

Cancer can be a great teacher. It not only teaches us about how our bodies work on both regulatory and cellular levels but also offers us a glimpse into how the human body is built and designed to heal. It may strike some as odd, even cruelly ironic, to discuss cancer, which the body produces, and the concept of self-healing in the same breath, but what I've learned is that profound healing is available even when a cure may not be; that radical, even transformational improvement in the quality of one's life and health are possible even in the face of serious illness; that a higher state of wellness can be reached, whether or not a medical cure is available.

I'm not suggesting that we don't seek a cure. Seeking out and following through on appropriate medical treatment is essential when treating cancer or any other serious disease. But what I want to discuss here and what I will be talking about throughout the book is how profoundly we can influence our ability to heal, which may enhance or even eclipse the whole concept of a "cure" or which will, most certainly, give us great agency on how close to a cure we may come.

What I hope is that all of us—especially those of us in the cancer care world—really begin to acknowledge the high costs of a "cure-by-any-means" approach to treating cancer and instead broaden our thinking around what constitutes good treatment and care. I'd like to see us in the oncology world take a broader view and look at the life of the patient and how the lifestyle choices a cancer patient makes influence or reflect the cellular activity of that individual's cancer or disease. I would like to see us incorporate positive lifestyle habits into larger treatment plans, knowing that they lead to better outcomes. To do this, we need to broaden our focus, to take in the whole patient, including her larger life, rather than just focus on the cluster of out-of-control cells inside the body.

If we can loosen our grip some on the quest for the Holy Grail of a "cure" and focus first on healing, we will approach treatment in a fundamentally different way. When we allow ourselves to open up to the possibility that our, or as doctors, a patients' behavior matters, something truly transformative may take place. When we emphasize healing instead of only curing, cancer becomes a human problem, not just a scientific one. My good friend and colleague Michael Lerner, PhD, who has been a pioneer in understanding the difference between healing and curing, especially as it relates to cancer, puts it like this: "Curing is what a physician seeks to offer you. Healing, however, comes from within us. It's what **we** bring to the table. Healing can be described as a physical, emotional, mental and spiritual process of coming home."[30]

This is an important distinction, because the truth is, many cancers simply cannot be cured—or at least they cannot be cured by medicine alone. Yes, they can be slowed. They might be controlled. They can be treated medically in ways that render them undetectable, possibly for a length of time, possibly even for a lifetime. But full eradication is not only relatively rare, it is also costly in terms of the toll it takes on the physical, emotional, and psychological well-being of a patient. In fact, aiming only to "kill" a cancer can cause irreparable harm to the body's natural ability to continue to heal itself and can make a patient vulnerable to a whole host of other health problems. This is where anticancer living becomes so crucial—harnessing our natural defenses to decrease the multiple side effects of treatment and improve outcomes. When we treat cancer only biologically and on a cellular level, we miss the cause in search of the cure.

Learning a New Language

Many in the medical community have chosen to use a lexicon of warfare when talking about cancer. Perhaps there is a well-intentioned but misguided belief that if we are enjoined to "fight," we won't let fear get the best of us, that if we're "armed" with the right "ammunition," we might actually "win" this "war."

I don't think these military metaphors serve us, however, because they imply that we must fight against our own bodies, instead of aligning ourselves to engage wholly with ourselves and others. The current language used in the world of cancer care separates us from ourselves, distancing our spirit and native insight from our physical body. But how can we heal when we are at war? How can we heal when we're expected to be constantly on high alert and battle ready? We now know that the use of this type of language is actually not helpful and can continue the state of fear while hampering engagement and empowerment. In 2014, researchers at the University of Michigan and the University of Southern California teamed up to conduct a series of studies looking at the impact of framing cancer as a hostile enemy in an ongoing war. Their findings suggest that war metaphors make people less likely to actively engage in behaviors to help reduce their cancer risk.[31]

Being "at war" with your body is not a healthy approach when you're trying to recover from or prevent disease. David Servan-Schreiber aptly pointed out that we all have cancer cells in our bodies, but not all of us will develop cancer.[32] The premise is not that our bodies are "harboring the enemy" or that we should live in fear of an internal uprising or even that our unhealthy habits are stoking the fires of war. On the contrary, our approach is about discovering and maximizing the healing powers in each of us that can keep our bodies in balance and allow them to work effectively (as they are designed and inclined to do) to prevent cancer cells from growing and spreading in the first place.

Cancer is terrifying because it's an inside job. It brings us into startling, close contact with our mortality because it's not happening to us, it is happening within us. It can be experienced as a particularly cruel form of betrayal. So how can we trust our bodies to beat this thing if it created it in the first place?

In the ongoing Comprehensive Lifestyle Study (CompLife) at MD Anderson, I have seen dozens of cancer survivors go through this process and come out the other side with a better understanding of what cancer is and how their daily choices influence whether cancer cells grow or wither within their bodies. When study participant and cancer survivor Jan C., who was sixty-two years old, finished the intensive six-week portion of the program, she wrote a note to future participants, expressing her thanks at being part of the study and, as she saw it, part of a fundamental change in cancer treatment and in the way survivors approach their lives. "In the beginning, I wanted to do it for my own health. I had already decided when able I would change my lifestyle," she wrote. "But when the program was presented to me, I realized it was so much more. I was able to help others in the future become healthier at the same time I was. Now that I have completed my six weeks' training, I WILL continue to the best of my ability and I am going to share it with everyone I know so they can live healthier, too."

Staying hopeful, even curious, is essential, despite all the doubt and fear that cancer brings with it. I've worked with many cancer patients, like Jan, whose lives were transformed for the better once they get over the initial shock of being diagnosed. In fact, many patients have told me that their cancer experience was the *best* thing that has happened to them, and that it took being diagnosed and going through treatment to finally be able to give themselves permission to make radical lifestyle changes and live the life they've always dreamed of living. Clarifying who you are and what you want out of life can be the unexpected positive side effects of a diagnosis. Tapping into our most authentic selves positions us to move into a powerful state of healing and well-being.

Take, for example, Lee C., a sixty-five-year-old psychologist who was diagnosed five years ago with stage III breast cancer. Before Lee discovered her anticancer lifestyle, she was at a low point in her life. She had trouble sleeping and taking care of herself, and she was unwilling to share the psychological burden of cancer with her three grown sons, who, she told herself, "have lives of their own to worry about." When she was introduced to the CompLife Study and what it entailed, Lee broke down and cried. "This is what I was looking for," she told us. "This is what I needed and I couldn't find it."

For Lee, an anticancer prescription that encompassed both her psychological and physical health helped her become more active and taught her to use meditation and yoga to both relax and let go. As a result, her sleep improved, and she became more appreciative of life. She discovered how to cook healthy foods like kale and spinach so they taste good, a skill she shared with her grown sons, who have in turn changed their own eating patterns. Her empowerment also gave her the courage to reach out and seek help, both from her family and her larger community. Here's how she explains her transformation: "I just really feel more centered and whole. The mindfulness has helped me stand back and just observe what's going on with me. What am I doing? What do I need to do? That helps me feel so much more in control. It's really helped me be more creative. I'm utilizing that in my daily life and it feels so much better." Now semiretired from her psychology practice, Lee has turned to creative work that has called to her for years.

I am humbled every time I interact with patients like Lee, people who, despite being in the midst of a tough, even painful round of treatment, or contending with a recurrence, or dealing with any number of the actual hardships of the disease, convey a strong sense of knowing exactly who they are, what they're dealing with, and what they want from life. With each of these encounters, I get to experience something of a "contact high," because these people radiate a special energy emanating from deep acceptance of life on life's terms. I've worked with patients who never gave their health a thought before, but when diagnosed with cancer became passionate about understanding how their bodies are designed to resist disease and how they can support their treatment. A diagnosis of cancer can often lead people to realize how meaningful and fulfilling—even enjoyable—taking great care of themselves can be. Anticancer living opens us up to a whole world of possibility.

Nothing impresses me more than seeing patients improve their level of self-care immediately on diagnosis. Some seem to just know, intuitively, that they will have a better outcome if they participate in their own care and can set aside a lifetime of behavior that does not serve them. (Lee is a great example of this.) On the other hand, I've also known lung and head and neck cancer patients who struggle with remaining tobacco-free even while they are undergoing treatment, despite knowing that their habits will likely worsen their outcomes. I've worked with overweight women with endometrial cancer who are unable to prioritize weight loss, even when told that this will reduce the disease's likelihood of recurrence. These patients may have such deeply entrenched difficulties that they strive in vain to give up behaviors that have been used for many years as survival strategies and coping mechanisms, even when these habits have reached their limits in terms of any benefit and have started to cause harm. Sometimes we use the language of addiction, and appropriately so; but addictions and the accompanying despair and hopelessness are very often intricately bound up with the pathways of disease.

Nothing feeds cancer or any other disease like a sense of hopelessness, because when we're hopeless, we stop trying. While they might not all say so on the record, oncologists have long sensed that mental outlook and emotional well-being are key to cancer survival. During my first month at MD Anderson, I told a surgeon about a grant I had just received to study the importance of stress management for prostate cancer patients. The surgeon responded, "You know, I know when a patient comes into my office who's kind of down and sad, pessimistic about their treatment and life, and they're alone—no friends or family with them at the visit—this patient is not going to do well. They're going to die sooner than my patients who fit the opposite profile."

When we work with this kind of despairing patient, we strive to help them shift their thinking, even if it's just long enough to get them to take a walk around the unit and have a cool glass of clean water. Even brief encounters with a caring health-care provider can begin a shift. Often, once they've taken even simple steps, I will see the tiniest glimmer of hope. Sometimes, all it takes is that one flicker of belief in oneself. All it takes is one or two moments when despair lifts long enough for a simple, healthy action to be taken. For some, there are deep-rooted emotional and psychological barriers that need to be addressed before true success can be attained. A critical step on this path is getting the right kind of support to start to work through any psychological obstacles and to have success in tackling the bigger issues.

A major part of our work with our CompLife Study patients is providing the emotional and social support they need to work through their fears and doubts and to step into meaningful and purposeful action, at whatever stage of healing and self-understanding they find themselves. We acknowledge the fears that naturally come with cancer, but we focus on building a sense of competence and capability among our study participants.

A cancer diagnosis can activate intense emotions that we may not be very familiar with or know how to handle. This can trigger feelings of isolation and loneliness at the point in time when support is what we need most. In this way, cancer is similar to common mental illnesses like depression or anxiety, which can leave a patient sensing that something is terribly wrong but unsure how to connect with others. As one patient once described it, "I felt like I had fallen into one of those hidden traps, like you see on TV, where a hole in the ground is covered over in leaves, and I couldn't find my voice and shout out for help." For other patients, feelings of isolation stem from a sense of stigma or of shame about their cancer, or a reluctance to "burden" their loved ones (like Lee not wanting to trouble her boys, who had their own lives and worries). A colleague told me that she recently attended the memorial service of a woman with whom she did volunteer work. Although she saw this person several times a month, she had no idea she was sick with colorectal cancer until she got a call inviting her to the service. "I wish I had had the chance to tell her how much I liked her, how much I enjoyed working with her," my colleague told her brother at the service. "It broke my heart when he told me that no one knew about it except for him and their older sister. It seems my volunteer friend felt ashamed about having this kind of cancer."

Becoming isolated from others is not only bad for us psychologically; it may also have a detrimental effect on our health. A 2012 study published in the *Journal of Clinical Oncology* looked at the effects of social attachment for 168 patients who underwent surgery for ovarian cancer.[33] The study was headed by my friend and colleague Susan Lutgendorf at the University of Iowa, one of the top research scientists focusing on the impact of stress and social support on disease progression and outcomes. Lutgendorf and her team focused on two types of support—emotional social support (close connections with others) and instrumental support (people who provide tangible assistance). They found that people who had strong emotional support survived significantly longer after surgery compared to women who reported less support. Based on this finding, researchers recommended that women planning to undergo surgery for ovarian cancer be screened for deficits in their social environment and that support activities and resources be offered as part of their treatment and recovery.

In *Anticancer Living*, Alison and I emphasize social connections and a mindful approach to life because we believe these components are the foundations that will allow other changes—converting to a primarily plant-based diet and increasing exercise and physical activity throughout the day—to take hold. The reason most diets and New Year's resolutions don't last is that they are conceived in isolation from overall lifestyle. The key to sustainable change is a structure that reinforces the change and provides support when willpower wavers and we are tempted to fall back into our old ways.

An important priority, of course, is educating oneself for the journey ahead. As Meg Hirshberg with the Anticancer Lifestyle Program points out, knowledge is power, especially where cancer is concerned.[34] We need to transform our sense of overwhelm into action, make meaningful connections with our medical providers, strengthen our bonds with our loved ones, and remain calm and present while we begin to understand what is happening inside of us and what we need to do to make ourselves feel healthy and well. Every decision needs to be one that will actively promote—and not harm—our health. Although you can read books, talk to doctors, and query your friends and loved ones along the way—the right answers will always come from you.

For those not currently dealing with a cancer diagnosis, now is the time to take the opportunity to look at your own lifestyle and begin to make healthier choices and adjustments to increase your odds of living free of cancer. Maintaining a healthy weight, exercising more, eating more vegetables, getting a better night's sleep—these are simple, straightforward actions that will have a profound impact on your body's ability to keep cancer, heart disease, diabetes, and other serious diseases at bay.[5,35-39] Often, the good results experienced from such changes are reinforcing enough to become transformative over the long term. However, if making these kinds of adjustments continues to elude you, it's time to take a look at deeper issues. Exploring possible emotional factors, whether from a past unresolved trauma or an ongoing issue could be key. Finding the right therapist or peer support network that can help resolve any emotional or psychological obstacles to your well-being will be a huge game changer, in fact a lifesaver. Here I would again take a page from David Servan-Schreiber's book and recommend being very honest when exploring and evaluating the care on offer. It may take some trial and error to locate the individual or group who can see and treat you as a whole person, in all your complexity, beauty, and individuality. There is no one-size-fits-all solution here. But as hard as it is sometimes to believe, help does exist; it can be found. And the commitment to the search is part of the healing journey.

Cancer or no cancer, we all have to get past fear. While many people first make life changes based on a fear of illness, what makes an anticancer lifestyle sustainable is what it offers us. That positive impact becomes the driving force behind new habits—literally, a new way of life. Feeling better, growing stronger, gaining confidence—these are the side effects of anticancer living that can start to tip the scale.

CHAPTER THREE

What Causes Cancer, Anyway?

Alison and I travel regularly to give talks about adopting an anticancer lifestyle to audiences that include both cancer survivors and those hoping they and their families will never face this daunting challenge. I present the scientific evidence linking lifestyle and cancer, and Alison shares strategies on how to make lifestyle changes permanent and sustaining, as she does in this book. After one of our recent talks, a young woman with breast cancer came up to the front of the room, shook our hands, and told us her story. The previous year, she had gone through a difficult divorce. While fighting for custody of her two children, she was laid off from her job at a local shipping company. Six months later, she was diagnosed with stage II breast cancer. "I had never been without work," she said. "That and the divorce, the stress from those two things, that's what caused my cancer. I'm sure of it."

We hear this level of certainty about what caused someone's cancer from at least one person in the audience at every presentation we give, no matter where we are, how many people are in attendance, and regardless of the specific focus of the talk. The first thing we should make clear is that if you get cancer, no matter what kind or what stage, the exact cause is almost never clear. While the recommendations in this book have been shown to reduce cancer risk, especially when practiced in combination, no one is immune to cancer, just as no one is destined for it.

If I were to ask a random sampling of people what they believe causes cancer, I'd get a broad range of answers, many of them correct. Some might say cigarettes cause lung cancer, which is absolutely true. Others might say radiation or environmental pollution or infection with a cancer-causing virus—all of which are also true. And lately, with our ever-expanding understanding of genes and how they work—specifically as they relate to cancer—more and more people would respond "our genes!" with an almost gleeful sense of certainty. This answer, of course, is also true, but it's also largely false.

Let me explain.

Malfunctioning genes are clearly the cellular mechanism that allows a cell to become what we call "cancerous."[1] But this complex process is most often triggered by something *external* to that cell—often something external to the human body—and this is the root of the confusion about whether the gene malfunction that prompts uncontrolled cell growth, leading to the formation of cancer, is mainly hereditary or externally triggered.[2–4]

It's fair to say that, given the amount of research funding pouring into genetic research, the gene has been a recent darling of the cancer world. Since the sequencing of the human genome in 2003, our understanding of the intracellular behavior of genes and how they contribute to the development of cancer has been nothing short of transformative. But our understanding of gene behavior, and especially of what influences gene behavior, is still in the very early stages. Nevertheless, there is a widespread misconception that inherited gene mutations are primarily responsible for most cancers.[5] The public believes that we are either born lucky, free and clear of inherited cancer risks, or unlucky, hardwired to get certain cancers based on the luck of the DNA draw. Nothing could be further from the truth. And for all of us—including those of us with inherited genetic mutations that increase the risk of cancer—this is actually good news.

We Are Not "Programmed" for Cancer

Only 5 to 10 percent of all cancers are caused by inherited genetic mutations.[6,7] Most experts feel that the number hovers tightly around the 5 percent range. For people born with genes that indicate a high risk of developing cancer (such as the BRCA-1 and BRCA-2 genes, which are associated with increased risk of certain breast and ovarian cancers), getting cancer is never a certain fate.[8] For example, women with the BRCA-1 mutation have a 55 to 65 percent chance of developing breast cancer by age seventy (the risk for women with the BRCA-2 mutation is 45 percent), relative to only 12 percent for the general population.[8] Similarly, the rate of ovarian cancer for BRCA-1 carriers is 39 percent (11 to 17 percent for women with BRCA-2) versus 1.3 percent for the general population.[8]

This focus on genetics and genetic mutations also veils an important truth: Up to 95 percent of all cancers are not caused by inherited genetic defects.[6,7] Some of course are due to chance. But most cancers are caused by something within our power to control—the way we live and the choices we make every day.[2,6,7,9]

Blue Cured

In 2010, Gabe Canales was on top of the world. A young entrepreneur living and working in Houston, Texas, he ran his own marketing and public relations firm, where his clients included high-profile restaurants, tech, real estate, and higher education companies. He was successful, very social, and in good health. During a routine annual checkup, he was given a spate of tests, including a PSA (prostate-specific antigen) screening. He got a call from his doctor saying that his PSA levels were a bit elevated. So he went back for a second test, and this one indicated an even higher PSA level. His urologist recommended Gabe have a biopsy, but when Gabe realized it was an invasive procedure (a probe is threaded up through the rectum and a microscopic knife slices samples from the prostate gland), he declined. The doctor followed up and pressed him, "Look, it's just going to be a pinch. Just a pinch and you can go back to work."

The procedure was much more than a pinch, as Gabe explains: "The topical numbing agent and the local anesthetic did not work, so I felt it every time this probe was threaded up through my rectum and a snippet of my prostate gland was taken. I felt like my body was imploding. It was the most excruciatingly painful experience I had had in my life to that point. I remember thinking, 'When will this end?' It was god-awful."

A week and a half later, Gabe was walking out of his house, gym clothes on, car keys in hand, when he got a call from the hospital. His urologist told him he had some bad news and some good news. "The bad news is you have prostate cancer. The good news is you'll be fine." All Gabe heard was, "You have cancer."

Gabe's urologist told him he needed surgery. "We need to take it out." The side effects of prostate cancer surgery included a period of erectile dysfunction and incontinence. "Here I was, a single, thirty-five-year-old guy with my whole life ahead of me. I needed a second opinion."

The next doctor told Gabe the exact opposite. He suggested a "wait-and-see" approach. Gabe imagined that he would think of little else aside from whether his cancer was growing and spreading inside his body. Did he really have only two choices—to undergo major life-altering surgery or to do nothing?

Gabe went to Memorial Sloan Kettering Cancer Center (MSKCC) in New York City to get another opinion. The MSKCC doctor, after a series of tests, also recommended "active surveillance." He explained that if they monitored the tumor closely, Gabe might not have to do anything for five, ten, or even fifteen years.

Less panicked, but still not totally satisfied, Gabe went to see one more doctor, Dr. Aaron Katz, chair of urology at NYU Winthrop Hospital and professor of urology at Stony Brook University School of Medicine (who at that time was an attending urologist at Columbia University). "That's when my life changed." Dr. Katz addressed an issue that had not been brought up before: nutrition. He recommended that Gabe radically change his diet—from meat and potatoes to a plant-centered, vegetable-heavy meal plan. "It's not that he recommended some crazy, unreasonable diet—it was just the opposite. He wanted me simply to make a conscious effort to eat less steak and potatoes, drink less beer and liquor, and eat more fresh vegetables and fruits—of which, at the time, I ate exactly none. I flew back to Houston and decided to take his advice."

Gabe began to educate himself, and he also started to lose weight and build lean body mass. When he went in for his first regularly scheduled surveillance visit, his blood work showed that his PSA level had gone down. "I had that aha moment when I realized that altering my diet as the doctor I had met in New York recommended was working. I knew, without a doubt, that I had some input over the outcome of this cancer. I needed to know more! So I began to really explore how lifestyle and cancer might be inter-related. One of my daily routines was drinking two to three large glasses of blended spinach, kale, cilantro, and jalapeno—just green vegetables."

Today, Gabe is a walking, breathing example of anticancer living and has become a close friend and colleague (I am on the medical advisory board of his nonprofit, Blue Cure). He will never know what "caused" his cancer, but he's found his purpose and he's now in the best health he's ever been in. Through his nonprofit, he's bringing the anticancer living message to young men and boys across the country, believing that prevention of prostate cancer—which is affecting younger and younger men—is a better alternative than needing to find a cure.

The Invisible Causes

We know that inherited genetic anomalies, though a great threat to a very small part of the population, aren't the main culprit when it comes to cancer.

When we get out of the laboratory and take a look around, we're actually confronted with two worlds. Off in the distance, moving farther and farther away from us, is the untainted natural world. Before the start of the Industrial Revolution, nature was able to provide us with everything we needed to live well: clean air, clean fresh water, abundant food sources, and beautiful terrain to move around in. Of course, there were diseases, famines, natural disasters, and other threats to human life, but the basics for healthy survival were there, too.

While our modern minds worked hard to make life easier and, where health care was concerned, prioritize longevity, we unintentionally shrouded the earth in a haze of pollutants that not only taint and harm the environment but also interfere with the ability of all living things to fully flourish—including us. It's undeniable that we are living longer, but we're also now faced with diseases that come with the longevity we've bought at the expense of disease prevention. What a terrible irony! The only silver lining in this is knowing that, since we've created the causes of so much illness, we can also eliminate them.

Alison and I grew up hearing the advertising slogan, Better Living through Chemistry. This was the bright, happy jingle of the DuPont Chemical Company from 1935 until 1982—when "through chemistry" was finally dropped. If you grew up during that period, you know that "chemistry" was supposed to encompass all the benefits and convenience that chemicals and additives brought to modern life. By the 1980s, however, when the slogan had come to be regarded as a cynical catchphrase, most of the world was finally catching on that perhaps living in a world chock-full of chemicals wasn't better after all.

Nowhere is the irony of this more obvious than in the realm of cancer care. Over the past thirty or so years, we've established a direct link between man-made chemical agents and the onset of cancer.[10,11] Yet we still mainly treat these chemically triggered illnesses with other chemicals in the form of chemotherapy. We get sick because of chemicals and we try to get better with chemicals. In the meantime, the costs to our bodies, our health, and our overall quality of life continue to mount.

What if there is a better way?

We now have some of the scientific data we need to make choices that sidestep many of the industrial and environmental chemical toxins laced into the foods we eat, the clothes we wear, and the products we use in our daily lives.

Here are just a few facts about factors that cause more than 50 percent of cancers:

- Diet, sedentary behavior, and obesity are responsible for 30–35 percent of all cancers in the United States.[12] It is estimated that almost 1 in 6 cancer deaths in men and 1 in 5 cancer deaths in women are associated with being overweight.[12]
- Tobacco is responsible for about 30 percent of all cancer deaths worldwide (though death rates from tobacco-related cancers in the United States have dropped significantly in recent years; tobacco-related deaths continue to rise in the developing world).[12,13]
- Viral infections, such as those caused by Epstein-Barr, HPV, and hepatitis, account for more than 15 percent of cancers worldwide. (Vaccines are now available to protect against infection from the types of HPV that cause cancer. Also, the Epstein-Barr virus causes cancer only in rare cases.)[12]
- Up to 10 percent of cancers are caused by radiation. This includes UV rays from the sun, which cause skin cancers, one of the fastest-growing cancers among young adults.[12,13]
- Alcohol is listed by the National Toxicology Program as a known human carcinogen.[14] The more someone drinks, the higher their risk of developing certain types of cancers including head and neck, esophageal, liver, breast, and colorectal.[15,16] In 2009, an estimated 3.5 percent of cancer deaths in the United States were alcohol related.[16]
- Environmental toxins that are known to cause cancers, such as asbestos, coal dust, and formaldehyde, to name just a few of thousands, are

widespread.[10,11,14] Scientists have no way of quantifying the link between specific environmental toxins and cancer onset, except in the most obvious cases (for example, coal miners have a higher-than-average incidence of respiratory cancers as a result of their exposure to the carcinogens in coal dust and asbestos, which cause mesothelioma).

Quitting Cancer

Tobacco use, of course, is the great example of a lifestyle choice or, if you prefer, an addictive habit, that is directly linked to cancer. Whether it's social, a secret vice, an anxiety release, or a style statement, for the past fifty years or so, we've known that tobacco, which contains more than 50 carcinogens, is a primary cause of at least fourteen types of cancer, including lung and head and neck cancers. Tobacco alone accounts for a third of all cancer deaths annually, and more than 80 percent of all lung-cancer deaths. What exactly happens when the substances found in tobacco interact with healthy cells is quite complex, but what is known is that when we don't smoke, or when we quit smoking, our risks for developing tobacco-related cancers decline significantly. There is clear evidence that quitting smoking has immediate benefits to our health and these benefits accumulate over time.[17]

The acute benefits of quitting smoking are realized quickly. The harms are such that surgeons will often not operate on active smokers due to the heightened complications and postoperative infections. However, most surgical oncologists will be able to operate on someone who has stopped smoking in as little time as a week before surgery. After ten years of being smoke-free, your risk for many tobacco-related cancers is cut in half.[16] Smoking cessation once someone has been diagnosed with a tobacco-related cancer improves the odds of survival and decreases the risk of developing a secondary cancer. For example, a meta-analysis of ten studies of people with lung cancer found that those who quit smoking at the time of diagnosis had a five-year survival rate of 63 percent and 70 percent for small-cell and non–small-cell lung cancer, respectively, versus 29 percent and 33 percent, respectively, among those who continued to smoke.[18] The same is true for a number of other tobacco-related cancers.[16]

What's truly fascinating is what happens when you combine smoking with another lifestyle choice, such as drinking alcohol. Those of us who've smoked in the past know how great a cigarette can taste when paired with a beer or a cocktail. What most of us don't know is that the carcinogenic effects of both tobacco and alcohol (which is independently linked to liver, breast, and digestive-tract-related cancers, among many others) are enhanced when they are combined.[15,19-21]

In other words, there is a negative synergistic effect when more than one cancer-related lifestyle factor is at play, and scientists cannot measure which substance is responsible for increasing the cancer-related risks when they are combined. What scientists do know, in the case of tobacco combined with alcohol, is that there can be a multiplicative risk of developing cancer.[19,20,22] If you smoke, drink, and are sedentary, your cancer risk increases. If you smoke, drink, are sedentary, and eat an unhealthy diet made up of mostly processed foods, your cancer risks rise even further.

The good news is that making changes in just one area of your life can significantly reduce your risk for developing certain cancers.[23-28] Making changes in more than one area will have a positive synergistic impact, reducing the odds of developing cancer or improving outcomes for those with cancer even more.[23-28] As Steve Cole, PhD, professor of medicine at the University of California, Los Angeles, wrote, "The old thinking was that our bodies were stable biological entities, fundamentally separate from the external world. But at the molecular level, our bodies turn out to be much more fluid and permeable to external influence than we realize."[29]

While we may never know what causes someone's specific cancer, we already have the answer for what reduces our risk and what changes we can actively make to slow cancer's growth and prevent it from spreading. Our knowledge of cancer's unique process can help us move forward in a more logical way, removing the veil of fear that prevents us from looking cancer in the eye. We know enough about this disease to confront it directly and take steps to confound its progress and take back control of our health.

CHAPTER FOUR

A Cell's Quest for Immortality

One cell. That's all it takes. One normal, microscopic cell goes haywire, a chain of events is set in motion, and over time this can lead to cancer.[1] Each of us is a walking constellation of 37.2 trillion complex, fragile cells. It's rather impressive then, that for roughly seventy-one years (the average global life span) these cells do what they're designed to do. But like stars in the vast night sky, it's inevitable that from time to time some of these cells will shoot out of alignment. How often do these cellular abnormalities occur? No one knows. But it's fair to assume that cellular corruption, or the molecular birth of nascent cancer cells, happens more frequently than we realize. Like shooting stars, these mutated cells appear and then our bodies respond, the abnormal cells either self-destruct or are destroyed through appropriate regulatory mechanisms. Meanwhile, we simply go on about our business, unaware these complex internal processes are keeping us cancer-free. Until one day, the DNA of one cell gets damaged, that damaged DNA begins to replicate, this triggers more DNA damage, and so on and so forth until this new cluster of bad cells takes hold and something imperceptible begins to grow uncontrolled within us. One, teeny tiny cell mutates, no longer following the genetically coded rule book, and we could be off to the races with cancer. Instead of gracefully dying off on its own or being subdued by our immune system, the cell proliferates.

We are not all going to get cancer, but we all have mutating, misbehaving, and abnormally growing cells in our bodies that have the potential to form the kind of a spreading mass that we call cancer. Why is it, then, that if we all have these mutating cells, we do not all get cancer? The answer is complicated, but it comes down to internal biological systems that keep cell growth in check. These include processes within the cells themselves, the surrounding cells, and substances in the microenvironment, as well as the response of our immune system and other systems in the body.[2,3] If a mutating cell is left unchecked, it starts to create a microenvironment that favors continued cell growth and makes it increasingly difficult for the body's natural defenses to do their job and keep cancer at bay.[4]

Cancer's Waiting Game

It takes time for a cancer cell to divide and grow to the size of being detectable—anywhere from five to forty years.[5] So, if it takes cancer half a lifetime to become large enough to be discovered, this means that the cancer we are diagnosed with in late middle age may have been hiding out in us since our early adolescence. I, for one, can only shake my head at all of the risky, careless behavior I engaged in when I was a teenager, but the fact that cancer can have such a long gestational period intrigues me because it indicates that cancer, though present, was not harmful to us when our bodies were able to inhibit its growth.

Following this chain of logic, then, if the body can contain cancer without being harmed, how might we extend its ability to engage those processes that control cancer's ability to proliferate and grow? What if we could help our bodies become more resistant and inhospitable to these proliferating mutated cells? What if, where cancer is concerned, a key part of prevention means keeping cancer quiet and benign in its behavior? What if it means somehow containing these first misfiring cells, like fireflies in a jar?

Catching cancer early is important because the longer a cancer can proliferate, the greater the risk of the cancer sending out "seeds" to other parts of the body, in a process known as metastasis (from the Greek *methistanai*, "to change"). If a cell detaches from its tissue of origin, it is supposed to undergo a process called *anoikis*—a form of programmed cell death. The term *anoikis* means "without a home." Anoikis ensures that cells stay close to the tissue to which they belong. However, tumor cells can effectively avoid anoikis as they stay alive and metastasize. Once cancer cells have avoided the body's natural process of cell death and transformed into freely circulating, adaptive cells, they are in search of a new home to "colonize." At this stage, treatment becomes especially complex and difficult, as now there are mutations of mutations of mutations to contend with. When cancer has successfully metastasized, it is not uncommon to see that the original cancer, which initially triggered the deadly progression, is vanquished, only for the patient to die of a later-forming variant of the disease. Preventing metastasis is why early interventions such as lifestyle changes and early detection are so crucial.

Early detection methods are at the forefront of this move toward early containment. As these tests improve, so do survival rates for many cancer patients.[6] Many laboratories around the world are working to develop blood-based tests to detect circulating cancer cells, proteins, or DNA for better earlier detection.[7] Post-treatment patients would benefit as well, as their remission could be monitored by a simple, low-cost blood test. For example, a team at Purdue is working on a test for cervical cancer that would use a simple strip of paper, much like a home pregnancy test, to reveal the presence of proteins associated with this often-deadly cancer, which responds extremely well to treatment when caught early.[8] This test, too, is being developed for use in detecting other cancers.

It goes without saying that the earlier a cancer is detected, the easier it is to control and presumably the better the long-term outcome. But what if we were able to prevent cancer in the first place?

It is time for us in the scientific community to put our focus on what we need to do to prevent that one lone cell from becoming corrupted or to control growth better once it starts to form.

A Brief History of Cancer and Its Treatment

A bit of context and history shows how very far we've come in understanding cancer biology and how this has changed our approach to treating cancer. The continuum is important to acknowledge as we enter what I hope will be an age of much greater understanding as to what anticancer living really is. We're on the cusp of truly understanding the personal influence we have over this confounding set of diseases.

Cancer has likely been with us since the dawn of humankind.[9] It was first named—*karkinos*, the Greek word for "crab"—by Hippocrates, the "Father of Modern Medicine" himself, sometime around 400 BC. Medical historian Howard Markel has noted that Hippocrates was wise in choosing the word *crab* to describe these malignant growths because it so aptly describes cancer in several ways: Advanced cancerous tumors, which are large crowded masses of cancer cells, are rock hard and brittle, and even often

EARLY DETECTION: A Mixed Blessing?

There is a controversial aspect to early detection, as it can lead to unnecessarily aggressive treatments for some nonlethal cancers.[10,11] Often, these illnesses are more accurately classified as "precancerous" states, and there is no scientific or medical evidence that these cellular anomalies would cause harm or contribute to a person's mortality if left untreated.[12] For example, there is currently a debate going on about the risks and benefits of early detection of prostate cancer.[11] Since most prostate cancers are extremely slow-growing, surgery or radiation or chemotherapy are often not required.[13] Once cancer is detected, however, it is our medical "norm" to cut, poison, or burn it out, regardless of the consequences to a patient's quality of life and overall health.[12] Recent research actually suggests that for men with low-risk disease, treating their prostate cancer may make no difference to how long they will live.[14,15] But those treated will certainly have to live with the unintended side effects of radiotherapy or surgery, such as the risk of permanent erectile dysfunction and urinary incontinence.[16,17] A similar challenging situation is starting to emerge for women diagnosed with a form of early-stage breast cancer (called ductal carcinoma in situ) for which we have no evidence as to whether the body's natural defenses will control the disease or if it will ever progress beyond stage 0.[18,19] In fact, British and American researchers are currently conducting a study to examine if it is necessary to treat low-risk DCIS.[20,21] Some breast cancer specialists are even beginning to suggest that these very early cancers not be classified as cancer at all. Perhaps "active surveillance" with an anticancer lifestyle prescription will become a more standard first-line treatment for very early-stage cancers as we gather more evidence that lifestyle can keep cancer in check.

bluish, like a crab's shell; the searing pain these masses cause as they crowd out healthy tissue is said to be as sharp and lacerating as the wincing pinch of a crab's claw.[22] In Hippocrates's day, cancer diseases often weren't detectable until masses burst through the skin of those who suffered. When doctors and curious scientists began to dissect these severe growths, they noted that the way the hard lava flows of tainted cells and the tributaries of blood vessels that fueled these cells sprawled and grabbed at healthy tissue mimicked the tenacious grasping of the crab.

The way that cancer has been viewed through the ages also gives us a vivid snapshot of how the general medical approaches to this cluster of cellular diseases has changed over time; but one fact remains: Cancer—despite so many truly impressive medical advances—is still one of the leading causes of death worldwide. It may be a cellular fact of the human experience, but it seems, given how furiously modern medicine has tried to keep up with it, that its persistence may have something to do with the way human life has evolved on earth. Given that certain cancer rates continue to rise, especially among young adults and children, it should seem obvious that the time has come to shift focus and look at how our daily choices might be making all of us more susceptible to these diseases.

Two thousand or so years ago, in ancient Greece, where Hippocrates lived, cancer sufferers were prepared for a painful, even cruel death. What we now refer to as palliative care, the compassionate management of pain and discomfort, was the primary, and in many cases the only, type of treatment available during that time. Surgical cures were sometimes attempted, but before the advent of anesthesia in the mid-nineteenth century and before the understanding of the need to use techniques such as sterilization to prevent infection, surgery was simply too barbaric and too risky. It is worth noting, however, that some ancient medical records found in Greece show that when surgery was attempted, patients who survived the excision of their tumors were encouraged to modify their diets and to engage in special exercise regimens in order to hasten recovery. This is the first evidence that, even before the advent of modern medicine, lifestyle was understood to have had a positive influence on patient outcome.

Surgical removal of tumors became the focal point of treatment once anesthesia was invented in the latter half of the nineteenth century. This brought in a nearly hundred-year reign of surgery as the treatment of choice for cancers, and this remained so, even when it became known that most cancers—even once excised—would one day return. Cancer surgeries tended to be radical. Surgeries were unapologetically aggressive with the singular goal of most cancer surgeons being to swiftly and surely excise as much diseased and surrounding tissue as possible. The thought was that the more radical the surgery, the less likely the cancer would be to come back. Unfortunately, this was usually wrong. Breast cancer patients, for example, lost not only the diseased breast, but also glands and lymph nodes and vital muscles and tendons. For other patients, cancer meant the loss of limbs or being maimed or disfigured and left unable to regain a meaningful quality of life. And yet the cancer would still come back.

At the dawn of the twentieth century, radiation was discovered, and it was soon known to be both a cause and a cure for cancer. Cancer cells, because they were so rapidly growing, were more susceptible to the effects of radiation than healthy cells. However, although radiation worked, it also brought with it much collateral damage as, inevitably, the healthy tissues around cancers were not spared. Early radiation patients suffered from severe burns—both internally and externally, and this caused a whole host of secondary illnesses, many of which were quite serious. Again, the quality of life for many of these patients was terribly compromised by the primitive, harsh early versions of this treatment.

After World War II, when it was discovered that the mustard gas used in chemical warfare kills cancerous cells, the age of chemotherapy began, and with it, new hope for prolonging remission (the length of time before a cancer returns at its original site) and preventing *metastasis* (when cancer spreads to other parts of the body).[23]

In 1971, the National Cancer Act was passed, which allocated $1.5 billion and three years to cancer research.[24] This was the first time that cancer was legislated as a national public health crisis, and the beauty is that we now have long-term studies, many patient databases, and an abundance of real data that have helped to shape our use of the treatment tools we have at hand. Over the past fifty years, our approach to various cancers has become much more nuanced, with the aims of minimizing unpleasant side effects or the onset of secondary illness.

For the next forty years, the three main treatment modalities of surgery, radiation, and chemotherapy, which are often used in concert, became the standard of care. With the adoption of this multipronged approach, we moved into an era when cancer survival rates surged and some cancers, such as certain childhood leukemias or early-stage thyroid cancer, even began to be viewed as curable. By the 1990s, many cancer rates were dropping, though some—especially gastrointestinal cancers (colon, rectal, and others) and virus-related cancers (such as liver cancer or oral cancers)—were rising, especially among younger adults. As more and more people are living longer with cancer and speaking more openly about it, our perception of how the disease affects us has broadened.

Now, in 2018, despite so many important advancements in our

understanding of cancer biology, the troika of surgery, radiation, and chemotherapy remain the blueprint for most cancer treatment. But there have been some important modifications and they are worth noting. The advent of the newly developed targeted therapies and immunotherapy has transformed the landscape of cancer treatment. Even surgeries have taken on a more nuanced approach. For instance, since the 1990s, when it became clear that less-invasive surgeries, such as lumpectomies, are every bit as effective as more aggressive surgical approaches, the rate of radical mastectomies has decreased. Even so, relative to the recent past, more emphasis is finally being placed on not just prolonging the life of a cancer patient, but preserving quality of life as well.

Gene Behavior as a New Focal Point of Treatment

After the successful mapping of the human genome was completed in 2003, we entered an exciting new era in treating cancer.[25] By looking specifically at gene biology and function, we're able to come at cancer from a much more sophisticated, nuanced, and, importantly, personalized point of view. Being able to actually "see" human genes in action has helped those of us in the cancer world to really wrap our heads around the fact that no two cancers are alike and that our trio of standard care options is woefully broad and rather random in its targeting. In other words, to say that in desperation we've been addressing a microscopic phenomenon with a sledgehammer would not be an overstatement; but this is more of a reflection about how impossible it was for us to understand the subtle genetic changes that make cancer possible before 2003.

Now, however, thanks to the complete map of the human genome, we can monitor gene functioning and identify the specific gene activities that are linked with many different chronic diseases, including some cancers. Scientists now understand that *gene expression* and *gene regulation* are responsible for allowing cells to replicate in an orderly manner and that faulty gene regulation is a primary driver of cancer. They have also begun to discover how lifestyle factors, including the six that are the foundation of *anticancer living*, influence gene expression and regulation and influence the mutagenic process.

The best minds in cellular medicine are now focusing on more precisely understanding and targeting the key biological processes that control cancer growth. This is, of course, an evolving field and there are new mechanisms and targets discovered constantly. However, reviewing some of the known key pathways to date will help us better understand how a mutated cell can become a group of mutated cells and ultimately threaten the host's life. This understanding will also show how our lifestyle choices can influence many of the cancer processes, allowing our bodies to be as inhospitable to cancer growth as possible.

While the mapping of the human genome was being completed, in 2000, Swiss researchers Douglas Hanahan and Robert Weinberg published an article that offered an elegantly simple theory about how cancer cells develop and progress. In their original thesis Hanahan and Weinberg identified six underlying key processes for cancer growth, which they call the "Hallmarks of Cancer":[26]

1. Sustaining proliferative signaling: cancer's ability to short-circuit normal controls and proliferate indefinitely.
2. Evading growth suppressors: circumventing growth suppressors to continue unrestricted growth.
3. Resisting cell death: cancer's ability to avoid the normal process of cell *apoptosis* (cell suicide).
4. Enabling replicative immortality: cancer's way of tricking our system by overexpressing an enzyme to allow a cell to become "immortal" and continue to proliferate (avoiding telomere attrition, which is part of the normal aging process).
5. Inducing angiogenesis: the formation of new blood vessels that feed the tumor.
6. Activating invasion and metastasis: processes that allow cancer cells to circulate freely through the body.

Several years later, Hanahan and Weinberg added two additional hallmarks to their model:[3]

• Reprogramming energy metabolism: the way cancer cells maximize their use of energy.
• Avoiding immune destruction: a process that lets cancer cells continue to grow and spread and not be controlled by the immune system.

They also added two enabling characteristics:[3]

* Genome instability and mutation: altering the genomic characteristics of cancer cells to protect them from "caretaker" genes.
* Tumor-promoting inflammation: cancer's ability to mimic inflammatory conditions that nourish the tumor and help it continue to grow.

For more details on each area, you can delve more deeply in the appendix.

Each area of the Mix of Six has been found to impact at least one, and usually multiple, cancer hallmarks.[27–42] In other words, the choices we make in our lives will likely influence the intricate biological processes determining whether cancer flourishes or withers in our bodies. Four hallmark processes that are influential on cancer growth happen to be also the processes for which there is the most data linked to our lifestyle: Proliferative Signaling, Activating Invasion and Metastasis, Immune Function, and Inflammation.[38–40,43–45] The goal is to transform our tumor microenvironment, the terrain in which cancer grows, whether it is the first cell that has mutated or a group of cells that have already formed cancer, and make it as inhospitable to cancer growth as possible.

The "hallmarks" model continues to change and be modified as our understanding of genes, gene expression, and cancer deepens. But it has provided a much-needed blueprint for researchers to begin to understand the basic mechanistic features of cancer growth that have allowed all of us to approach cancer treatment with more effectiveness.

It is important to note that there is not consensus among scientists as to the relative importance of each of the hallmarks for different cancers. One of the challenges is that cancer is a heterogeneous disease, even within organ-specific cancers (e.g., breast cancer). As such, different biological processes may play a more or less important role. It is also hard to differentiate the biological processes, gene abnormalities, and gene functions that are the true "drivers" of disease versus processes that are happening alongside disease development—the "passengers." In addition, our understanding of cancer is changing rapidly, and what was thought to be critical in the past is now set aside; what was unknown, ignored, or dismissed is now accepted; and new biological processes are continually being discovered and explored as treatment options. This is the scientific process.

As an example of how this lack of consensus looks in real life, Judah

Folkman gave a keynote speech at the 2007 annual meeting of the Society for Integrative Oncology, where he described what it was like trying to get funding for his early work in angiogenesis, which is the ability of cancer to stimulate the formation of new blood vessels in order to create a sustaining nutritional supply. He showed us his grant reviews from the National Institutes of Health review committee, wherein one reviewer said: "There is only one person in the world who believes such a crazy idea as angiogenesis and that is the principle investigator of this grant application." Needless to say, the NIH did not fund the grant. But that did not stop Folkman. He went on to prove that the process of angiogenesis was critical for a number of cancers to thrive, and his discoveries led to the development of multiple drugs that successfully treat several different cancers and other diseases, such as cardiovascular disease and macular degeneration.[46] Folkman's discoveries gave much-needed credence to the cancer hallmarks thesis and it gave the cancer research community a great model for pursuing cancer research from a cellular, mechanistic point of view.

The Recent Shift to More Targeted Treatment Approaches

Discoveries and treatment breakthroughs are now happening on many fronts as our understanding of the individual causal triggers of cancer growth becomes more sophisticated. This more individualized approach is so important because cancer is a master at variability, and this is why our one-size-fits-all approaches to treatment—especially eradication—have fallen short.

A new range of drug therapies, collectively known as targeted cancer therapies, are showing tremendous promise.[47] These therapies work on a molecular level and offer a more precise kind of treatment by targeting specific abnormalities unique to the cancer cells to limit their growth. What they are "targeting" are certain genetic abnormalities unique to cancer and the proteins that regulate gene behavior that are the "drivers" for that cancer. By working at a targeted cellular level, these precision therapies appear to work without harming healthy cells as much as conventional chemotherapies. Yet even these targeted approaches have unwanted side effects, from minor problems such as skin conditions to more severe issues such as heart disease and metabolic disorders.[48]

Targeted therapies include *hormone therapies*, which stop the growth of tumors that are stimulated by specific hormones. Hormone therapies show great promise in treating breast and prostate cancers, although they come with side effects, including bone loss, chronic pain, "chemo" brain, hot flashes, and weight gain.[49] Other types of targeted therapies are *signal trans-duction inhibitors*, which block signals from one molecule to another to break up the relay of signals that cancer cells need to continue their un-abated division and replication, as well as *apoptosis inducers*, which force cancer cells to abandon their quest for immortality and die.[50,51] *Monoclonal antibody therapies* bind to the cancer cells and prompt recognition by the immune system, while *angiogenesis inhibitors* successfully block access to the blood vessels that feed tumor growth, thereby cutting them off from their nutritional support.[52,53] Often these targeted therapies based on an

THE MICROBIOME AND CANCER

Another focal point of scientific interest in how cancer works is the grow-ing understanding of how the microbiome—which refers to the bacterial flora found in and on our body—may be part of the cancer development puzzle.[54] There are theories being developed that suggest that altering gut bacteria may make a person respond better to treatment, especially immunotherapies.[55] Research in this area suggests that the microflora of people with cancer is different from those without cancer—though the implications of this are still unclear.[56] Additionally, we know that certain microbes, such as the helicobacter pylori bacteria, are known causes of cancers, so looking further into whether bacterial microbiota play a role in carcinogenesis makes great sense.[57] Since 2011, there have been several studies that point to this relationship, and one in particular, conducted at the European Molecular Biology Laboratory, stands out. In 2014, re-searchers discovered they could detect the presence of colorectal cancer based on the presence of a certain type of bacteria in stool samples, with nearly the same level of accuracy as the standard screening tests.[58] This is just one of several compelling studies (including one recently conducted here at MD Anderson[55]) that are beginning to draw meaningful conclu-sions about the causal link between certain types of bacteria and the cellular corruption that leads to cancer. More on this, and how to create a healthy microbiome, in chapter 11, "Food as Medicine."

individual person's tumor's gene abnormalities are combined with conventional chemotherapies for a multipronged approach.

While targeted therapy is a promising field, success can be limited if the cancer doesn't depend on just one targetable mutation.[59] There are more than forty thousand gene mutations affecting over ten thousand unique genes with 500 genes classified as cancer drivers. It is still difficult to differentiate the aberrant genes that are the true drivers of the disease from those that are merely passengers.[60] However, the Cancer Genome Atlas project is making progress in this area, and new discoveries suggest that for some cancers the number of "driver mutations" could be as low as one or two. The greatest challenge for medicines targeting specific genes is cancer's ability to transform and express new mutations, often leading to resistance or a recurrence of cancer in patients who undergo targeted therapies.[60]

Another type of cancer treatment, *immunotherapies*, supercharge the immune system so that it can successfully destroy cancer cells or remove the brakes that are put on the immune system, or a combination of the two, resulting in true cancer cures in a small subset of patients who previously would have died of their cancers.[61] Most recently, research is examining combining the targeted therapy approach alongside immune therapies, but the efficacy of these efforts has yet to be proved. What we don't know yet is how to identify which patients will respond to these immunotherapies.

A VACCINE THAT PREVENTS CANCER

The human papillomavirus (HPV) is so common that 9 out of 10 sexually active Americans will contract it at some point in their lives.[62] Ten years ago, a vaccine was created that prevents infection of the strains of the virus that are responsible for causing cervical and other deadly cancer diseases. The success of these vaccines has been nothing short of astonishing, as onset rates of the targeted viruses have been effectively cut in half.[63] The American Cancer Society recommends that children become vaccinated between the ages of 9 and 14, before they become sexually active.[62,64]

"In the past several years, studies have shown the vaccine is even more effective than expected," said Debbie Saslow, PhD, senior director, HPV Related and Women's Cancers for the American Cancer Society.[65]

There are many reasons to postulate that lifestyle factors that impact the immune system could improve response to immunotherapy, and that is an area we are actively investigating.

Meanwhile, vaccine therapies actually prevent cancers known to have a viral origin, including cancers caused by the human papillomavirus (HPV), such as cervical, penile, and head and neck cancers, as well as those known to be caused by hepatitis B or C, such as liver cancer.[62]

Last but not least are the recent forays into *gene or biological therapies* in which the cells of a cancer patient are extracted, their genes altered, and then reintroduced to the body.[66] In a very few cases, the results have been extraordinary, but the financial burden is staggering and repeating this success has proved difficult, at least at this very early stage of our understanding of the behavior of genes in cancer cells.[67] Perhaps the lack of focus on lifestyle factors is a variable that keeps this kind of "personalized" approach from working more broadly.

The medical world is moving swiftly toward treating cancer on an intercellular level. Until the dawn of the targeted cellular approach, the overarching goal in developing drugs in oncology was to create drugs that could be given at maximum dosage in order to kill as many cells as possible without killing the patient. The collateral damage to this approach was, and remains, high and costly. The goal of this more targeted approach is to use drug therapy to restore something, rather than destroy it, and this sea change in our thinking about treatment objectives alone is going to bring great relief—and I believe radically improved prognoses and quality of life—to countless cancer patients in the near future. With every breakthrough in our understanding of how DNA and RNA—and thus, our genes—respond to a cancer signal, the closer we come to understanding how to prevent the onset of cancer in the first place. Meanwhile, exciting scientific evidence is showing how lifestyle modifications directly influence some of the biological hallmarks of cancer and the genes controlling these cancer processes in positive ways—sometimes in the same ways as chemical interventions, but without unwanted side effects.

CHAPTER FIVE

The Epigenetics of Prevention

There is no doubt that the complete mapping of the human genome has profoundly and fundamentally deepened our understanding of cancer biology, which has, in turn, pointed us toward developing and using much more nuanced, less harmful screening and treatment approaches. The pharmaceutical industry is rushing to develop new chemical forms of intervention to inhibit or stop cancer cell mutation and proliferation. As those focused on finding a cure through treatment keep their gaze on the genome, those of us interested in prevention, as well as eradication, are making great strides due to the emerging sciences that fall under the generalized field of epigenetics. Epigenetics broadly refers to the processes that drive gene expression (the behavior of genes), but which do not alter the actual DNA sequence that is housed within that gene.

Epigenetic processes are quite natural and necessary: Without them, our cells would literally be dormant. Epigenetic processes control the minute changes in our DNA that cause what are basically identical cells to behave quite differently. For instance, how is it that one cell acts as a liver cell while another acts as a skin cell even though these two cells both contain identical strands of my DNA? Every facet of cellular differentiation is due to the behavior of the cell or the epigenetic processes that influence those identical strands of DNA to behave differently. *Epigenetics* means what is "above" or "on top of" basic genetics: It's often referred to as "the science of change," as it looks at what causes variations in genetic expression. Epigenetics drives all cell behavior—good, bad, and otherwise.

What, then, are the epigenetic factors that cause a normal cell to behave in ways that allow it to grow out of control and become cancer? There are both external and internal factors at play. It is believed that the external factors may play a more important role in these processes than internal ones.[1] *What external factors are driving the epigenetics of cancer development and proliferation?* Are they environmental (toxins), dietary (nutrients), behavioral (stressors), or one of other countless sources, or any combination of several of these, any or all of which might cause a cell to become dysregulated?

Answering this question, I believe, is what will lead us to the missing piece in the cancer prevention and treatment puzzle. We now know that cancer mutates so spectacularly and so unpredictably that each new cancer cell is different from the last and no cancer is ever the same in one individual when compared to another, even when they have been diagnosed with the same "type" of cancer.[2] Despite this, we've gotten incredibly close to "curing" cancer, but we can't quite seem to get there. Even when we are able to eradicate 99 percent of the cancer cells in a tumor, often the surviving 1 percent of cells that elude us will reemerge, this time, more powerfully driven to mutate and change with a fierce, potent diversity that will render new drug therapies equally ineffective.

We are now seeing breakthroughs across many disciplines that connect how we live in the world with how our cellular biology behaves. What we're learning, at a faster and faster pace, is that lifestyle factors do, indeed, directly influence the gene behaviors necessary to regulate healthy, homeostatic, cellular growth—maintaining orderly and appropriate cell growth.[3-5] We are seeing that these external factors influence the gene regulatory processes of the *cancer hallmarks* and beyond.[3,6-12] What is so very exciting about all this is how much control we have over these dynamic epigenetic influences.

With each new discovery on how lifestyle influences gene expression, we're adding to an important new kind of genomic map: This has been christened the "epigenome." This gathering of information will provide us the scientific guidance we need going forward to begin to make significant inroads into actual cancer prevention.

The Sweet Science of Social Genomics

Social Genomics is the study of how everyday life circumstances influence gene expression. Our lives are infinitely complex and ever changing, but the work that is being done by researchers in this area is clarifying how certain aspects of our lifestyle influence either the prevention or proliferation of many diseases, including cancers. Social genomics offers us a way to view genetic behavior through an incredibly hopeful and optimistic lens where cancer is concerned because lifestyle factors are something that we can change, regardless of our current circumstances. This is the area of scientific research and inquiry upon which anticancer living is built.

Elissa Epel, a renowned social scientist, described her interest in epigenetics to me in a recent conversation. "I'm interested in how the psychological and social world is transduced . . . how it gets under the skin . . . to affect the different systems in our bodies that regulate our health, such as the immune system, our metabolic systems, our eating, hunger, and appetite: there's this whole realm of personal choice that really impacts our health on so many fundamental levels."

Social scientists like myself, Steve Cole, Epel, and many others have spent our careers looking at how environmental factors (including social, physical, and emotional factors) influence gene behavior by somehow permeating the barrier between our experiential selves and our cellular selves to promote both health and well-being or possibly trigger the onset of any number of diseases, including cancers. Research from my laboratory and others is showing how factors like stress and depression modulate key gene expression pathways in ways that will increase our vulnerability to cancer.[13,14] Practices like yoga, tai chi, or other stress-management techniques not only improve aspects of quality of life but also modify these gene regulatory pathways leading to better cellular control.[15-17]

Steve Cole, who is considered the founder of the new field of social genomics, has done some incredibly compelling research on how the chronic stressors in life can adversely affect our health.[18,19] Cole and his team at UCLA discovered that people who live in neighborhoods marked by poverty, high unemployment, loneliness, social isolation, and fear (high-crime areas) have changes in gene expression that may make them more susceptible to developing cancers and other diseases. The good news is that these effects—though they have the potential to alter gene behavior over the course of several generations—are demonstrably reversible.[20] This means that we can actually change the course of our own cellular evolution by simply improving aspects of our lives.

Cole made the following discoveries:

* Removing a person from a stressful environment—even late in life—will allow their genes to return to a state of balance.[20] That means our health has huge potential to rebound.
* Early interventions to improve a child's situation can fortify a child in ways that prime their bodies for appropriate gene expression over time—even if these interventions are short-lived.[21]
* Looking at the epigenetic impact of these life stressors on a biological level will help us identify lifestyle changes we can make that will allow us to act before genes malfunction or cancer manifests.

What Cole began to realize is that taking lifestyle factors into account when looking at gene expression really means looking at gene behavior through an utterly new lens. His is a beautifully unifying vision that acknowledges that there is a psychological component, a physical component, and a chemical component in the epigenetic processes that lead to cancer

THE EPIGENETIC COST OF CHILDHOOD EXPERIENCES

Scientists are understanding how trauma gets written into the body in ways that have a cascading effect on our health and well-being. Working with one's history of trauma and the patterns of thought, behavior, and biology that have developed as a consequence can lay a new foundation for emotional balance and a new mind-set around wellness.

Studies show that those who suffer from adverse childhood experiences (ACEs) have higher rates of many diseases—including cancers.[22-24] Finding help for overcoming these early traumas (abuse, neglect, etc.) is essential for engaging in healthful behaviors and regaining a high quality of life.

The good news is that these early childhood challenges, though they may have influenced gene behavior early on, are not life sentences. They are reversible.[20,25] The pillars of anticancer living, along with focused psychological treatment, can heal lifelong wounds and put us on the road to real freedom and agency.

development.[18] With this awareness, we can then take daily actions that either fortify the body's ability to keep genetic expression balanced, or we can live in ways that weaken this essential homeostasis. The good news, especially for those of us burdened by stressors that may, practically speaking, be inescapable, is that the proactive actions we take can be as simple as acknowledging that we're in a stressful situation and engaging in behaviors to change or diminish the harms of the stressors. This kind of psychological awareness alone can activate the kind of biological fortification and systemic regulation that work to keep diseases, including cancer, at bay.

THE HUMAN EPIGENOME PROJECT (HEP)

Back in 2003, right around the time the Human Genome Project was being completed, a group of international scientists created the European Epigenome Project.[26] This group, headed by Andrew Feinberg, a geneticist at Johns Hopkins School of Medicine, in 2005 launched the U.S. Human Epigenome Project, a sister project that would pursue complementary (rather than overlapping) data.[27] Combined, the two groups hope to create a comprehensive map of genes as it relates to epigenetic activity and tagging—which means literally tracking the changes in gene expression that become heritable, or passed from a cell to a daughter cell—without changing the inherent DNA sequence in any way. My former colleague at MD Anderson, Jean-Pierre Issa, MD, who is now at Temple University and is also a founding member of the Human Epigenome Project, said, "Cancer, atherosclerosis, Alzheimer's disease—they are all *acquired* diseases where environment very likely plays an important role."[28] Feinberg believes that cancer is a much simpler cellular process than current gene theories promote. He believes that with these kinds of databases, we are nearing the ability to identify premalignant conditions and positively influence them by making changes in lifestyle, which would mean that we can stop cancer before it begins simply by making modifications in our daily lives.

How Experience Becomes Imprinted on Our Genes

A fascinating study published in 2008[29] looked at stress levels in survivors of the Holocaust and their offspring and discovered that the descendants of survivors have a unique stress hormone profile that may predispose them to anxiety disorders at a higher rate than their nonaffected peers.[29] Rachel Ye-huda, a researcher in the growing field of epigenetics and the intergenera-tional effects of trauma, and her colleagues at the Icahn School of Medicine at Mount Sinai and the James J. Peters Veterans Affairs Medical Center in the Bronx, measured the levels of the stress hormone cortisol and found that the Holocaust survivor offspring had lower levels of cortisol than the control group.[29] When they looked further, they found that this group had higher levels of an enzyme that breaks down cortisol. They reported that the offspring of the Holocaust survivors had specific changes in stress-related genes linked with PTSD and depression.[30] This indicates that these individ-uals' inherited genetic abnormalities as it relates to producing the stress hormones needed to react to trauma, and these may have been affected in ways that can be passed from one generation to the next. This is supported by extensive animal research showing that the negative effects of stress ex-posure are passed down through multiple generations, even among those multiple generations removed.[31] We are starting to see the same phenomena with the heritability of obesity-linked gene regulatory factors influencing offspring even seven generations removed from the original source.[32-34]

Elizabeth Blackburn, who was awarded the Nobel Prize in Medicine in 2009 for her work on telomeres, discussed this phenomenon in 2012, where she and her colleague, Elissa Epel, realized that violence, poverty, and abuse—epigenetic factors—tore away the "protective cover" that shielded an indi-vidual's genome.[35] This has prompted great fascination and interest in understanding the evolutionary aspects of epigenetic experience as it relates to illness and disease. Is this just a one-way street in terms of the lasting effect of such stressors and the ensuing lifestyle factors?

The answer, at least with emotional epigenetic factors, appears to be a resounding no, because epigenetic changes are what we think of as "mallea-ble," or mutable, influences. There is a dynamism at play with epigenetics that rattles all of our assumptions about gene behavior either being the re-sult of heredity or bad luck. Understanding the reversibility, the changeabil-ity of epigenetic influence offers a radically new way to understand how differently we can approach treating diseases like cancer when we open our-selves to concepts like reversibility or redirection as it concerns our gene behavior.

The question of "reversibility" is more complex when it comes to chem-ical sources of epigenetic influence. One of the most notorious examples of this are the daughters and granddaughters (and sons and grandsons) of women who took the drug diethylstilbestrol (DES), an estrogen-based compound that was meant to prevent miscarriage.[36] The drug was widely prescribed in the United States in the mid part of the twentieth century, and the CDC estimate that anywhere between five and ten million American women took the drug between 1938 and 1971, when it was finally pulled off the market. The daughters of these women who were, themselves, exposed to DES while in utero, are prone to developing a particularly rare kind of vaginal cancer and to have problems conceiving and carrying a pregnancy to term, while the sons of these women, who were also exposed to DES while in utero, are prone to a particular set of diseases, including certain cancers.[37] More startlingly, the granddaughters of these women who used DES during pregnancy had an increased risk of ovarian cancer.[38] These studies are also supported by animal research showing that the epigenetic effects of DES exposure are apparent two generations later, showing a clear transgenerational effect carried through the genes.[39,40]

Changing the heritability of this kind of chemically induced genetic disruption takes a more focused medical intervention than reducing stress or modifying lifestyle factors, but knowing that you have this exposure in your family history and sharing that information with your physician gives you the chance to take early intervention measures that may prevent the onset or proliferation of the diseases associated with this kind of gene-modulatory exposure.

My colleague Janet Gray, PhD, who is at Vassar College, has become fascinated with exploring the intersection of the environment and women's health—particularly as it relates to breast cancer. In 2017, she was the lead author with her colleagues on an update on the evidence linking breast cancer to environmental exposures.[41] Recently, she's begun to explore the connection between the plastic compound bisphenol A, or BPA (a chemical that stimulates estrogen), and its epigenetic role in breast cancer.

Cancer as an Evolutionary Response to Modern Life

In 2016, at Yale University, the results of a very unique study were released. The investigation applied the tools traditionally used by evolutionary biologists to reframe how we think about cancer tumor metastases in an effort to shed light on how we might develop more effective treatments.

The study, which was led by Jeffrey Townsend, was published in the *Proceedings of the National Academy of Sciences.*[42]

Beginning with the idea held by many scientists that cancer is an evolutionary process, Townsend and his team gathered tumor tissue from normal, primary, and metastatic tumor cells from a range of individuals with either no disease or with various types of cancer. Using evolutionary biology methodologies, they created a "tree" that would map the evolution of the cancers among this group by pinpointing the genetic mutations found within the gathered samples. What they found was that their maps revealed relationships between tumor chronology and genetic changes. From this, they were able to identify three key properties that all the cancers they sampled shared: First was being able to see that metastases originated along differential paths within the primary tumors and then spread out in a "branchlike" pattern, rather than in a linear fashion (as earlier models assumed), suggesting that single genetic changes are unlikely to be necessary or sufficient for metastasis. Second, they found that this metastatic process can genetically differentiate itself much earlier in the life of the primary tumor than previously thought—*and even occur before a primary tumor is diagnosed.* Third, they found that the metastatic process is linked to the "driver mutations" that give selective (or evolutionary) advantage to certain mutations over others—and this propels the metastatic process.

These discoveries are significant because they will allow us to focus on the genes where this kind of "evolutionary," or "driver," mutation is occurring and target therapies that will halt the metastatic process—even perhaps before we begin to tackle the primary tumor.

Ultimately what this helps us understand is how tenaciously cancer vies for survival: we need to know, as Townsend points out, "that cancer simultaneously evolves along multiple trajectories" and that "the oncologist of the future is going to have to understand this evolutionary biology in order to outmaneuver the disease."[43]

For decades, the idea that cancer was primarily an evolutionary response was a cornerstone theory of cancer science. Then, in the 1970s, the molecular revolution shifted our focus away from this "bigger picture" framework and our focus stayed small, until, ironically, the recent breakthroughs we've made with the human genome project and the genomics revolution we're in the midst of right now. Scientists are rapidly realizing that the only way to manage all this data is to use the tools of evolutionary science and an evolutionary perspective to reach the next levels of effective treatment and move more decisively toward prevention.

Cole also sees cancer proliferation as an "evolutionary" adaption and explains it by adding the social science piece to the equation by noting that our bodies are designed to react to acute stress (think running from a predator or fleeing a burning building), but they just aren't designed to be under the chronic stress and the multiple unhealthy behaviors that characterize modern life. I fully share this view with him and I've seen over the course of my career how helping patients get out from under their unhealthy lives is essential to healing and regaining a sense of health and well-being.

We must constantly remember that cancer cells are cells that have lost all balance, all semblance of normal behavior. In fact, they are cells that have become genetically programmed to continue to morph and change, with the sole purpose of being able to escape any kind of homeostatic regulation or any kind of evolutionary constraints—be they biological or lifestyle. We see that these cells also hijack multiple systems within our body, modifying gene expression with the sole purpose of allowing them to stay alive. This is why treating cancers has thus far been so confounding: Cancer cells are constantly changing because of factors that cannot be addressed with surgery, radiation, or drugs. We simply won't have effective treatment if we don't bring the massive lifestyle component of cause into play.

Cancer, it seems, has figured out how to outpace, even outwit what we consider normal cellular evolutionary behavior, and scientists are beginning to see a clear parallel between the accelerating of cancer onset with the expanding and ever-changing raft of socioenvironmental stressors and lifestyle factors in which we are all steeped.

Our Genes Are Not Our Destiny

Visualizing how the accumulated unhealthy exposures of modern life show up when we plot the negative aspects of epigenetics on a graph alongside the increasing incidence of cancers worldwide over time invites a new kind of understanding and dialogue. And we need that in order to empower and activate our patients and ourselves. Our social histories are actively and continuously written into our DNA in ways that we can come to better understand and influence. In fact, we can change the biological narrative by changing the way we live.

We're now learning that our genes are not our destiny—nor is evolution, when it comes to cancer. Now we know that we have great power over both of these factors—much more than we ever thought imaginable. What this means—despite the almost fifty-fifty odds that we currently face—is that cancer is not inevitable. We now know that we can contest and challenge the statistics.

For optimal success in preventing and controlling cancer once diagnosed, behavioral risk reduction needs to take place. For those with cancer, this needs to happen *alongside* targeting the abnormal genes and stimulating the immune system. Modifying as many of the factors that we know influence the healthy gene expression and balancing the cancer hallmarks will help to create a body that is as inhospitable to cancer as possible. While high-tech, multimillion-dollar studies continue to explore cancer hallmarks and targeted interventions, the low-tech solutions of living a healthier life and engaging in comprehensive lifestyle change remain a powerful, effective antidote to avoid or survive cancer. And you don't have to wait for this prescription to be approved by the FDA or travel halfway across the country or around the world to find a doctor who can help you implement it.

In fact, all you have to do is keep reading.

CHAPTER SIX

Synergy and the Mix of Six

In *Anticancer,* David Servan-Schreiber focused on four key components of lifestyle that he knew were helping him to heal while he had cancer. They comprise of diet, environment (toxins), exercise, and stress. In *Anticancer Living,* Alison and I have added two new pillars of healthy lifestyle to these components, and they are social support and sleep. David himself knew how crucial the close connection of his family was to his survival, and he likely understood the importance of sleeping well, too. Researchers around the world are adding valuable studies and data to the growing bank of science that validates and fine-tunes our understanding about the healing powers of these daily habits. In summary, here are the six areas, which I will cover individually in more detail:

Connectedness Counts: We human beings are not meant to go it entirely alone, and so we start, create, and choose families; find friends, tribes, and allies; join teams, communities, and groups; in general engage in activities where we get a boost of social interaction. Even the introverts among us need connection, balanced with solitude and quiet. Companionship in all its varieties shields us from stress, loneliness, and vulnerability. We have seen a growing body of research on the power of love and social support to heal—it's so important that Alison and I have given it top priority among the "Mix of Six" lifestyle factors.

Let Stress Go: We all need some kind of life friction to get us up and out of bed in the morning, but our lives should be defined by how energized we feel, not how stressed-out we are. Stress is known to stimulate cancer proliferation, not to mention that it erodes our well-being in a multitude of ways.[1-3] Chronic stress is corrosive and wears away our ability to experience health on both social and biological levels.[4] It is the great instigator of so much disease that we've given it high priority in this discussion.

Sleep as a Supernutrient: Sleeping well is profoundly healing; a vital "activity" in which we must engage to foster well-being. Virtually nothing else can change your outlook on life and your ability to heal as much as sleep does, and there's a lot to be said about what goes on biologically during these hours, too.[5-7] Anticancer living means prioritizing this highly productive healing time, and addressing any obstacles or difficulties. Your body will thank you!

The Joy of Movement: Our bodies are designed to move. When we are sedentary, the internal rhythms and tides of the chemicals and fluids that govern the processes that keep us healthy and robust can become silted, sluggish, and ineffectual. We need to honor the body's design and stretch, reach, walk, run; to move in order to fortify and activate our innate healing processes. Physical activity is essential to keeping disease or illness at bay—and for recovery as well (though this may seem and, at times, feel counterintuitive).[8] Cancer diseases pose specific challenges in terms of keeping our bodies in motion. But we need to think about physical activity as a healing modality, as a source of nurturance and enjoyment for our biology. Just as there is a time for us to rest, there is a time for us to be in motion. It's an essential part of the healing balance.

Finding the Food that Heals: The human body is designed to sustain health when our weight is kept in a range that allows us to feel well, strong, agile, and energetic. We know we are at a comfortable (which means healthy) body weight when we sleep well, eat moderately, and can participate in all the activities we enjoy. This is such a simple concept, but because we are all buried under an avalanche of misinformation, as well as highly processed and unhealthy foods, the whole topic has become vastly overcomplicated. So, back to the basics on eating for health and wellness.

Toxin Patrol: We are all surrounded by environmental toxins that we mostly cannot smell, taste, or touch—both at home and out in the world.

Much of this exposure is beyond our control, but not all of it. We're on the cusp of a sea change in our understanding about environmental toxicity; initiating proactive steps now will serve everyone in the long run. Shifting our consciousness in this area is a cornerstone of anticancer living.

Each area of the Mix of Six has been scientifically linked to one or more key biological hallmarks necessary for cancers to form, grow, and survive.[9] Research also suggests that these lifestyle factors interact with and reinforce each other in both positive and negative ways.[9] For example:

- A solid and supportive network reinforces our good habits. Information sharing, partnering to achieve health goals, and just plain love activate our healthy biology. Without it, we tend to flag, lose hope, and become overwhelmed.
- Chronic stress actually *decreases* the beneficial effects of healthy foods while heading us toward poor food choices. And it diminishes interest in exercising, disrupts sleep—all of which, in turn, can come to burden our relationships. Learn to short-circuit this vicious circle.
- Sleep disruption modifies food preferences, changes nutritional metabolic pathways, and reduces energy for exercise.
- Conversely, consistent exercise helps us reduce stress, eat more moderately and better metabolize nutrients, and sleep better.
- Exposure to environmental toxins can unduly stress our bodies and sap our energy—coming to influence our weight, metabolic processes, and ability to change the way our bodies and brains develop.

The interrelationship between the Mix of Six factors allows the shared synergy to support us when we have a "bad day." For example, people tend to punish themselves for going "off a diet" by eating nothing the next day and engaging in the guilt-shame cycle. As an alternative, in addition to being more careful about food choices, you can also increase your mind-body practice. Find relief from the harms of stress and the unhealthy food by increasing meditation or yoga. Exercising more after such a lapse can also decrease the "harm" of those choices. In anticipation of such a lapse, and we are often aware of them in advance, engage in extra exercise, stress management, and healthy sleep prior to and then after inevitable slipups on your road to a healthier lifestyle. Make yourself stronger and more grounded so you can go into your life with greater clarity and awareness.

I've found with our patients at MD Anderson that experiencing the self-reinforcing qualities of the Mix of Six changes people in ways that are often surprising, unique to each person, and nothing short of miraculous. Becoming aware of these lifestyle factors and the relationships between them, realizing that so much is in our control, wakes us up to the most basic yet most overlooked purpose we all have in life, and that is to live so that our body enjoys maximum health and well-being. And to do so whether cancer is present or not.

Hashmat E. has spent her professional life caring for others in her human rights work, in particular with disabled children around the world. Her work has saved thousands of lives and touched inestimable numbers of others. The cost, though, which is not uncommon in such professions, has been neglect of her own health due to long hours and the high stress of being faced with so much pressing need. While out in the field in Pakistan, she found a lump in her breast. By the time she was able to see a doctor and was diagnosed with cancer, the lump had quadrupled in size.

After she was diagnosed with breast cancer, Hashmat needed to discover ways to put herself first—for the first time. Like our other CompLife participants, she found she needed to home in on the "Mix of Six" and adjust virtually everything—from her diet and exercise routine to her sleep pattern and daily stress management. In her case, she did have a strong network of support, and that proved to be a good foundation for the changes she had to make. First, she modified her diet to limit her sugar intake, as she'd become reliant on sugary snacks to keep her going when she was overly tired from jet lag or just wiped out due to overworking. Then she started counting her steps and tracking her fitness. To learn to relax, she took advantage of our meditation and yoga classes and she told me that for the first time in years, she was getting really restful sleep at night.

Then something unexpected changed: She discovered the word *no*. Learning to say no, to set limits on demands, and to delegate more effectively to the support that was available to her was Hashmat's turning point. She credits her daily mind-body practice with increasing her awareness of how she responds to others, and to their needs, even when urgent. As she put it: "I've felt I'm happier now. Because of that, I'm enjoying life more. I have a better relationship with everyone and I'm able to think. Even people who worked with me, they were telling me, 'What did they give you at the hospital? You are wiser now.' I don't overreact to the things that used to upset me."

For Hashmat, the added stress of her cancer diagnosis and treatment was a real wake-up call for other sources of stress in her life. Managing the emotional side of the cancer experience was critical. In fact, she had tended to ignore those aspects of her life before joining the CompLife Study. Now she is empowered to put what's best for her health at the top of her priority list every day. What she found was that this enabled her to better meet the needs of others—though she now does it differently. Despite what she's been through, she says she feels better today than she ever felt before being diagnosed with cancer. As she told me, "I check my steps every day and I feel really good about it. I go to sleep on time, and I tell myself, 'It's okay if this thing is not done today. It can wait.'"

Synergistic Healing

We have known for some time now, thanks to the pioneering work by top scientists around the world, that certain lifestyle adjustments can profoundly affect the trajectory and outcome of cancer. Much emphasis has been placed on individual lifestyle factors such as diet, exercise, and reducing stressors (both psychological and biological), but an increasing body of research shows that the benefit of each lifestyle factor is enhanced and heightened when we make changes in more than one area.[10–12] This is what makes anticancer living so dynamic and, from a research standpoint, somewhat tricky.

Despite these challenges, several landmark studies have shown the dramatic impact of comprehensive lifestyle change. Research headed by Barbara Andersen, PhD, at Ohio State University in Columbus examined the long- and short-term effects of a comprehensive lifestyle intervention on women with stage II or stage III breast cancer who had undergone surgery.[13] Patients in the intervention group attended eighteen weekly sessions covering techniques to reduce distress and improve quality of life, improve health behaviors (diet, exercise, smoking cessation), and make sure they stuck with their treatment and made it to follow-up appointments. Andersen and her team taught patients progressive muscle relaxation and helped them recognize stress and learn to respond to it differently. After the initial eighteen weeks, the intervention arm had eight monthly sessions to help them maintain their changes with a focus on social support, where participants identified people in their lives whom they could ask for help.

Eleven years later, women who participated in the intervention had a 45 percent lower risk of cancer recurrence than those in the control group, and they were 56 percent less likely to have died from breast cancer, compared to women in the control group. Intervention patients were also 49 percent less likely than women in the control group to die from any cause.[14] When women in the intervention did have disease recurrence, they lived longer after recurrence than women in the control group.[15] The findings also indicated that women who took part in the intervention had significantly improved psychological, behavioral, and health outcomes, as well as improved immune function compared with patients in the control group.[13, 15–17]

Meanwhile, at the Preventive Medicine Research Institute and UCSF in San Francisco, Dean Ornish, MD, and his team have published incredible

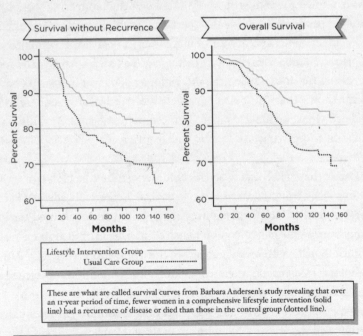

Impact of Lifestyle Intervention on Breast Cancer

> Survival without Recurrence <   > Overall Survival <

Lifestyle Intervention Group ——————
Usual Care Group ·······················

These are what are called survival curves from Barbara Andersen's study revealing that over an 11-year period of time, fewer women in a comprehensive lifestyle intervention (solid line) had a recurrence of disease or died than those in the control group (dotted line).

Adapted and reprinted by permission from John Wiley & Sons, Inc.: B. L. Andersen, H. C. Yang, W. B. Farrar, et al., "Psychologic intervention improves survival for breast cancer patients: A randomized clinical trial," *Cancer* 113, no. 12 (December 2008): 3450–3458.
   Adapted in collaboration with Laura Beckman.

outcomes for studies looking at the effects of comprehensive lifestyle change on heart disease and prostate cancer (www.ornish.com). In his revolutionary 2005 study, Ornish recruited ninety-three men with early-stage prostate cancer undergoing active surveillance, a situation in which men have confirmed prostate cancer but it is clinically appropriate to hold off on surgery.[18] Half the men were randomized to undergo intensive lifestyle change and the other half were simply followed over time with no intervention. This design enabled the researchers to assess the effects of comprehensive lifestyle changes alone, since the randomized control group was not undergoing any treatment. The participants in the lifestyle group were counseled on following a whole-foods plant-based diet low in both fat and refined carbohydrates, encouraged to exercise thirty minutes six days a week, manage their stress for an hour a day using yoga and meditation, and take part in weekly support group meetings for one year.

At the end of the study, participants in the intervention group had a 4 percent decline in PSA (prostate-specific antigen) levels compared to a 6 percent increase in the control arm.[18] Furthermore, blood taken from men in the intervention arm suppressed human prostate cancer cell growth 70 percent better after the intervention than before (the control group only had a 9 percent improvement in the blood's ability to control prostate cancer growth in a petri dish).[18] When Ornish examined all the men in the study and classified the amount of lifestyle change, he found that the greater the change, the greater the reduction in PSA levels, and the better the blood cells were able to control prostate cancer in vitro.[18] After two years, only 5 percent of men in the intervention group had undergone conventional prostate cancer treatment (radical prostatectomy, radiotherapy, or androgen deprivation), compared to 27 percent in the control.[18]

In a remarkable 2013 follow-up, Ornish replicated the same study, reducing the intervention to three months.[19] His team discovered increased telomere length (a reflection of our biological age) in the prostate cancer survivors five years after they underwent the intervention, compared to decreased telomere length in a control group. Longer telomeres reflect a reversal of cellular aging.

In both of Ornish's studies, the greater the amount of lifestyle change, the better the outcomes.[18,19] In addition, levels of telomerase, a protein in the nucleus of cells that helps to maintain telomere length and integrity, increased from pre- to post-intervention after only three months. Ornish and his team also conducted prostate biopsies before and after the intervention and found that 501 genes were altered.[20] Genes that promote cancer and affect chronic inflammation and oxidative stress were down regulated, or turned off, in the intervention group, while beneficial genes that protect us from the cancer hallmarks were up regulated, or turned on.

What these initial results tell me is that comprehensive lifestyle change can improve clinical outcomes and has substantial impact on key cancer hallmarks. As Dean puts it, "We're learning more and more that these mechanisms are much more malleable than we had once realized. That in turn gives many people new hope and new choices that they didn't have before."

THE KEY PRINCIPLES OF ANTICANCER LIVING

- It is never too late—or too early—to adopt an anticancer lifestyle.
- The anticancer living plan is built around the Mix of Six lifestyle factors that most directly affect the body's ability to ward off or fight disease.
- The Mix of Six work together in positive ways, as they are all interrelated, and success in one area will help foster and sustain success in other areas.
- We must first harness and build our social support network to create a foundation for other lifestyle changes.
- You can achieve health, healing, and increased longevity—without being cured.
- Healthy behaviors are contagious—share your anticancer living habits with others.
- You will feel freer and more able to experience life with joy and love when you make anticancer living lifestyle choices.
- Anticancer living is a way of life, not a quick fix, and it is dynamic, fluid, and unique to each individual.

A Life-Changing Diagnosis

One cancer survivor who is living proof of the synergistic effects of the Mix of Six is Glenn Sabin, the only documented patient ever to recover from chronic lymphocytic leukemia without undergoing conventional cancer treatment. When Glenn was diagnosed in the fall of 1991, he was a healthy,

RAISING KIDS THE ANTICANCER WAY

With three growing children, Alison and I have worked hard to instill the general principles of anticancer living. We've done this mostly by example. As most parents (especially the parents of teenagers) know, it's the only way to really get a message across. "Do as I say but not as I do" rarely works. Alison brings her teaching techniques into our home and tries a variety of approaches to implement healthy living into our daily lives, everything from the "three-bite rule" to "no cell phones in the bedroom" with varying degrees of success. The important thing from our perspective as parents is that we are always trying. We don't get discouraged if a certain approach doesn't work, if our efforts are sabotaged by other parents, or if our teenagers find sneaky ways to get what they want, even if it's not good for them. We try to stay the course, encourage them to make healthy choices, and make those same choices ourselves so we are modeling anticancer behavior and are sufficiently alert, present, and rested to face the next challenge as parents.

So, become a model for your kids on how to be attuned to cancer prevention. Explain why you're making certain food choices but also make them consistently—and have enough on hand to serve the whole family. Wean everyone off sugar and junk food! Tell them that you want them to get adequate rest because sleep helps the brain and the body fight disease, will lead to better academic and athletic achievement, and you want them to be as healthy as possible for as long as possible—then avoid late-night binge television yourself, or adopt a family-wide no-screens hour before bedtime. To really get their attention, tell them you want them to defy the current statistical models that say they won't live as long a life as you will! But try not to be too dogmatic, and focus on helping them to make their own connections between their choices and how they feel. They may have some surprising wisdom to share. Remember that life is not perfect, and neither are we. And neither are our kids.

physically active twenty-eight-year-old newlywed. He went in for his annual physical and came out of it diagnosed with a type of blood cancer that is considered incurable but survivable. (His own father, with whom the doctor first discussed Glenn's prognosis, was told his son likely had only six months to live.)

At the time of diagnosis, Glenn's spleen, an organ that filters blood and is involved in regulating immune function, was so engorged with cancer cells that it was nearly four times its normal size and was visibly pressing through the skin of his abdomen. Such a diseased spleen had to be removed, but beyond this, the only other standard medical treatment available to Glenn at this time was a bone marrow transplant. To undergo this procedure meant that he would have to endure chemotherapy to kill the cancerous cells in his own bone marrow, then be given a donor's bone marrow and hope that it "took" in his own body. Not only would this treatment be somewhat grueling and painful, but fully 20 percent of those who underwent the procedure actually died. For Glenn, this was a medical version of Russian roulette he just wasn't ready to play, so he opted not to have the procedure.

His remaining option? According to his doctor, "Watch and wait." Glenn opted for this approach, but with one crucial difference: Instead of passively watching and waiting, he began to educate himself. He got busy learning about the biology of his disease and the changes he could make to his lifestyle that would keep the cancer as quiet and inactive as possible while enhancing his overall general health. He called this "proactive observation." As he explains, "My goal was to try to be the healthiest cancer patient I could be."

He immediately set about improving his diet, drinking the cleanest water possible, using dietary supplements, adjusting his work life so that his stress load was reduced, and upping his daily exercise, knowing that the physical activity would also improve his psychological and emotional wellbeing. "I use relaxational exercises, like swimming or walking, to relieve stress and to enhance my sense of calm," he told me. He also began to focus on getting deep, restorative sleep, and he credits his wife (whom he's known since childhood) with providing him with the kind of love and social support he needed to conquer the fear and anxiety that naturally comes with being diagnosed with a chronic disease. She helped him stay grounded while he stepped with purpose onto his anticancer living path.

For the first twelve years following his diagnosis, Glenn's cancer remained in check. Though it was still detectable, it was not proliferating, and so his doctors encouraged him to continue doing whatever he was doing. Then, in 2003, he was hit with an acute episode, which included an unrelenting low-grade fever, night sweats, and severe anemia. His blood counts, in his own words, were "an absolute mess." At this point, he consulted with additional doctors at Johns Hopkins in Baltimore and Dana-Farber Cancer Institute in Boston and the clear consensus was that he needed to be treated with chemotherapy, steroids, and other potent drug agents. Despite how sick he was, Glenn decided he didn't want to go this route, given that these treatments, which come with serious side effects, didn't offer "durable remissions" for most CLL patients. Instead, he took a break from work and looked for ways he could improve his new healthy lifestyle even more. "I wanted to see if I could continue the healing I'd been generating for myself for twelve years, *to see if I could affect the underlying biology of my disease,* and I needed to do this in a very controlled way."

Glenn refused treatment, but he didn't fire his superb medical team. Instead, he made an agreement with them. He would continue to tweak his lifestyle and make regular visits to the doctor's office several times a week to have his blood work closely monitored. "What we wanted to watch were the trending patterns of my leukemia, to see if we could actually witness some 'cause and effect' with what I was doing. I became an n-of-1 experiment—in my case, an informal study of one patient going back decades—and we decided that we'd gather data in a very organized and controlled way."

Although he was exhausted most of the time, Glenn continued to exercise, swimming outside under the sun and taking daily walks that helped him regain his strength and keep his mind clear. After several weeks, his anemia cleared, the night sweats stopped, and his blood levels stabilized. Two months later, his blood counts were back to normal.

In 2014, a pathology report showed no evidence that Glenn had ever had a lympho-proliferative disorder. As he explains, "My bone marrow and blood were absolutely clean. In plain English, this means that there was no evidence that I had ever had CLL."

After being diagnosed with a chronic leukemia when he was twenty-eight years old, Glenn Sabin is now a disease-free man of fifty-four. His remarkable journey and improbable recovery have been documented through the Dana-Farber Cancer Institute and Harvard and are now part of the medical literature.[21] His case is also captured in his own book *n of 1*, coauthored with oncologist Dawn Lemanne, MD, MPH.[22] Interestingly and importantly, however, Glenn does not consider himself cured. What he does acknowledge is that the anticancer lifestyle he adopted helped him to heal and to achieve a high level of health and well-being, despite his having lived with cancer for nearly half his life.

As Glenn's story illustrates, lifestyle changes when made together can have a synergistic effect. As you make your way through the chapters that follow, you'll begin to see that there is an amplification of the healing factors within the Mix of Six. Healing ourselves is what anticancer living is all about. Making cancer prevention a reality instead of a pipe dream is the Holy Grail of anticancer living, and it is what drives all the research in lifestyle medicine that is currently being conducted around the world and in our own CompLife Study, with patients like Hashmat. Our goal has been to gather the data that scientifically legitimize the Mix of Six so that including lifestyle medicine in cancer treatment and prevention becomes the gold standard of patient care. Once we aim our sights on preventing cancer in the first place, we will finally move away from a model of disease care to one of true health care. This is the goal of anticancer living.

PART TWO

• • • • • •

The Mix of Six

CHAPTER SEVEN

The Foundation Is Love
and Social Support

We might debate which of the six pillars should lead off because they are all key. Although to some it might seem an unusual choice, we have chosen to put social support in the top spot. While diet and exercise are critical, of course—along with the other pillars— what Alison and I have found is that support is the backbone on which all other lifestyle changes will either succeed or fail, whether it is logistical (having someone take care of the kids while you attend a new yoga class), motivational (to help overcome entrenched eating habits), or psychological (to uncover deep emotional issues that keep you from being the person you want to be). The people you enlist to support you are key to your success. Establishing an effective, personally tailored support network is where anticancer living begins, not where it ends. It is the root required for the tree to stand, the foundation upon which the house can be built, and the stability that will ground and balance you as you move forward.

This is not how we are taught to think about our lives. Western culture tends to emphasize individual accomplishments, a do-it-alone attitude that dismisses or diminishes the support that helped enable and empower some-one to reach their goals. We tend to focus on results, not on process. The same is true with lifestyle change—people tend to start with what they think they can do on their own (i.e., change their diet, workout more) with-out realizing that those changes will teeter on flimsy ground if they aren't upheld by a solid framework of love and support. Just as the magic ingredi-ent of the Mix of Six is the connectedness and synergy involved, so connect-edness among us lends a hand often in marvelous ways.

One of the most inspirational stories I know when it comes to the power of social support is the remarkable journey of our friend Susan Rafte, who has survived for more than twenty years with advanced metastatic breast cancer. When Susan was initially diagnosed and treated for stage IIIB invasive ductal breast cancer in 1995, she was only thirty and a new mother to Marika, who was nine months old. At that point, Susan had her whole life mapped out. She had quit her job as a legal assistant on the day she went into labor with Marika and planned to have two more children and raise her family with her husband in Houston. When she found a sensitive lump in her breast, her father, a pediatrician, diagnosed her over the phone. A biopsy confirmed their worst fears. Before Susan could fully process and recover from her original diagnosis, the cancer spread to her bones and she underwent a risky procedure that involved removing her stem cells, hitting her body with high-dose chemotherapy, and then returning these cells to a cancer-free environment. Luckily, the surgery worked, but it was not an easy process and far from a smooth road to recovery. Her family, each with their specific caregiver roles, were beside her from the get-go and throughout her treatment and recuperation. Her sister Jane, a dancer in New York, was so moved by Susan's illness, she started a nonprofit called Pink Ribbons Project to raise money for cancer research. Eventually, Jane left New York City and moved to Houston to help her sister full time. In the initial transition, Jane put her career on hold. When Susan regained her health and strength, Pink Ribbons Project came to life in Houston. Jane also incorporated her dance skills into her activism, creating a group called Dancers in Motion Against Breast Cancer that put together performances and raised money for cancer awareness and research.

Susan credits the support of her family and friends with her ability to survive intense treatment and to emotionally recover from a lingering fear that she wouldn't live to see her daughter grow up. But beyond her family and friends, Susan had trouble finding survivor groups that focused on the unique challenges and emotional stressors faced by young mothers diagnosed with cancer. "At the time, those support groups weren't out there," she explained. "I was sitting in a circle with grandmothers thinking, 'I've got a baby. I'm trying to live to see my daughter make it to kindergarten. You're talking about grandkids.'"

Susan decided to fill an important void in Houston's cancer support community and provide support for young women with children, with particular focus on women with advanced cancer. She teamed up with another survivor and formed the Pink Ribbons Volunteer desk at MD Anderson Cancer Center, which has grown to a group of eighteen women who help guide patients through cancer treatment and all the emotional ups and downs involved in the process. "We meet patients where they are, whether they're starting chemo or just coming for the first day or they come from the outside and they're metastatic," Susan explains. The group has been nicknamed "the Flashers" because, when patients are struggling to decide what type of surgery to undergo, Susan and other volunteers sometimes take them to a back room, take their tops off, and show what the surgery results really look like after different procedures.

As a twenty-year survivor of stage IV metastatic breast cancer, Susan gives other women hope by her example and her enthusiasm for life. Patients with metastatic breast cancer are often a forgotten group, because few oncologists expect them to survive. Susan and a small group of patients took major steps to correct that oversight by creating a metastatic breast cancer support group. While getting cancer at a young age was rare when she was diagnosed in the '90s, today it is not as uncommon, a fact that speaks to the importance of doing everything we can to both prevent cancer and improve our chances of surviving a cancer diagnosis. Many of the women in Susan's metastatic support group are young women and moms with young children. The average age is forty.

Part of the beauty of social support and its impact on our health is that it works in both directions—giving and receiving. Just as having the support of others is vital for cancer survivors and the rest of us, mounting scientific evidence shows that giving our time to support others also sustains us physically and emotionally, and may improve our body's ability to prevent and overcome disease.[1-4] A 2013 review of forty different studies found that volunteer work reduced early mortality rates by 22 percent.[3] Those who volunteered at least an hour a month had reduced rates of depression and reported that they were more satisfied in life. Although this review did not focus on cancer patients, and it may sound counterintuitive for someone struggling with cancer and cancer treatment to volunteer and help others, where possible we know this can have a profound positive effect on the person providing the support.

Sure, doing good makes you feel good, but can it really impact your health in a measurable way? Several years ago, Barbara Fredrickson and her team at the University of North Carolina in Chapel Hill ventured to find out. They conducted a study involving sixty-five members of the university's faculty and staff and found that people who increase their feeling of social connectedness actually improved their vagal tone.[5] The vagus nerve regulates how your heart rate changes with your breathing and is connected with the parasympathetic nervous system, the part of our nervous system that helps us to relax.[6] The vagus nerve is also tied to how well people connect with one another—how our ears tune in to human speech and how we regulate emotional expression.[7,8] In terms of biology, the better your vagal tone, the greater your heart-rate variability, which has been linked to lower heart disease, better immune function and glucose levels, and lower all-cause mortality.[9–11] In terms of our social interactions, the greater your closeness to others and the greater your altruistic behavior, the better your vagal tone.[12] Connecting on a deep level with people you encounter through volunteer work and altruistic behavior leads to good vagal tone, which means that as you help others you are keeping your own body well regulated.

Although I haven't measured Susan Rafte's vagal tone, I imagine that it is very good indeed. Through her volunteer work (as well as her professional work with the Pink Ribbons Project), she has found purpose in her illness, which has increased her social connectedness and helped to keep her positive and engaged.

Meanwhile, the Pink Ribbons Project that Susan's sister founded (and which Susan later chaired) raised $6 million for cancer research before finally closing its doors in 2016. Some of that early money went toward the development of a drug called Taxotere, which helped keep Susan's cancer in remission so she could go through with her stem cell transplant in 1997. So, on multiple levels, her social support network helped to save her life.

Mutating Cells Divide and Unite Us

Cancer, by its biological design, is an illness that wants to separate us out. No two cancers are ever alike, and so it's an illness that, on a very profound level, can only be experienced by the individual. As it tries, in its silently aggressive, cellular way, to keep the patient all to itself, it also serves as a rallying cry, bringing those who care about the patient to attention and ready to act (like Susan Rafte's sister). All the effects of cancer, beginning with the treatment and its aftermath, have the power to change everyone who loves and cares about the patient. In this way, one person's cancer really does become a community health issue and presents a great opportunity for all affected to evaluate and change their lifestyle habits. Education of course is key. When we understand why something is helpful—or not—we can make informed, healthier choices. This is where the powerful, curative, and preventative powers of the Mix of Six really come into play. When we, or a loved one, are diagnosed with cancer, we can make lifestyle changes that will promote the health and well-being of everyone around us.

I see this effect in the transformed lives of the remarkable women who have been through the CompLife Study. After they learn how to live healthier lives, they are eager to spread the word to the people they know and love, so they, too, can feel great and avoid chronic disease. Anticancer living spreads in the other direction as well. The loved ones of our CompLife patients want to help their mothers, wives, or sisters survive, so they tend to take up the cause and change their own habits as a way to actively show their support and to improve their own health. What's more, many of the study participants are, like Susan Rafte, mothers of young and growing children, so their changing habits become a new healthy living model that influences their children and could last for generations. Many people would mistakenly classify these changes under diet (if a whole family changed the way they ate to support their mom through cancer treatment), exercise (if a couple started walking together after the husband was diagnosed with early-stage prostate cancer), or mind-body (if a family started doing morning yoga or meditation because dad needs to reduce his stress). But in all these examples, it is important to recognize and understand that they truly start with social support. It is only through these loving connections that these changes take hold, and research actually shows that this solid base is what has the potential to make them last. Whether you are joining a running group to support a friend, learning healthy cooking techniques from a sibling, or trying to manage your own stress after a colleague has a health scare and decides to slow down, sustainable change begins with help and inspiration from others.

For those facing a cancer diagnosis, love and social support are especially essential. We all know how bad it feels when we embark on something new and terrifying that excites us. When we share our hopes and desires with others, we know how devastating it can be when we experience our goals as being met with either distracted indifference or worse, outright criticism. Conversely, we know how wonderful it feels when we are really heard and our wishes are met with respect and interest. I know for myself that I can be fortified to pursue something new, complex, and rigorous with seemingly insignificant gestures of support such as an affirming nod, a smile of recognition, or the simple words, "Tell me what you need."

The Importance of Staying Connected

We now have an impressive body of research that shows how the more firmly one stands in the face of cancer, in terms of staying closely connected to loved ones, friends, work colleagues, a faith community, networks of support—the better one will fare.[13-17] A 2014 study of 164 breast cancer survivors by researchers at The Ohio State University College of Medicine in Columbus found that women who reported lower levels of social support prior to cancer treatment experienced higher levels of pain and depression.[18] In addition, their blood work, taken before treatment as well as six months later, showed increased levels of a gene linked to inflammation, which we know is closely tied to cancer growth and progression.[19,20] Based on these findings, OSU researchers concluded that "early interventions targeting survivors' social networks could improve quality of life during survivorship."[18] In other words, accessing and building your anticancer team is essential as a first step in the cancer journey, just as it is essential for all of us hoping to make changes that fortify our bodies and improve our lives.

Research shows that when we stay connected to those we love and those who want to help us, cancer is less likely to progress, lives are extended, and overall health improves. Our bodies maintain their natural defenses and we are better protected from the proliferation of mutating cells and the formation and progression of tumors. A 2017 study of women with breast cancer found that those with the most social ties were less likely to die from cancer and less likely to have a recurrence.[21] For that study (the largest of its kind to date), Kaiser Permanente researchers tracked breast cancer survival and recurrence in patients in the United States and China for up to twenty years. Over that time period, women with fewer social connections were 43 percent more likely to have a recurrence and 64 percent more likely to die from breast cancer.

But most important of all—whether the disease remains active in us or not—a higher quality of life is experienced when we stay in close community with others.[22,23] By enlisting others to help us stay present, grounded, and active, we have, the scientific research shows, the best chance of sustaining and even improving the quality of our lives, whether or not we have cancer.

The Roseto Effect

In 1964, scientists ventured to Eastern Pennsylvania to analyze the culture in the small mining village of Roseto. The reason? The inhabitants exhibited a much lower rate of heart disease than the national average, and even among their closest neighbors.[24,25] Researchers wanted to find out if this community of Italian immigrants was engaging in a unique diet or some other kind of lifestyle behavior that explained this phenomenon. What they discovered shocked them.

The Rosetans, as they came to be known, worked in the same toxic slate quarries as their neighbors from nearby Bangor and Nazareth and so were exposed to toxic dust and fumes as well as to workplace accidents. They also smoked hand-rolled, unfiltered cigars loaded with nicotine and tar and drank wine with their meals, which often consisted of fried meatballs and sausages and salamis and cheeses.

So what made the difference in their health and well-being? Their strong familial and social ties. Family was everything to the Rosetans.[25] They lived, worked, played, and died together. Each household contained three generations, and in this culture, age and wisdom were valued and respected. The wealthier inhabitants of Roseto lived as their neighbors did. There was no ostentation, no social-class discrimination. The intense social support they enjoyed lowered their risks not just for heart disease but other diseases as well.[24] They lived an orderly, quiet life that did an excellent job of *not internalizing stress.*

Over time, as the younger generations began to adopt a more "American" lifestyle, the Roseto effect began to fade. The social fabric of Roseto began to fray and with it the health benefits of their stress-reducing, family-centered lifestyle.

The Blue Zones

This same sustaining social fabric as with the Roseto effect may be at the heart of "Blue Zones," regions of the world that have the highest percentage of centenaries (individuals who live to be one hundred or more).[26] What Blue Zones seem to have in common are relatively small communities, strong family units, and a supportive community structure. Take, for example, Okinawa, Japan. The elderly of Okinawa pride themselves on having not only the longest life expectancy but also the longest good-health expectancy. The Okinawa Centenarian Study, which began in 1975, found that one-hundred-year-olds on the Japanese island were extraordinarily lean, healthy, and energetic and had remarkably low rates of heart disease and cancer, including stomach cancer, which is common on mainland Japan.[27]

One of the age-old practices of Okinawans is the creation and maintenance of *moais*—small groups of friends that commit to each other for life.[26] The idea originated with farmers who met and discussed crop-planting techniques and committed to help other members of the *moai* if their crops should fail. Today, the groups serve as an extended family, pooling resources, helping each other problem solve and manage crises, and supporting each other through times of grief and loss. As people age, they are not only supported by the younger members but they also maintain a sense of purpose supporting family and being active members of their communities well past the traditional age of retirement.

Having a strong community that goes beyond someone's immediate family and household seems to have a dramatic impact on human health and longevity. This effect may also come into play for cancer survivors who have a wider and deeper support network. A 2005 study by researchers at George Washington University Medical Center found that women with stage II or III breast cancer who had a greater number of "dependable, non-household relationships" tended to live longer than their less supported counterparts.[28] In fact, the study, published in the *Journal of Psychosomatic Research*, concluded that women with greater support outside their homes were 60 percent less likely to die from cancer a decade after their initial diagnosis.

Watch and Learn

In 2007, during a routine physical on his forty-sixth birthday, Josh Mailman's GP felt under his rib cage and said, "Something feels a bit different. I don't know what it is, but I'd love it if you'd get an ultrasound so I can figure out why." Since Josh's blood work and other routine tests were all normal and he felt fine, there was no sense of urgency. But being a good doctor's son, he followed up and had the ultrasound a few months later. That's when, as Josh puts it, "all hell broke loose." There were lesions in his pancreas and his liver, and after a biopsy he was diagnosed with a very rare form of neuroendocrine cancer. His was classified as "nonfunctioning" because he had no symptoms, yet the disease was advanced as he had a 70 percent tumor load in his liver and a softball-size tumor in his pancreas. Josh later asked his doctor how she had "intuited" something was off, how she had sensed such a serious internal change when he was symptom-free. "I have this mental image of what a healthy liver feels like and I just remember that yours didn't feel quite right." Her blind pickup of the disease changed the course of Josh's life.

As Josh rushed to educate himself on his disease and learn about his treatment options, the feedback and responses he got were consistently negative. He was not eligible for surgery and the only drug on the market was not designed to fight his type of tumors. His only option it seemed was to watch and wait for several months so doctors could observe and better understand the nature of his unique and rare cancer.

Thankfully, Josh did not take this as a sign to become passive or to isolate himself from his community or from professional resources. He was referred to the integrative oncology department at the University of California in San Francisco, where he met Dr. Donald Abrams. In those early meetings, Abrams never asked about Josh's cancer: His focus was solely on Josh's quality of life. Abrams wanted to know where Josh was in his life (he was a successful tech entrepreneur, married, with a baby at home); what his hopes and aspirations for his life were (to live a long and productive and healthy life); and, crucially, what his body needed to best support him while they got to the root of his disease. Thanks to this healthy, loving professional support (support that focused on Josh as a person, not on his cancer), Josh was able to change his lifestyle and become more empowered to heal himself. "I put the focus on myself, rather than the disease," he told me. "With Donald's help, I really began to focus on what I was eating, how I was living my life. I began to check in with my body in wholly new ways and began to sense that I needed to rebalance things in my life. So I began to make changes."

A scan three months later showed no changes in Josh's cancer. This was remarkable, given the advanced stage of his disease. Six months later, the same. Something seemed to be halting the progression of the cancer— which defies the very nature of the disease. Now his oncologist and her team on the other side of the street were intrigued. They wanted to know what kind of lifestyle changes he was making. For his part, Josh was mostly just focused on educating himself and learning all he could about his disease. He continued to bike daily and had modified his diet some and had begun taking probiotics and other supplements, but otherwise he'd made no radical changes. He also joined a support group, which he described as helping him to transform "watch and wait" into "watch and learn."

"I wanted to use this time of reprieve that my body had given me to educate myself as best I could so that when I did finally have to act, I would be able to do so in non-panic mode." A year after his diagnosis, Josh traveled to a large international patient conference in Toronto, where he learned about a form of nuclear medicine being successfully used in Germany to image and treat his type of cancer. He approached the doctor who had given the presentation, and three weeks later, he went to Germany for his first round of a treatment called Gallium-68. This was in 2008.

In 2009, with his cancer now progressing, he was briefly hospitalized, and yet still there was no viable treatment for him on the horizon. So he called his doctor in Germany and went back for three more rounds of treatment. This and his focus on lifestyle kept his disease stable for another six years. In 2016, he went back for another round of treatment and today, in 2017, he continues to live a full, active, and productive life while also having advanced neuroendocrine cancer. It was only by staying socially connected, reaching out instead of isolating himself, that Josh was able to educate himself, find a treatment when it seemed no treatment was available, and (against all odds) slow the progression of his advanced disease.

"I am by no means a perfect example of the anticancer lifestyle guy," Josh told me. "But I do focus on re-centering myself and I focus on how I want to feel in the long run. It's about balancing my life, despite the disease. It's there, but it's not running the show. I'm certainly not fighting it; instead, I am successfully living with it."

Josh's story illustrates the importance of social support on multiple levels. His doctors were open enough to connect with him with love, and as an individual. They listened, observed, validated, and showed great empathy as

CHOOSING YOUR BEST MEDICAL TEAM

The moment when a cancer diagnosis is first delivered by the doctor sets the tone for this crucial relationship, and it can even predict how well a patient will comply with and respond to treatment.[29] An empathic doctor will break the news of a diagnosis to a patient in person whenever possible; will explain what it means in an informative, straightforward, and kind manner; will calibrate the delivery of this news to best mirror the rate of comprehension and the emotional reaction of the patient; will offer to talk to loved ones on the patient's behalf. A doctor who looks you in the eye rather than keeps his head down buried in the lab work or who only focuses on the X-ray images in hand is likely not the person you will connect with. You should choose to work with people who instill in you a sense of calm, of availability, and of concern for the larger implications the disease will have for your life.

Even when a cancer is caught early, the news at diagnosis can be very traumatizing.[30] It triggers all kinds of emotions, not the least of which is fear. A compassionate doctor knows this and will frame the diagnosis in the most realistic, yet least threatening way. "I have news. You have this disease. We will gather information and I will share it with you and we will figure out the next steps together." A doctor who instills a sense of calm and trust is putting the patient before the illness. This is both reassuring and empowering.

A good primary care physician, which in the case of cancer diseases is usually an oncologist, will not underestimate the emotional impact of the diagnosis, and she will not rush a patient into any kind of treatment decision while in distress or under duress.

In fact, the best oncologists always put the patient first, making sure that he or she is the first to know when there is new information (test results, new treatment options, etc.) and striving to allow the patient to take the lead in terms of making decisions about their treatment, including whether or not to get a second or even a third opinion or even finding a new primary oncologist. A good oncologist knows it's not his skin in this game—it's yours.

they calmly and patiently allowed the nature of Josh's disease to reveal itself. This seemingly paradoxical approach is what, data and research show, leads to the most positive outcomes possible, because the emphasis is put on healing the person rather than just simply curing the disease. For Josh's part, he stayed curious and hopeful and did not cut himself off from the resources around him. By connecting with a support group, he learned firsthand about his disease from others who were experiencing the same things and also found out about a conference that led him to try a promising new treatment.

A major component of his success is having people around him who truly love, support, and nurture his health and well-being. The support he fostered was at the heart of his lifestyle changes, as well as his cutting-edge cancer treatment. From this solid base and with the proper attitude about reaching out into the world and not shutting himself off from it, research shows that Josh is more likely to continue to survive and thrive, even as he continues to live with cancer.

What Health-Care Providers Can Do

Doctors and other health-care providers can and should play a central role in helping cancer patients (and others facing a health challenge) engage their social support network to best help their chances of survival and recovery. This should be as central to treatment as scheduling follow-up appointments or prescribing medication. Doctors have a great deal of authority that they can leverage to help patients reach out and not try to go it alone:

- Add a love-and-support assessment when gathering a routine health history. This should include finding out who lives at home with the patient and getting the names and contact information for one or two other supportive and reliable friends and family members. Simply asking for an "emergency" contact is not enough.
- Tell patients that their overall treatment and recovery will be more successful if a supportive loved one attends all appointments, procedures, and treatment sessions. It does not have to be the same person each time, but it must be someone who listens well and enhances the patient's sense of well-being. Patients are often too stressed to take in and remember the recommendations and advice of health-care providers. Having someone at their appointments who can help to retain and

record information and instructions can help keep patients on track to better manage and maintain their health.

- Keep an updated list of various cancer-related support groups and make this available to patients early on in treatment.
- Provide patients with a list of organizations that are close by (the cancer center, the YMCA, a senior center, the library, etc.) that offer programs that will enhance social connectedness, including classes and groups that include information on improving lifestyle and overall health.
- Above all, keep an open mind and remember that a motivated patient will bring invaluable information and insight to the treatment process and so increase the probability for a positive outcome.
- Determine if a patient is suffering depression or anxiety due to chronic loneliness, and refer them to treatment with a therapist or psychologist. There is good evidence for the use of cognitive behavioral therapy, while other forms of therapy such as acceptance and commitment therapy or longer-term psychotherapy may be helpful as well.

How Cancer Affects Our Loved Ones

Coming to grips with a cancer diagnosis takes time and emotional energy. Many newly diagnosed patients are so overwhelmed with the concept of cancer that they don't quite know how to discuss it with their loved ones.[31] I hear from so many patients that they are concerned that the news will cause emotional harm to those they love, and so they automatically adopt a stoic stance, believing this will protect others from the terror and uncertainty of their illness. But believing that we have to "go it alone" may actually have an adverse effect on our most important relationships, and significantly, on our cancer outcome.[32,33] Cancer allows all of us to face the realities and the limitations of the human body, to accept and honor the fact and reality of our mortality, and to work together to figure out how to live well now, as opposed to dwelling on the past or worrying about the future. The path we take forward should not be one we take alone.

Having the Talk

For many cancer patients, looking a loved one in the eye and saying, "I have something to tell you. I have cancer," is the single bravest, most vulnerable statement of fact they will ever make. What comes after that moment is hugely important—not only for the patient, but also for his loved ones. We all need to be able to talk about our fears, share our hopes and dreams, and support each other, and when we have to bring cancer into the family dialogue, we have a unique opportunity to become closer.

For both the patient and for family members, learning to listen well to one another is also crucial. We all tend to want to rush in and make things better, but jumping from hearing the news into a pep talk short-circuits the chance to just let the news sink in and for this new reality to be processed. This is especially true with patients who have to break the news to young children, where the tendency to start with "Mommy will be fine!" can cause confusion if it's clear that mommy is actually quite scared or visibly unwell. The best way to discuss a new cancer diagnosis with children is the same with trusted adults and that is with appropriate candor, empathy, and a hopeful curiosity about where this will lead everyone in the family. As a cancer patient steps into treatment and the demands placed on him shift, open communication will keep family members and loved ones from having to try to "guess" what kind of support might be needed and therefore how best to take care not only of the patient, but of themselves. So listen. Listen when your loved one talks about his cancer experience and listen to your family members when they want to talk to you about their experience of your diagnosis and what feelings it brings up in them. Then keep your eyes open.

Actions Speak Louder Than Words

If your loved one, the patient, begins to withdraw, take note. He or she may be suffering from the intense emotional or physical effects of the disease— or both. Wherever you can step in and take some of the chores of daily life, you ought to do so—but not before checking in with the patient. Sometimes just acknowledging what they're going through is enough to energize them to keep up with some tasks of daily living. Or, they may be grateful for the offer to help and may ask you to do more than you'd planned for. Either way, it's all about communication.

Where children are concerned, actions definitely speak louder than words, as children may not be able to verbalize the complex feelings that come up for them. Observe how your child reacts to your news: they may become more affectionate or more withdrawn, or they may be more emotional than you're used to. Cancer affects all of us, not just the family member who has it, and we need to be gentle and kind with one another as it changes us.

With so many feelings and new experiences, including, for the cancer patient, a likely reduction in energy levels during treatment, we need to be validating of each other's experiences. There is no right or wrong way to be or do cancer—the only mandate is that we continue to love one another.

Lastly, we need to up our empathy game. This does not mean we indulge in either self-pity or pity: Empathy in anticancer living terms is actually the opposite of allowing cancer to victimize us or strip us of our power and make us passive. True empathic listening and attention is energizing and empowering. It puts complex intangibles like feelings or worry about the future in perspective and allows us to be present and involved.

Cancer is, indeed, a family disease, but it can bring us closer to one another and often brings out the best in everyone. We are given the rare opportunity to discover hidden strengths, address hard truths, and ultimately bring our focus to anticancer living.

But the love and support of a family isn't the only way to have strong social support working in your favor: studies show that having the loving, consistent support of at least one person can make all the difference in a cancer outcome.

In Sickness and in Health

A Harvard University study looked among 750,000 American patients suffering from ten different types of cancer who were diagnosed between 2004 and 2008.[34] Those who were married had a 20 percent better chance of surviving than those who were either single, divorced, or widowed. The biggest improvement in survival rates was among married patients who had non-Hodgkin's lymphoma or head and neck cancers. The study concludes that patients who are partnered are more apt to catch the disease early, get the right treatment, stick with their treatment protocols, report changes in their health, and make lifestyle changes that will enhance their overall health and well-being.

The good news is you don't have to be married to benefit from this kind of partner support if you have cancer. A committed friend or family member who understands your diagnosis, attends appointments with you, helps you do research, and makes sure you are well cared for during treatment can have an equally positive effect on your outcome and overall sense of well-being.

Loneliness Can Be Lethal

Chronic loneliness or social isolation contribute to illness and premature death at rates comparable to or higher than obesity or smoking fifteen cigarettes a day, research that analyzed three million adults under the age of sixty-five shows. The study, which was led by Brigham Young professor Julianne Holt-Lunstad and published in the journal *Perspectives on Psychological Science*, frames loneliness and social isolation as serious public health issues, ones that the medical community needs to address.[35] This is especially true as direct physical, social interaction gives way to digital communication in all areas, from shopping to banking to education. Add phenomena like online bullying and trolling on social media to the mix, and we've got a real recipe for stress, too.

Loneliness can be caused in part by increased sensitivity to social cues. People who feel lonely tend to read ambiguous social cues negatively and further isolate themselves as a result.[36] Shifting our default response from negative to positive, toward gratitude rather than blame, self-criticism, or judgment, is becoming basic mental health "housekeeping" for many of us. Recent research suggests that this can have a cascading effect that impacts our sense of social connection and integration. When we default to the positive, as opposed to the negative, our self-confidence grows. We are more likely to reach out to others, to connect with people on a deeper level, and make choices that are more health supportive in the long term.

Strong Social Support Slows Cancer Progression

Over the past twenty years, researchers have gathered correlational data that show that cancer patients with strong social support survive longer than those without it.[15-17] Additionally, the stress that comes with loneliness or a lack of social support has been found to trigger the proliferation of tumor cells by affecting the behavior of genes linked with inflammation, immune function, and other cancer regulatory genes.[32,33,37–42] Cancer patients with strong social support show lower levels of stress hormones that activate the production of cancer cells, and this is helping all of us to better understand the processes that lead to disease proliferation and metastases.[43,44]

In her work with ovarian cancer patients, Susan Lutgendorf, PhD, at the University of Iowa and with funding from the National Cancer Institute, has conducted studies that show the powerful influence of social support on mortality.[45,46] Her work revealed that patients with ovarian cancer who have low levels of social support lose approximately one year of life when compared to patients with similar disease who have strong social support.[47]

Working with my colleague Anil Sood, MD, a research scientist and surgeon at MD Anderson, Lutgendorf found that patients who reported higher levels of social support had lower levels of two key tumor-promoting factors—interleukin-6 (IL-6), a marker of inflammation, and vascular endothelial growth factor, or VEGF, a measure of angiogenesis.[46] Stronger emotional relationships were associated with lower IL-6 and VEGF levels. This and other research links social support to reduced levels of the cancer hallmarks of *sustaining proliferative signaling, inducing angiogenesis, activating invasion and metastasis, avoiding immune destruction,* and *tumor-promoting inflammation.*[18,28,32,33,38,45,48–57]

Lutgendorf also discovered that women with ovarian cancer who had lower levels of social support had higher levels of norepinephrine, a stress hormone that has been connected to inflammation and tumor growth.[58] The research showed increases in these harmful hormones and inflammatory factors at the tumor site itself at the time of surgery.

Steve Cole, PhD, from UCLA, has worked closely with both Anil Sood and Susan Lutgendorf. Cole has been able to visually track the way social isolation "lights up" cancer genes in ways that stimulate proliferation by using heat maps.[59–62] These three scientists looked at the ovarian cancer patients with the highest psychological risk—those who were not only socially isolated but also felt depressed. These patients showed greater expression of genes supporting tumor growth compared to patients with high levels of social support and low depressive symptoms.[63,64]

The research being conducted in this area of social influences on "stress biology" is helping cancer biologists and oncologists begin to understand the crucial relevance of systemic influences that lay beyond the tumor and its microenvironment.[65-67] Cole, Lutgendorf, Sood, and others are conducting groundbreaking research that is helping those treating cancer patients to look beyond the cancer microenvironment and into the patient's macroenvironment to more fully understand how lifestyle behaviors influence cancer activity. This understanding of the influence of lifestyle on cancer progression forms the scientific basis for anticancer living and confirms the importance of social support (as well as the other lifestyle factors included in the Mix of Six) in successfully treating cancer and other diseases.

The Healing Power of Groups

The renowned psychiatrist David Spiegel, MD, and his team at Stanford University Medical School have been at the forefront of studying and understanding the great psychosocial and emotional benefits cancer patients experience when they connect with others dealing with a similar diagnosis in a formal group setting.[68-70] When Spiegel first started psychotherapy groups for cancer patients forty years ago, there was a common belief that allowing patients to talk about their disease would exacerbate their anxiety and fear. Skeptics thought that putting cancer patients in a room together would somehow compromise their well-being and their treatment success. Spiegel had a hunch that just the opposite would happen, and his work has highlighted the important benefits of putting cancer patients together to share their experiences with one another. When patients can share their fears and concerns with others, especially those grappling with similar issues, reports show an improvement in their overall health, particularly where their emotional well-being is concerned.[71-73] And in some cases, being part of these support groups leads to longer survival with advanced cancer.[74-76] As Spiegel explains: "The power of group support makes tremendous sense to me. We're social creatures and the brain enables us to form connections with others and build networks of support that help us stay alive, that help us deal with threat, that help us nurture our young, and create stable and relatively safe cultures. And that social connection, especially in the face of illness, I think, is a very powerful ally. It helps us manage our stress responses, helps our bodies do better, and helps one another get through life-threatening situations."[77]

Support groups offer a forum for regularly sharing and disseminating information, too. I heard one patient say she prefers to call her support group her "action team," and she told me that the energy boost she gets from being with her "action buddies" provides her with the lift she needs to keep going through difficult treatments. For Josh Mailman, being part of a support group exposed him to new treatments for his rare type of cancer and helped him avoid potential pitfalls based on the experiences of fellow survivors. In terms of the patient with her "action buddies," the group provides deep and empathic support that helps her keep her emotional reserves full, which makes her relationships at home with her husband and children more rewarding. The focus on education and action keeps her motivated to continue taking care of herself, in both body and mind, no matter where she is in her treatment or recovery.

The power of this kind of social support unique to cancer groups reflects the experience of our friend Dorothy P., too. A longtime breast cancer survivor, Dorothy is part of a group of survivors who call themselves "the Pink Posse." The women in the group share intimate details about every aspect of their treatment with each other, and they've shown up for each other whenever a hand is needed, and as they are able. They've become so close that one of them intervened when she saw Dorothy slipping into depression after Dorothy's husband was also diagnosed with cancer, and she insisted on taking her to meditation classes. Another "chosen sister" gave Dorothy the gift of a couple of sessions with a therapist when it became clear to her that Dorothy was on the verge of complete burnout. Dorothy credits these interventions with changing her life and keeping her remission going. And, she confides, this is not something she might have been receptive to had it come from a family member or someone in another area of her life. Getting some therapy was just what she needed to learn to slow down and regain her balance and fortify her anticancer way of life.

The Health, Happiness, and Safety of All

In 1976, Michael Lerner and two colleagues founded a remarkable healing community on the rugged Pacific Coast of Northern California. They christened their endeavor Commonweal, a name that reflected their vision of creating a learning community that focuses on three key areas of community: health and healing, education and the arts, and the environment and justice.[78] Over the past forty years, Lerner has experienced the power of community in healing, particularly where cancer is concerned. One of his endeavors has been to partner the Commonweal Cancer Help Program with a cluster of Healing Circles, centers that offer low- or no-cost groups that provide a serene, engaged community for those contending with cancer or any other health challenge. The goal of these healing circles is to provide a place where people can communicate openly, share information, educate one another, support each other emotionally, with the goal that each individual will grow toward wholeness and health. One of these Healing Circles was cofounded by Diana Lindsay, the longtime lung cancer survivor whose story we shared earlier. Her chapter of Healing Circles is in the town of Langley on Whidbey Island in Washington State. Their mission is to provide easy, open, and ongoing access to the local community, and since opening in 2015, they log an average of six hundred visits a month, despite how tiny the town of Langley is (it has a population of roughly one thousand). "When I got well, we [Diana and her husband, Kelly] just wanted to give back to our community. We wanted to create a place where we could guarantee that there would be social and emotional support available to anyone in our community who wants it. I'd done a lot of reading of the scientific literature that showed that having strong emotional and social support improves health outcomes in so many different areas: dementia, heart disease, cancer, mental health—you name it. Conversely, negative social support is detrimental to health and has been proven by studying good and bad marriages." She goes on, "We see the Healing Circles as just a big giant community experiment, a conscious effort at building strong social support networks. It's been very meaningful to me and I know that feeling of purpose has done great things for me and kept me alive."

Finding Healing Communities Online

There are some ways that technology, with care and conscious use, can help us stay connected to others, and find nontoxic two-legged companions, especially when we have cancer. There is so much useful information to be found online: the challenge is what to believe and what to leave behind.

I don't think it's ever wise to try to self-diagnose by poring over random websites late at night or reading one person's blog about how they treated their disease by eating only one fruit or using daily coffee enemas improperly to advise your choices. You get the idea. But there are some excellent resources out there to help us stay connected to those we love, and to find support if we are isolated and alone.

One of my favorites is CaringBridge, a nonprofit online platform that allows cancer patients to document their experience.[79] Patients invite friends to join the site and to check in on their progress or to offer various forms of assistance. This keeps a patient who may be undergoing rigorous, depleting treatment from having to answer individual emails, return phone calls, or spend limited energy reserves repeating relevant, important information to members of his broader community. What's so brilliant about this setup is that it is designed to encourage people to move toward the patient rather than putting the burden on the patient to reach out to others. Similarly, there are calendar apps that allow friends and neighbors to set up "meal brigades," in which a schedule for meal delivery to the home of the patient is established. These websites allow the patient to set a schedule that works best (every Monday, Wednesday, Friday, for example), explain dietary needs and preferences, indicate how many people in the household need to be fed, and so forth. This kind of help and community support is invaluable and is made super easy for all involved by these well-designed digital platforms.

There are also online forums devoted to specific types of cancer where patients can ask questions and the community members chime in and share their experiences with one another. There are medical research sites, patient blogs, and, of course, there are many hospital, medical center, cancer center, and university websites that not only provide information on current research and data but also provide links to community-based support groups, educational programs, and more.

A Purposeful Life

People who have a purpose in life tend to be happier and healthier than their counterparts who are less purpose driven.[80] They also tend to be more connected to their community and to form deeper bonds with friends, which research shows has an effect on their health down to the cellular level.[81,82] For most of us, our relationships and support of others is a key aspect of our life purpose. The Harvard Study of Adult Development has followed several hundred Harvard graduates and working-class men for the past eighty years.[83-86] (It is one of the longest-running studies ever conducted.) One of its key findings is that the happiest and healthiest participants in both groups are those who maintained close, intimate relationships throughout their lives. As study director Robert Waldinger explains, "Taking care of your body is important, but tending to your relationships is a form of self-care, too. That, I think, is the revelation."

The diagnosis of cancer, or any life-threatening illness, can often lead people to reconnect with loved ones, reprioritize their lives, and discover and define a clear life purpose. Patients who derive meaning from their illness have better quality of life and lower stress hormones.[87] One of the benefits of mind-body practices such as yoga and cognitive behavioral stress management is that they increase a patient's ability to find meaning in their illness experience.[88-91] As with focusing on the positive and learning to be grateful, purposeful living leads directly to improved social connections and a sense of belonging, two essential components in building your anticancer team.

You'll see throughout this book that the stories of patients who focus on healing while living with cancer all tend to share this one fundamental trait: Each one, in his or her own way, decided to move away from fear and despair and dedicate themselves to cultivating a more authentic sense of purpose by living an anticancer life and *sharing what they've learned with others*. All these people work hard at cultivating their health and wellness daily, and all of them work to maintain a purpose in life. It can be challenging to see the positive in a life-threatening experience like cancer, especially for those whose prognosis is grim. Viktor Frankl, the famous Viennese psychiatrist and Holocaust survivor, addresses this issue eloquently in his book *Man's Search for Meaning* when he says: "In some way, suffering ceases to be suffering at the moment it finds a meaning."[92]

Research by Susan Lutgendorf and her team at the University of Iowa examined the different biological effects of two broad categories of well-being or happiness: (1) eudaimonic well-being, wherein people's well-being is derived from a sense of purpose and meaning in life, engaging in activities that support their core values and are aligned in accordance with their "true self," or "spirit" (what the ancients Greeks called the *daimon*) and (2) hedonic well-being, wherein well-being is derived from activities that maximize personal pleasure.[93]

In healthy individuals, the deeper sense of well-being (eudaimonic) has been linked with decreased inflammatory gene signaling compared with those who reported higher levels of immediate satisfaction and material success (hedonic well-being), although both aspects of well-being were associated with lower levels of depression (see box, page 106). In ovarian cancer patients, Lutgendorf and her colleagues found that women who scored higher on eudaimonic well-being had lower levels of stress hormones at the tumor site.[94] The same effect was notably not seen with patients who reported high levels of hedonic well-being. This aspect of social connection down regulates key cancer hallmarks, including *sustaining proliferative signaling, evading growth suppressors*, and *inflammation*. In other words, having deeper connections with other people and a deeper sense of purpose in life could help us avoid or overcome cancer.

Many of the studies to this point, showing connections between social ties and genetic expression, have been correlational. In other words, we can say these things are related, but we can't necessarily conclude that one thing caused the other. However, a 2017 study by Sonja Lyubomirsky at the University of California in Riverside and her colleagues (including Steve Cole) actually shows that a certain type of kindness causes changes in the profile of genes that are turned on and off.[95] Lyubomirsky and her team assigned 159 healthy men and women to one of four groups: (1) performing acts of kindness for others; (2) performing acts of kindness for the world in general; (3) performing acts of kindness for themselves; or (4) a neutral control activity. After engaging in their assigned tasks for just four weeks, differences in gene expression profiles emerged only for those who were engaged in performing acts of kindness for others relative to the control group. These individuals had gene profiles reflective of reductions in inflammatory gene signals and increases in genes linked to antibody responses. For the first time we now have scientific evidence that kindness toward others impacts our genes in ways that could prevent disease. As the authors concluded, "These findings demonstrate a causal effect of prosocial behavior on leukocyte gene regulation, and they contribute to a growing body of literature mapping the molecular pathways that may link prosocial behavior to physical health."[95]

Even Pets Help Us Heal

Stewart Fleishman, MD, while at the Continuum Cancer Centers of New York at Beth Israel Medical Center in New York City led a single-group study to see if having therapy dogs in the treatment areas or hospital rooms of a few dozen patients undergoing intense and challenging treatments for head and neck cancers had any beneficial effect.[96] These patients were already suffering from the severe adverse effects of their diseases, such as pain, fatigue, difficulty speaking or even swallowing. The treatments (concurrent chemo and radiation) would invariably cause their physical symptoms to initially get much worse, and usually the major indicators of emotional and social

WHAT KIND OF HAPPY ARE YOU?

In the first study of its kind, researchers from UCLA's Cousins Center for Psychoneuroimmunology and the University of North Carolina examined how positive psychology impacts human gene expression.[81] What they found is that the source from which you derive your happiness has surprisingly different effects on the human genome.

People with high *eudaimonic* well-being—the kind of happiness that comes from having a deep sense of purpose and meaning in life, an awareness of the bigger issues of life, and engaging in these kinds of activities—had favorable immune cell gene expression and low levels of inflammatory gene expression as well as strong antiviral and antibody gene expression.[81,94]

People with high levels of *hedonic* well-being—the type of happiness that comes from the emotions we experience when we do something pleasurable and fun for ourselves—had high inflammation and low antiviral and antibody gene expression relative to those with high *eudaimonic* well-being.

Neither type of happiness is better than the other and people should enjoy both types of happiness. However, one type of happiness has a much more positive effect on which genes are re-turned on than the other.

Steve Cole, one of the authors of the study, wrote, "People with high levels of hedonic well-being didn't feel any worse than those with high levels of eudaimonic well-being: Both seemed to experience the same high levels of positive emotion. However, their genomes were responding very differently." He continued, "What this study tells us is that doing good and feeling good have very different effects on the human genome, even though they generate similar levels of positive emotion." The longer-range do-good eudaimonic happiness clearly has a more salutary effect. "Apparently, the human genome is much more sensitive to different ways of achieving happiness than our conscious minds."[97]

well-being track negatively in parallel with the intensification of adverse physical side effects. The patients receiving pet therapy, upon completion of the roughly seven-week treatment protocol, reported the predicted negative physical effects. Surprisingly, however, the group reported elevations in their emotional and well-being metrics after spending time every day with the therapy dogs and their handlers. One patient even told Dr. Fleishman that he would have quit the tough treatment protocol but did not because he "wanted to see the dog." As a beautiful additional benefit, the center staff on duty during this study also reported elevated mood and job satisfaction and credited it to the happy, relaxed presence of the dogs. In the few short years since Fleishman published his findings in 2015, it's now common to find therapy dogs helping patients at cancer centers across the country. The unconditional love and loyalty our pets offer stands as an interesting counter-example for us humans—which undoubtedly explains the cultural trend toward renewed appreciation for the four-legged friends in our lives.

When it comes to one another, we might take an example from our animal companions. The seriousness of a cancer diagnosis often cuts through our relational issues and can help us to either make significant, positive changes in our relationships or prompt us to get out of those that do not support us. Complacency, ancient resentments and grudges, disappointment, and unmet expectations: Cancer shakes up all of these dynamics and offers us an opportunity to examine all of our relationships, from intimate to casual. Separating ourselves from the "two-legged toxins" in our lives might be as important as choosing our own anticancer medical and wellness team moving forward. We know intuitively how people make us feel. It's important to tune in, respect those feelings, and head for what supports health and healing.

The Healing Power of Faith Communities

While spirituality has not been found to directly impact cancer outcomes, belief and a sense of deeper connection with the world play a big part in quality of life, happiness, and helping to avoid depression and social isolation, all factors that have been linked to disease and the cancer hallmarks. What I see over and again working with cancer patients is a sense of awakening that comes with their diagnosis, to the point where some survivors believe that God gave them cancer in the sense that everything happens for a reason, and their new purpose in life is to face and overcome the challenge of their diagnosis. Others who were not actively religious or spiritual may become more so through their cancer journey. Cancer has a way of clearing away the minutiae of life and allows survivors to fully consider their larger purpose, which is often felt as a spiritual purpose.

When our friend Molly M. was hit by a recurrence of her brain cancer only six months after her initial diagnosis and surgery, she told me that she had come face-to-face with her own mortality and accepted it in an odd, calm way going into her second surgery. *Perhaps my time is up in this life*, she thought. The last six months had not been pleasant, to say the least. She had gone through periods of paralysis and suffered frequent debilitating (and terrifying) seizures. "I remember thinking, 'This is it. I'm just not going to get out of this one.'"

But midway between arriving at the hospital at 6:00 a.m. and her scheduled surgery time later that morning, Molly felt a visceral wave wash through her. She realized, in that moment of clarity, that she was going to be fine. She told her husband not to worry—she was going to live. He was stressed but trying to hold it together for her sake.

As with her first surgery, she would be awake during the procedure. Molly asked the surgeon to videotape the procedure for her biology students, but he said he was unable to at such late notice. At the end of the procedure, Molly tried to get up and walk out of the operating room on her own. The team insisted on putting her in a wheelchair, but she spent only a few hours in the recovery room before she was released.

What Molly did not know when she was in the waiting room, was that the 450 students at the school where she taught were gathered at the morning chapel sending her healing energy and prayers. Molly is absolutely convinced that this energy directed her way by her very caring community made all the difference in terms of her ability to survive her second surgery. "Something powerfully healing happened between me and my kids that day," she says. "It was the most profound experience. And one that I'm certain influenced my survival. It solidified my belief in the power of the mind."

That was a pivotal moment in Molly's turn toward anticancer living, which has likely played a role in her ability to survive and thrive for the last eighteen and a half years. She decided to do whatever she could to prove the doctors wrong, and worked fastidiously to rewire her brain and retrain her body. She credits the support of her husband and a team of "angels"—family, friends, social workers, hospice volunteers, medical staff at the hospital and brain tumor clinic, her herbalist, and massage therapists for achieving such surprising results. As Molly likes to put it, "Miracles take a lot of work!"

Molly operates from a central belief that where there is life, there is hope. She also believes that we all have the capacity in our minds to heal. "The best way to live an anticancer life is to embrace whatever healing modalities are best for you," she explains. "Use the mind to center yourself with whatever form of meditation works best for you, while balancing rest, exercise, a healthy organic lifestyle and eating practices." Through being positive, boosting our immune system, incorporating healthy foods, and using techniques developed by our ancestors thousands of years ago, Molly believes it is possible to ward off cancer. The evidence suggests she might be ahead of her time in realizing how deeply our thoughts and actions influence our health. Alison and I are continually inspired by her example. For us, she is a living, breathing embodiment of the transformative possibilities of anticancer living.

Molly believes fully in the healing energy she receives from her community. For those who have a stronger connection to more organized religion, the place of worship can be a source of community for people who might not have family, at least not in their immediate area. Rabbis, imams, priests, and pastors provide their congregants a form of unconditional love and support. For Jana L., a sixty-year-old research nurse, her diagnosis with stage III breast cancer led her to become more involved with her church, which became a bigger part of her social support network. As part of her sixtieth birthday celebration, Jana is training to take part with her daughter and her daughter's husband in the Camino de Santiago, a monthlong pilgrimage on foot across northern Spain that ends in Santiago de Compostela, where, legend has it, the body of St. James is buried. This is a great example from our perspective because it shows not only the importance of spirituality, but also how social support can act as the basis for making other healthy lifestyle changes. In this case, Jana is getting in shape so she can accompany her daughter on a spiritual pilgrimage across the Spanish countryside. Her faith and social support are enhancing her physical fitness.

Of course, faith and healing have a long history—almost as long as the story of mankind. But in modern medicine, which is so utterly focused on data, statistics, and scientific proof, it's hard to factor faith and its effect on cancer outcomes or healing in general into the equation. But that's not the case for everyone.

Church Health in Memphis

There's an extraordinary health center in Memphis run by Scott Morris, MD, one of the few doctors I know of who also has a master's degree in divinity from Yale University. At Church Health, a nonprofit that Scott started twenty years ago in a dilapidated building he rented for one dollar a year, he and his team have seen over seventy thousand people.[98]

As a minister, Scott has long understood that the link between health and faith is inextricably entwined. "Have you ever wondered why so many hospitals are named for saints or religious orders? The call to heal is all over the Bible—virtually on every page. I understood early on that our body is truly a gift from God, and it's our responsibility to honor that gift and care for our bodies as though our life depends on it—because it does."

Church Health is a model of meeting people where they are, which, in this case, is in the midst of a community that is "poor" by most standards but which still, to this day, stuns Morris with the abundance of "spiritual capital" spread among his patients, neighbors, and friends. Morris objects to the Platonic notion that our body and spirit are separate. "A broken heart won't show up on an X-ray," he tells me. "But if I make a counselor or a minister available to talk about what is ailing someone's heart, their blood pressure may improve, or their shortness of breath may give way to cleansing tears. Pills can't touch what human connection and the acknowledgment of God and the Spirit can."

Morris is a maverick when it comes to understanding the value of anticancer living. "First, being healthy is not about the absence of disease," he tells me with conviction. "It's about helping people live a life well-lived. Who cares if you live two years longer if you're alone in a nursing home? Everything we do here is built around a passage from Colossians that says, 'You are the children of God, therefore as God's chosen people holy and dearly beloved, clothe yourself with gentleness, kindness, compassion, humility, patience, and above all put on love, the harmony which binds all.'" What this says to me is that compassion and love are at the heart of Morris's practice. He is not focused on statistics or "outcomes" per se but rather on a deeper sense of health that addresses the whole person, not just their disease or symptoms.

To achieve wellness, Morris and his team have created what they call the Model for Healthy Living. It focuses on seven components of equal importance: medical care, faith/spiritual life, nutrition, movement, family and friends, the emotions, and lastly, work.

Morris understands that all these components work in a kind of harmony and that most of them come together most powerfully in community.

"Church—any church—is not just a place of worship. It's a haven for the local community. This is where we're baptized and married and eulogized—in the presence of our loved ones and neighbors," Morris tells me, then adds, "We're designed to be healthiest when we share the best of ourselves with others. At Church Health we understand that striving to live a healthy life is a lifelong prospect, and so we have programs aimed at young children, preschoolers, all the way up to seniors. It's all about educating people and bringing them together to celebrate and actualize healthy lifestyle choices. I see it everywhere: If you eat well with your family, you share that with your neighbors, and they share that, and so on. Wouldn't you much rather walk through the neighborhood with friends and learn about how they're getting healthy rather than stand on a Stairmaster alone? It's so evident to me that community is what really heals us. And if you don't believe me, just check the Bible. It's something God feels pretty strongly about, too."

The last thing he wants me to know is something that every doctor who truly wants to be part of the anticancer living movement needs to acknowledge. "I need these people as much as they need me. We puzzle over tests, we make tough decisions, but mostly, we pray. I for them, and they for me. We are all in this together. I would never leave here because I'm learning how to be a more spiritually fit person by doing this work. I'm being healed just as much as my patients are." But he is quick to add, "Everyone is welcome at Church Health. I have no interest in converting anyone or preaching to nonbelievers. But I do believe the spiritual dimension of our health is as important, if not more so, than the physical aspect of it and I'm not shy about sharing this. I think it's only beneficial to acknowledge the divine wholeness of the individual, no matter what you believe."

Social Synergy

Whether it's the support of Dr. Morris's Church Health or the devotion of a family member to be by your side during cancer treatment, social support plays a central role in every aspect of lifestyle change, from stress management and sleep to diet and exercise. What's more, researchers have found a clear relationship between social connectedness and physical health within each stage of life—from adolescence to old age.[28, 82–86] The work of Anil Sood, Susan Lutgendorf, Steve Cole, Barbara Fredrickson, and others has shown that social support is closely tied with stress, and appears to have a direct impact on multiple cancer hallmarks.

You can see the interplay of social support with other areas in some of the stories we've shared. When a member of Dorothy's Pink Posse group saw she was overextended, she pushed Dorothy to focus more on her mental health and not just her physical health, which in turn improved Dorothy's sleep quality and allowed her to stop relying on sleeping pills. Jana's increased spirituality and deeper involvement in her church not only reduced her stress, it led her to train for a pilgrimage across Spain with her daughter. Through social support, she has increased her physical activity, lowered her stress level, and become more aware of what she eats and how much sleep she gets to better sustain her during her training for a monthlong walk. As Gabe Canales, whom you met in part 1 explains, social support plays a key role in accountability and helping to sustain healthful changes: "Changing lifelong habits can be challenging, and you need a strong support system: a significant other, spouse, friend, coworker or a nutritionist/dietitian, a support group—someone who you can be open with about what you're trying to achieve, someone who can help encourage you to stay on track."

Meg Hirshberg, founder of the Anticancer Lifestyle Program that is offered both in-person and online, introduced in part 1, is a model for how to bring the anticancer living message to the larger public.[99] Meg, a two-time cancer survivor herself and a friend of the late David Servan-Schreiber, describes the healing power of the groups she's designed and led like this:

> When you put people together in a group, miraculous things happen and they start to laugh and bond, which is also a really important part of our program. We do everything we can to encourage that camaraderie. Participants are assigned to call a different person each

week so they connect with each member of the class one-on-one, outside of the larger group.

Sometimes they grumble about that in the beginning, but by the end, they all love it.

These are very hardworking people, and a lot of times some of their family members have issues with alcohol or drugs. They, themselves, are working really hard, and they already have serious life challenges, and then they get hit up with this cancer diagnosis and they're just devastated. As one person who went through our class put it, "When I joined this class, I felt like someone had thrown me a life raft."

This kind of emotional support is so empowering, so important. These classes and that kind of peer support help these people plan their futures with a degree of psychological well being and support that they didn't have before they got sick. It's powerful to watch this kind of healing happen first hand.

The power of the group to heal is rapidly becoming recognized as a cornerstone of anticancer living. Within our own CompLife Study, we've witnessed that patients, who are often the caretakers of their families, experience true emotional and psychological support for the first time, allowing them to transform their lives and, despite the cancer, begin to thrive instead of just survive.

I recently ran into someone who fits this bill to a T—Michelene H., one of the first CompLife participants. At first, I must admit that I didn't quite recognize her. Michelene had lost at least fifty pounds since I saw her last. But that was only part of what made her look so different. She was radiating positive energy. Her brown eyes were beaming, and she nodded her head as I took in her transformation, like, *That's right. It's Michelene.*

She had undergone a double mastectomy and breast reconstruction and had been cancer-free for three years. Michelene told me around her surgery she controlled her pain using meditative breathing techniques. She said she was reading food labels and avoiding nitrate-enriched foods, and she was still exercising and meditating every day.

Michelene is not someone who came from an environment where such practices were common or even in the realm of everyday experience. She grew up poor in North Philadelphia and left a violent home environment as soon as she turned sixteen in search of a better life. She moved to Houston in part to get as far as possible from the toxic energy of her family, determined to break the cycle of abuse and provide her own young children with a healthier life. Being part of the CompLife Study introduced Michelene to every aspect of anticancer living, and I could see three years later that she was healthy, vibrant, and strong.

Michelene is now volunteering in a program called Cancer Connection and mentors other women facing the same diagnosis she was given—triple-negative, stage III breast cancer. As a triple-negative survivor, Michelene is a unique and inspiring volunteer. She tells the other cancer patients that there is life after cancer, even when facing a challenging diagnosis. Her daughter, who was her primary support during her cancer treatment, was so inspired witnessing her mother's journey that she has returned to school to become a registered nurse. I am always gratified when I run into CompLife patients, because even though the study is ongoing, I can see in women like Michelene that our model is working. Here was someone who was not merely doing *well* after a challenging cancer diagnosis, she was *thriving*. She was not just taking care of herself, she had transformed her physical appearance and mental outlook. She was literally glowing with pride and strength. Michelene had gained enough confidence to reach out to help others, which the latest research shows further improves our health and longevity.

But another thing that Michelene said caught me off guard and made me fully realize the importance and impact of having and maintaining a strong support network. After the intensive portion of the study ended, after six weeks with all that support, she felt let down. She was upset at us for taking her social support away. Here she had this wonderful team teaching her how to live a healthier life, and then, just as she was adjusting to these new, healthier habits with coaches to keep her on track, the intensive portion of the study ended. She continued with her counseling sessions for the next year, and then those sessions ended, too, and she was on her own.

Indeed, the loss Michelene felt is something that's easy to understand. As she put it, "In looking at how far I had truly come, I don't often realize how powerful my journey has been until I am reminded of the path, obstacles, and blessings I experienced. I have to pinch myself and ask . . . , 'Did I really have cancer?' Now, looking back I did have those feelings of abandonment, but my sticking to and learning as much as I could to live a healthier lifestyle far outweighs those past feelings. The team taught me how to live again . . . better than before cancer, and for that I am eternally grateful!" In our lives, most of us will never be part of such an intense program of lifestyle change. The question is, how can you accomplish the same transformation in your own life?

What we have learned from the science and from our combined experience making these changes is that the traditional model of lifestyle change is flawed. Trying to improve your health by going on a diet and signing up for a half-marathon do not get to the core issues that influence behavioral changes. Before any of that, you need what Michelene felt the loss of so keenly—an anticancer team.

THE ANTICANCER LIVING GUIDE TO LOVE AND SOCIAL SUPPORT

So many people Alison and I encounter in our talks across the country skip the vital step of building a solid support network and jump right into the latest diet or fitness routine. But without the foundation of social support to hold up these other changes, what they are trying to build is likely to collapse at the first challenge. It's time to shift our thinking about what makes and keeps us healthy to better consider the influence of our friends, families, coworkers, caring professionals, chosen communities, and teachers. They are at the heart of a sustainable anticancer lifestyle. It is also important to engage in activities that foster eudaimonic well-being, where your wellness is derived from a sense of purpose and meaning in life. Paradoxically this can grow out of our steepest challenges, as we have shared in this book.

Building Your Anticancer Team

Before you can start building a team, you need to recognize and evaluate the people you have around you. If you have been part of a community for a long time, you may be able to draw upon an extensive network. If not, then this is the moment to look at what you have and how to put together the help and support you need. The most important relationships in terms of our health are with people who are close enough to us emotionally to provide spacious and empathic caring. While it's important to have someone to drive you to a doctor's appointment, or watch your kids while you are there, the most crucial support might be from that person who is able to help you through the emotional part of whatever health crisis or life challenge you're facing.

FIVE SUPPORT AREAS

1. Practical Support: Those who support you in practical, tangible ways. People you can count on during difficult times to drive you to appointments, organize care rotations, help with meal planning and prep, etc.

2. Informational Support: Those from whom you can get informed advice, and talk through options and decisions. People whose opinion you trust and who you know have your best interest at heart.
3. Motivational Support: Those who support your worth in this world, see the importance of the changes you are trying to make, and help keep you motivated to keep at it. For those with cancer, these are the people who remind you of your qualities as a whole person—not just a patient.
4. Community Support: Group connections and social integration provide both a sense of belonging and the ability to assist others, which reinforces your own value in the world.
5. Emotional Support: Those with whom you can share your deepest troubles and joys and who offer unconditional love and comfort.

Think about different types of support as pillars that help to keep you level as you move forward. *In what areas are your pillars of support less stable? Where do you have enough and where might some more assistance be welcome?*

BUILD UP YOUR WEAK SPOTS

- Look for people and groups that could help fill out your team and balance your support. One person, even an intimate partner, however caring, simply cannot provide support in all areas. Diversifying your support base is crucial. Caregivers risk burnout, too, and everyone's needs must be balanced.
- In terms of social integration: Is there a group you could join related to something you enjoy doing, such as a hobby, activity, or sport? Could you join or become more involved with a church, spiritual group, yoga center, library, walking group, musical group, etc.?
- If you're lacking a sense of nurturing and being nurtured, is there a place where you could volunteer and find strength by connecting with and helping others, and find such help in turn?
- If you don't have someone who provides you with emotional support, could you find a therapist who might help you work through issues or a support group that is made up of people with whom you share a common background or issue?

When taking stock of your community, consider who you are in touch with and who you haven't talked to in a while, or even a long time. Don't be afraid to include someone from your past or whom you have lost touch with on your list. He could end up being the most important person in your anticancer network.

Enhancing Your Eudaimonic Well-Being: Step One—Discovering Your Core Values

Core values are the lens through which we evaluate what we see, feel, and hear around us. They are not descriptions of what we do for a living or how we accomplish our goals. They are the values that underlie what we do, how we interact with others, and the choices we make. It is important to identify and be aware of what they are, and where your daily actions are at odds with your beliefs. This is an important step to move toward a more purpose-driven life and to have your daily decisions align with the person you want to be in the world. This exercise, that I learned as part of the Stagen Leadership Academy, is a first step on the path of fostering eudaimonic well-being.[1]

When considering your own core values, think about words/terms that point to what is most important to you as a person and that reflect your highest priorities in life.

As an example, here are the phrases I use to explain my core values:

- Be Present
- Be Healthy
- Have Compassion/Empathy
- Be Honest/Have Integrity
- Make a Difference
- Maintain a Sense of Wonder

I start with how I want to be in the world, what's important to me, then move to how I hope to impact others. My core values underlie the work I do and the attitude I try to maintain—an openness to new ideas and feelings—as I meet new people and experience new things.

WHAT ARE YOUR CORE VALUES?

Directions:

- Write down words that you think fit your core values.
- Limit yourself to no more than twenty key words.
- Edit it down to ten and then finally to a maximum of five to six key words or phrases.
- Make sure each word/phrase matches your way of living and viewing the world.

PUTTING YOUR CORE VALUES IN MOTION

When put into the context of our lives, core values become guiding principles that can help us be true to who we are in everything we say and do and get us closer to leading the life we choose rather than one that's "driving" us. Now that you have identified the words/phrases that speak to your core values, construct sentences that explain how those ideas take shape in your life. Here are some examples based on my own core values:

VALUE	ACTION
Be Present	I try to stay connected to the moment and examine who or what is driving my thoughts and behaviors.
Be Healthy	I eat health-supporting foods and minimize health-depleting foods. I exercise my heart and muscles daily. I nourish my mind to foster calm within myself.
Have Compassion/Empathy	I listen and truly connect with people where they are in the moment. My actions and behaviors take others into consideration.
Be Honest/Have Integrity	I am true to my word. I am responsible and dependable.
Make a Difference	I will leave the world a better place than how I found it. I am actively engaged every day in helping others.
Maintain a Sense of Wonder	I am open-minded to all new experiences. I continue to learn new things and look at the world and the human experience in new ways.

HOW DO YOU EMBODY AND EXPRESS YOUR CORE VALUES?

Directions: Construct a sentence or two explaining each of your core values, what they mean to you, and how you plan to act on those values in your life moving forward. Consult your core values when making decisions and try to align your daily choices and behaviors with your core values.

Enhancing Your Eudaimonic Well-Being: Step Two—Providing Support to Others

Whether it is friends, family, colleagues, or a casual acquaintance, we all need and benefit from the support of those around us. We know that providing support to others is both a gift for the recipient and for the giver. As we are evolutionarily wired to psychologically and biologically benefit when we help others, taking on the role of listener and supporter is a positive step in fostering eudaimonic well-being.

Volunteering has been connected to longer life, happier life, and increased satisfaction. A review of forty studies that looked at the health effects of helping others found that volunteering on a regular basis reduced early mortality rates by 22 percent.[2] And volunteering doesn't have to be your life's purpose to impact your health. Researchers reported health impacts for participants who volunteered for as little as one hour per month. David Servan-Schreiber talked about cancer in terms of terrain and making your personal terrain as inhospitable to cancer as possible. Think about giving in the same way. You are creating a terrain of positivity that will improve your outlook on life and help sustain and grow a healthy social network. Giving to charity and helping others is fertilizer for your social support terrain.

Volunteering Online—The United Nations has a variety of online volunteering options that can connect you with people from other countries and other continents, doing anything from translating documents to creating videos or designing infographics. The job-listing site Idealist has an entire section of its Volunteer Resource Center devoted to Online Volunteering, and the group Volunteer Match lists more than six thousand "virtual volunteer opportunities." The possibilities for volunteering in the digital era are truly limitless and cross every boundary, religion, interest, and ideology.

THE ANTICANCER LIVING GUIDE
SOCIAL SUPPORT SUMMARY

Create Your Anticancer Team

List people in your support network who fall into the support categories mentioned in this chapter and consider where and how you could find someone to build up that particular pillar.

Identify Your Core Values

Think about eudaimonic, purposeful living and where your own experience varies. Identify five to six words or phrases you want to live by and formulate a sentence or two about your core values and how you might better align them with daily actions.

Give the Gift of Support

Don't underestimate the life and health benefits of supporting others and receiving support in turn. Consider teaming up with someone in a group or your community and volunteering together for a couple hours a month.

CHAPTER EIGHT

Stress and Resilience

Everything that occurs in life—from the inception of a cell to daily events, big and small, to the dying breath of every living thing—is the result of a certain kind of friction, of interaction, and we can call this kind of stimulation *stress*. When we define the word this way, as a form of interactive energy, it's possible to look at it with some neutrality, as just a fact of life (if not the central fact), without the negative connotations we tend to heap on it. It's important to do this because, in the short term, the stress response is very much a motivator of life, of action, and certainly of interaction. However, when stress becomes chronic, when our life challenges surpass our ability to effectively cope with them, it becomes problematic for our psychological, emotional, and physical health. At that point, stress can grow into an unrelenting burden on our body, mind, and spirit and it has the capacity to undermine our health, exacerbate disease, and shorten our life span.

Stress is woven into the very fabric of life and we have a physiological response that is hardwired into us—the fight-or-flight response—that keeps us out of imminent danger. But when stressful events become overwhelming and switch from being an acute daily occurrence into a chronic issue, the change can trigger not just negative psychological and emotional reactions but it can also cause physiological damage. A growing body of scientific research shows how stress impacts all aspects of our lifestyle and all aspects of our physical health.

In terms of stress and cancer, we now know that stress modulates key biological processes linked with cancer risk and progression, and that chronic stress is associated with worse outcomes for those with cancer.[1] In fact, chronic stress dysregulates the immune system, decreasing our body's natural defense against cancer, and leads to increased inflammation.[2] At the same time, stress promotes tumor growth by releasing into the bloodstream proteins and hormones that help tumors enlist the body's resources for cancer's singular purpose—to grow.[3,4] Most frightening is that we now know stress has the capacity to modulate key cellular processes, literally down into the nucleus of every cell in our body, and modify genetic pathways that make our bodies more hospitable to cancer growth.[5]

While increasing research points to the health dangers of stress, the good news is that stress is not genetic. None of us are condemned to live a stressful life. In fact, stress is something we can actively control and manage. Researchers at UCLA found that caregivers, who often face intense levels of chronic stress, were able to change their inflammatory profiles by engaging for twelve minutes a day in a specially designed yoga meditation.[6] What's more, the directed meditation had a dramatically greater effect on their biomarkers compared to having caregivers rest and listen to calming music.[6]

In my own research with breast cancer survivors undergoing radiation therapy, I have found that yoga does more than simply fight fatigue and improve aspects of quality of life (which are important for cancer survivors undergoing chemotherapy and radiation).[7] Patients who incorporated yogic breathing, relaxation techniques, and meditation with their yoga practice improved their general health while reducing their stress hormone levels. So, while chronic stress poses serious health risks, the solution is readily accessible, free of charge, and the only side effect is that it also makes you feel great.

The Unique Emotional Stress of Cancer

There is nothing that can bring on acute mental, emotional, and physical stress like a cancer diagnosis. One minute you are living your life and the very next, all of it is up for grabs. For many people, especially if the diagnosis is of advanced cancer, you are thrust into acute awareness of your own mortality. Very few things in life are more stressful than this.

The shock of a cancer diagnosis can even be quite traumatic.[8] Like a tsunami that makes landfall without warning, it can flood a patient with high levels of anxiety that literally washes over every aspect of life: Will I live? Will my children be okay? Will this bankrupt my family? Will my spouse or significant other carry on without me? Will I still be able to work? Will I be disfigured? Who will take care of my pets? A wave of shock rushes in upon us, and we may be catapulted into a full-blown state of traumatic stress. At the very least, we'll be awash in feelings that we may have spent a lifetime avoiding or we may experience new, tough feelings for the first time.

Psycho-oncologists are beginning to study the emotional trauma that cancer can bring with it. Initially, the emotional trauma cancer patients experience can be acute (what the *Diagnostic and Statistical Manual of Mental Disorders*, or DSM, classifies as "Acute Stress Disorder," or ASD).[9] If this is dealt with right away, the patient is then able to work through the other feelings that ride in behind the initial trauma. The traumatic response, however, can often be delayed and then shows up as longer-term PTSD, or post-traumatic stress disorder.[10] PTSD has been studied in patients with melanoma, Hodgkin's lymphoma, and breast cancer, among others. Taken collectively, these studies (which use the full DSM-IV diagnostic criteria) show a range of 3 to 4 percent of early-stage patients suffer some form of psychological trauma, while up to 10 to 15 percent of cancer survivors can suffer from some type of clinically defined mood disorder such as depression or anxiety during or after treatment.[11] When a less clinically conservative measure of mental health is used, such as depression screening measures that have been linked with biological outcomes and survival, the numbers balloon, with more than 35 percent of early-stage patients exhibiting signs of trauma and up to 80 percent of those with recurrent cancer showing signs of this kind of psychological stress.[11–15]

Successfully addressing the trauma of cancer is a crucial first step in a patient's journey: only when the overwhelming psycho-emotional stress of the disease is acknowledged and treated can the patient begin to work on building the emotional resilience that is needed to build an anticancer life.

The Emotions of Mortality

We live in a culture that encourages the suppression of emotions, where stoic silence is prized over honest, open emotional expression and sharing. Perhaps nowhere is this truer than in the context of cancer care, where a patient is encouraged to "fight" and "battle" the disease and to "live strong" in order to survive. This expectation for battle readiness, for a certain kind of emotional hardness, is not the most beneficial approach to dealing with cancer, nor is it even possible for the newly diagnosed.[16,17] Certainly every cancer patient must have the courage to face the unknown, but before there can be courage, there must be acceptance, and before there can be acceptance, there has to be an honest willingness to express and process the complex feelings that cancer brings with it.

It is important that the primary medical team a cancer patient works with understands the emotional and psychological implications of the diagnosis. This is where integrative oncology becomes so crucial.

Every cancer patient must be encouraged and allowed to express his or her fears, hopes, and desires, ideally even before any treatment decisions need to be made. But this isn't always easy: How does a young mother express her fear of dying without terrifying her young children? How does a single man approach his parents for financial support while he has to cut back on work during chemotherapy? How does a woman express her fear that her husband will no longer find her attractive after a double mastectomy?

These questions are valid, honest, and important, and it's our job as cancer care professionals to become aware of the need for patients to find or develop the tools they will need to work through the complex emotions that cancer brings. Otherwise, straightforward feelings like sadness may morph into chronic depression or unaddressed fear might turn into chronic, debilitating anxiety. Dealing with the authentic, necessary, and very human emotions that come to the surface not only prevents the onset of serious mental illness, like those I just mentioned, but also fortifies the patient to focus on healing.

First we have to help cancer patients identify the emotions they are experiencing. This can be done by an empathic oncologist or an experienced nurse and certainly by loving and supportive family members and friends. But sometimes just lending an ear is not enough, and throughout this chapter, I will discuss the ways that cancer patients—and the rest of us—may cultivate peace of mind, which is the essential ingredient to successfully making any significant and lasting lifestyle changes. When we identify, express, and work through our emotions, we are then able to tap into our "gut," or what I think of as our body's innate intelligence, and make decisions with this intelligence in mind. This is especially crucial when one is dealing with a serious disease such as cancer. When we've acknowledged and dealt with our feelings, we better position ourselves to make decisions that reflect our true values and desires, rather than making decisions based on the fear or anxiety that stress brings. Being in emotional balance allows us to make healthy lifestyle choices that will enhance our ability to heal.

THE EMOTIONS OF MORTALITY

Here is a list of some of the common emotions related to a cancer diagnosis or other life circumstance that puts us in touch with our impending mortality. Which ones have you experienced, whether you've had cancer or not?

- Anxiety
- Fear
- Anger/rage
- Depression
- Denial
- Helplessness
- Regret
- Guilt
- Loneliness/alienation
- Broken
- Shame
- Confusion
- Overwhelmed

Was there someone you could share these feelings with? Were you able to acknowledge, honor, and process these feelings so that you felt more emotionally integrated and able to face the reality of your situation? In terms of your emotional life, do you feel understood and respected? If you have cancer, is your medical team aware of your feelings and working in a way that includes your emotional concerns? Are your loved ones also aware of the emotions you are grappling with?

The feelings that come up in life are tough and intense, but absolutely natural and necessary. Acknowledging them within yourself, and openly with others, will prepare you for the unavoidable stressors that come along with life's challenges, including a cancer diagnosis, in ways that will provide lasting benefits.

Developing emotional magnanimity is essential to keeping at bay the stressors that are known to aggravate cancers and other diseases. In this chapter, Alison and I will discuss the groundbreaking research that's been done on the link between stress and cancer proliferation and we will offer practical tips for how to reduce stress in your life in ways that will help keep cancer contained as well as improve your overall sense of well-being and health.

It is important to note that stressful events themselves, the stressors, which seem unavoidable in our current culture and climate, are not what cause the harm. It is our reaction to the challenges in our lives that does the real damage. To prevent disease and live as healthfully as possible, it's imperative that we learn to manage our stress, which means managing our reactions to stressful events and exchanges in our daily lives. Only when we've got stress under some control can we make the kind of positive lifestyle changes that make up anticancer living.

Embracing Reality

Some cancer survivors describe being diagnosed with cancer as "the best thing that ever happened to me." But not Molly M., the woman you met who has lived for the past eighteen and a half years with the most lethal form of brain cancer. "Getting cancer was awful. But it forced me to slow down and really listen to my body. I had to leave my students and the teaching job I loved, but, ironically, my new full-time job became educating myself so I could heal myself and help others. I would never describe cancer as the best thing that happened to me, but I will say this: It has made me wiser. The bottom line is, I had a choice: I could let cancer be in charge or I could be. I decided I was more important than the disease and now I'm focused for a significant portion of every day on anticancer living." Molly describes the kind of fierce pragmatism that cancer can bring out in us. A cancer diagnosis or other life-changing events have the capacity to ground us firmly so we can step with purpose onto the anticancer living path. But first, we have to deal with our feelings and find some emotional equilibrium so that we fortify ourselves against the inevitable distractions life will try to throw at us. When we develop the skills we need to keep stress at bay, we can begin to make lifestyle choices that prioritize health and well-being over stress and disease.

Is a Positive Attitude Helpful?

One of the really surprising sources of stress I hear cancer patients discuss is the pressure they feel under by well-meaning family and friends—even strangers. Being told to simply "Stay positive!" or dismissed with "You've got this!" or worse, things like "I read this is an easy one to beat," puts unnecessary pressure (stress) on the cancer patient and can also make them feel dismissed or diminished, though this is usually the last thing the person who said this intended. Being asked to adopt a peppy mind-set isn't the same thing as being encouraged to find your way to an optimistic outlook. I realize this is a somewhat subtle distinction, but I've seen too many cancer patients, especially those who face a recurrence, blame themselves for somehow not having the right "positive" attitude. As a psychologist, I've come to realize that not everyone knows what to say when they find out someone has cancer, and some people, even close friends and family, don't have the capacity to be as supportive or present as we might hope. The important thing for cancer patients is to focus on bringing people into their lives who are capable of being more emotionally supportive and empathetic.

Michael Lerner, PhD, has been exploring the subtle messages we convey when we think we're being supportive and cautions that telling people with cancer, "You'll beat this if you just stay positive," puts the emphasis in the wrong place. It forces the patient to fixate on the cancer rather than on building a joyful and purposefully healthy lifestyle around the cancer.[18] "People need to be allowed to experience whatever it is they're experiencing," he recently said to me, "whether it's fear or anxiety or depression or an opening to the beauty of the world or love." He went on, "When one practices being joyful, being happy, being in touch with the vast mysterious beauty of the world, this is quite constructive and can be powerfully transformative. I've known people who have fallen madly in love for the first time even as they are dying of cancer. I can't think of a more positive life experience than that."

Lerner, like many at the forefront of the anticancer living movement, emphasizes that forced optimism can be toxic and that the goal is to become relaxed and skillful with handling our emotions. When we do this, he believes, it will naturally lead to a more positive outlook on life, greater intimacy with our fellow mortals, and a keener ability to live in the here and now.

Getting out from under the vast cloud of stress that seems to blanket our world (or what Elissa Epel, a leading health psychologist and the coauthor of *The Telomere Effect*, refers to as leaving "the house of stress that we all live in") is a key step onto the path of healthy living.[19] It involves a turning inward (toward the calm, knowing center that we all have inside) and consciously accepting all the feelings that our morality awakens in us. As David Servan-Schreiber put it in his memoir, *Not the Last Goodbye: Reflections on Life, Death, Healing, and Cancer,* "One of the best defenses against cancer is finding a place of inner calm."[20]

Glenn Sabin, the longtime cancer survivor whom we introduced in part 1, also credits his ability to find inner peace with his capacity to move beyond the initial emotions of his diagnosis. "Being in a calmer frame of mind provided me the mental means to dig deeper for answers to how I might manage my disease in a meaningful way. How I could create health in spite of disease. The foundation to my health was achieving an unfettered mind."

What is quite remarkable, and I believe has the power to imbue a cancer diagnosis with a profoundly human kind of "opportunity," is that each of these remarkable people made the decision to remain hopeful in the face of life's great uncertainty. This hopefulness allows a person (whether cancer is present or not) to step out of fear and into action. Moving past fear allows us to approach life with renewed awareness and curiosity and to focus on the deeper rewards life still has to offer us, regardless of our prognosis. When we surrender to the truth of our (health) circumstances and turn inward for answers, we are then able to tap into our innate, powerful sources of healing.

I recently asked Diana Lindsay what was the key to her miraculous recovery. "I would have to say that I don't know," she responded. "I entered the world of not knowing and I remain in the world of not knowing. But if I had to try to articulate it, I'd start by saying, 'First of all, you have to pick yourself up off the ground when you get a prognosis like mine and you have to be willing to hope, to take the risk of hope.' I made a complete commitment to healing, gave everything up, and just completely dedicated myself to it. I learned to listen to my body and discern what it needs, and now I do everything I can to help my body stay well."

Monastic Mind Control

Western doctors have long been both intrigued and suspicious of claims that the mind can have such a dramatic impact on our bodies and our health. In the early 1970s, Dr. Herbert Benson, a Harvard physician, took a team of scientists to Northern India, where he had heard of a group of Tibetan monks who, through meditation, claimed they could control aspects of their physiology. The prevailing Western belief at the time was that physiological processes such as heart rate, blood pressure, and skin temperature were not under the control of our minds. What Dr. Benson found astounded him. The monks had exquisite control over their own physiology. Using only meditation, they were able to lower their heart rate, decrease their blood pressure, and decrease or increase their body temperature to specific parts of their body.[21]

Subsequently, Richard Davidson at the University of Wisconsin brought some of these same monks and others into the laboratory to study how their brains worked.[22] He found that the monks who had been meditating for extensive periods of time had distinctly different brain function than the general population, and they responded to stressors in a very different way than nonmeditators or novice meditators, with reduced heart rates, lower metabolism, and slower breathing.[21,23,24] They were more in control of their reactions, physiologically and psychologically, and able to maintain a state of calm even during stressful situations.

Almost forty years ago, Jon Kabat-Zinn, the creator of the Stress Reduction Clinic at the University of Massachusetts Medical School, started a clinical and research program that developed a practice he called mindfulness-based stress reduction (MBSR).[25] MBSR is typically an eight-week program incorporating a combination of different practices from Eastern traditions, with an emphasis on Vipassana meditation, a form of mindfulness meditation. Through decades of research, Kabat-Zinn and his team have discovered that, even after just eight weeks of MBSR, patients showed distinct changes in the electrical activity of the brain.[26] Brain regions that process positive emotions increased in activity, and brain regions that process negative emotions decreased in activity. Their research also reveals a direct correlation between changes in the brain due to meditation and how well the immune system functions. In one 2003 study, Kabat-Zinn, Davidson, and their team studied the electrical activity in the brain of meditation-naive participants who went through the eight-week stress-reduction program compared to a control group that was waiting to take part in the program. At the end of the eight weeks, both groups received a flu vaccine. The people who had been through two months of MBSR experienced an enhanced immune response that allowed their bodies to respond better to the vaccination. What's more, researchers found a dose-response effect in the relationship. In other words, the more someone meditated, the more effective the vaccine.[26]

Dr. Sara Lazar at Harvard University took Kabat-Zinn's research a step further and measured, using MRI scans, whether there was a change in the actual anatomy of the brain after the eight-week MBSR program.[27] She found a decrease in the size of the amygdala, the part of the brain responsible for

MEDITATION

There are many kinds of meditation, but some common features include focused and controlled regulation of breath, and, to some degree, control over one's thoughts and feelings. This is not really "control" in the traditional sense. The intent is to allow thoughts and feelings to float by without allowing them to lead your focus astray.

Focused-Attention Meditation

A focused meditation usually starts with the breath and could be followed by reciting a syllable or phrase, or a simple prayer. You also could focus your attention on a burning candle or on an image that affects you.

Mindfulness Meditation

With mindfulness meditation, thoughts, feelings, and emotions may be coming and going, but the key is not to focus on them and to let them freely come and go. This takes practice and can be more challenging than focused meditation. If you get distracted or start fixating on a thought or object, don't get upset with yourself. Just bring yourself back to your breath and try again.

Compassion-Based Meditation
(Also Called Loving-Kindness Meditation)

Loving-kindness meditation is essentially about cultivating love. Start by cultivating the feelings of love and compassion you have for someone close to you. Then send that loving-kindness toward yourself and foster self-compassion. Then shift to family, friends, and close loved ones. In the third phase you may choose to focus on a challenging person in your life with whom you are having a conflict or struggle. And finally focus on strangers and send out loving-kindness and compassion to everyone.

the fight-or-flight response, and an increase in the size of the hippocampus, the part of the brain related to memory. So, just like we exercise to improve our heart function and increase the size of our muscles, the same thing can be done with mind-body practices—we can exercise our brain to change the way it functions.

The Surprising Benefits of Meditation

Research published in the past ten years clearly demonstrates that meditation not only changes our lives but also modifies brain function and anatomy, reduces inflammation, modulates key biological processes right down into the nucleus of cells, changes gene expression, relieves anxiety, improves memory, and lowers stress hormones in the bloodstream.[28–33] At Wake Forest, researchers found that if they trained people to meditate, they could reduce the experience of pain (in this case a 120-degree hot pad placed on their right calf for six minutes) by 40 percent.[34] In comparison, morphine and other pain-relieving pills typically lower pain by 25 percent. Psychologists now train U.S. Marines to meditate as a way to keep them focused and alert in war zones. Researchers found that if marines meditated for at least twelve minutes a day, they increased their ability to maintain attention and retain working memory when facing life-or-death situations.[35] African refugees suffering from post-traumatic stress who were taught meditation techniques were able to dramatically reduce their anxiety, replicating previous findings showing that meditation reduced depression, insomnia, and alcohol abuse in Vietnam veterans.[36,37]

I know from my own experience that, for the breast cancer survivors who go through the CompLife Study, learning a mind-body practice is often what they cite as the most life-changing benefit they take away from the intervention.[38] As part of the study, patients learn a form of seated meditation and a yoga-based movement practice ("sun salutations" for those of you familiar with Vinyasa yoga). Patients are asked to increase their daily practice (over the course of six weeks) to twelve sun salutations a day, a brief relaxation technique, and up to twenty minutes of guided meditation. In our exit interviews, participants consistently point to the stress-management component as key to helping them change their outlook, improve the quality of their lives, and engage in healthful diet, exercise, sleep habits, and relationships.

These women do not come from privilege and they did not run away from their lives or quit their jobs as a way to find peace. They simply change their reaction to the stressors they face on a daily basis. Take Brucett M., for example. Brucett works as a merchandizer in Houston, setting up displays in stores. She's on her feet most of the day and then comes home to a bustling household that includes her husband of sixteen years, two grown children, and two teenagers. She was only forty-three when she was diagnosed with stage II breast cancer. For Brucett, like so many of the people I've encountered, finding a way to manage her stress was key to her long-term survival and to enjoying her life. She tended to let things get to her—encounters she had during the day, exchanges with her kids that seemed rude, times when she wished she had said something but hadn't. Meditation made her more aware of herself and more conscious of her reaction to stressors. Here is how she described the change to me, "I don't know if anyone has ever felt like this. To have so many questions, but the answers are trapped in you. That's how I've felt for so long. Well, I've come to realize that through meditation

YOGA, MIND-BODY PRACTICES, AND RELIGION

Many mind-body practices originate from Eastern countries such as India, Tibet, and Japan and from religious practices (e.g., Hinduism or Buddhism) thousands of years old. The Western Christian tradition also includes such practices as contemplative prayer. Humans on every part of the planet have found ways to focus inward on oneself, on one's connection to others, to a higher power, and to the world as a whole. Engaging in a mind-body practice is a time to seek calm, when we can slow down and bring awareness to the moment. Fostering and expanding one's spirituality and life purpose is an important aspect for achieving optimal health and well-being. People can modify the practices to meet their own individual needs and to ensure that they remain aligned with their own religious practices. Indeed, we work through these issues often with our own patients. For example, one of the CompLife patients with a deep Christian practice had some initial concerns of whether the yoga and meditation would conflict with her practices and beliefs. In fact, the opposite occurred. By making subtle modification in the language used in the yoga and meditation, the patient expressed later that she had never felt closer to her God than in the mind-body sessions.

and deep relaxation that my answers are flowing. I can honestly say that I've never been in such deep thought about my life."

Brucett's transformation and a growing body of research point clearly to the power of our minds to help us through stressful times, such as a cancer diagnosis, and maintain our focus and purpose through every challenge we face. My only question is this: when the benefits of meditation appear so extensive and varied, why aren't all of us taking fifteen to twenty minutes a day to focus on our breath to rejuvenate our mind, body, and spirit?

The Stress and Cancer Proliferation Loop

Though there is no scientific data to indicate that stress causes the onset of cancer diseases, there is a growing body of research that does link chronic stress with cancer growth and proliferation.

Anil Sood, MD, my colleague who works in the department of gynecological oncology at MD Anderson, has for nearly twenty years been conducting groundbreaking research on how chronic stress, which includes psychosocial factors like chronic depression, anxiety, and social isolation, has a direct influence on cancer's ability to grow and spread.[39-41]

The major cause of all cancer deaths is metastasis, when cancer spreads from its original site in the body. When metastasis occurs, cancer cells break free of their original tumor, travel through the blood system, lodge in different areas of the body, adapt, adopt a new blood supply, and flourish. When a cancer has progressed into this process, it becomes extremely difficult to treat. The steps of metastasis include angiogenesis, proliferation, invasion, embolization, and evasion of effective immune system surveillance. Research has shown that chronic negative affect in a patient is linked with the sustained (or chronic) activation of these proliferation processes.[3,39]

One of Sood's most telling experiments involved a group of mice that were injected with a specific amount of ovarian cancer cells.[42] He exposed some of this population to two hours of restraint stress daily for three weeks (mice get stressed when they cannot move) and let the others go about their business. The animals that were restrained had tremendous growth of their cancer and in the spread of the disease throughout their body.

Sood found that the main culprit in causing the tumors to grow and spread was the stress hormone norepinephrine. When he blocked the effects of norepinephrine (he used a common beta-blocker called propranolol, but in humans we can use meditation or other stress-management techniques), the effects of stress on tumor growth totally disappeared. The animals that had norepinephrine blocked and were exposed to stress had the same outcome as the animals not exposed to stress.[42]

These experiments on the effects of stress on cancer growth have now been replicated in other animal studies and clearly show that stress leads to biological changes that make the tumor microenvironment more hospitable to cancer growth.[3,43-45] Sood and others have clearly demonstrated that chronic stress, and the cascade of stress hormones that ensue, can influence ALL the cancer hallmarks and other biological processes linked to cancer growth.[1-4,31,42,46-49]

Additionally—and stunningly—what Anil Sood and others have discovered is that as cancer proliferates and spreads, tumors secrete inflammatory products called cytokines that can actually affect the brain.[50] As Sood recently explained, "Think about that: We know now that people experiencing excess stress have higher levels of inflammation, and, in parallel, an active, proliferating tumor releases these same inflammatory factors that can actually stimulate a stress response in our brains that will change the biobehavioral state of the patient, which may lead to increased depressive symptoms." In other words, cancer not only causes psychological stress, but it may actually influence our mood through biological changes it causes in our bodies. As Sood explains, "There is a bi-directionality here that shatters the myth that there is a disconnect between our affect (what we think of as our emotional state), in regard to chronic stress, and how cancer behaves." There is now also evidence from Sood's laboratory and others that not only do tumors create their own vasculature to keep them well fed with blood and that stress enhances this process, but tumors also develop their own nerve supply. Again, this tumor-based neurogenesis is facilitated by chronic stress and the release of stress hormones.[3,41] What this research shows us, unequivocally, is that chronic stress and cancer create a bi-directional loop that supports the proliferation of the cancer and may influence the state of mind of the patient.[1-4,42,49]

Another important area of research demonstrating that chronic stress can reach into the nucleus of every cell and create damage is work we touched on in chapter 4 on telomeres and telomerase. Telomeres are on the end of chromosomes, which are found in the nucleus of every cell in our body. Telomeres protect the structural integrity of the chromosomes. As telomeres shorten, we develop what is called chromosomal instability. When cells that have chromosomal instability multiply, it can lead to mutations. If left unchecked, chromosomal instability can lead to cancer. Within the nucleus of our cells we also have an enzyme called telomerase that helps keep the telomeres "healthy." With each cell division there is a slight decrease in telomere length, something called telomere attrition. As we age, our telomerase decreases and our telomeres shorten. Telomere attrition is, in fact, part of the normal aging process and telomere length is thought to reflect a person's biological age.

Researchers Elissa Epel and Elizabeth Blackburn tracked the mothers of healthy children and compared their telomere length to the telomeres of mothers who were caring for children who suffered from chronic illness. The mothers who were caring for sick children had shorter telomeres and lower levels of telomerase.[49] In addition, the length of time they had been caring for their chronically ill children was reflected in their telomere length. The longer their caregiving, the shorter their telomeres. Chronic stress was literally speeding up their aging process.

TAKING CARE OF YOURSELF SO YOU CAN TAKE CARE OF OTHERS

Because we are living longer, more people are forced into roles of caregiving who do not have training as nurses or aides. Informal caregivers now account for 80 percent of the long-term care provided in the United States. Caregivers face an incredible burden and it is vital that they don't take on this burden alone.[51] The stress of caring for a loved one can become chronic and lead to reduced immune function, increased inflammation, and disease and earlier death in the caregiver.[52-55] If you are providing care for someone, here are some steps you can take to manage and control your own stress so you don't get sick, too:

1. *Don't go it alone.* Social support is key to maintaining your sanity and your health. This might mean reaching out to friends and loved ones and/or joining a caregiver support group where people can relate to what you're going through. The added benefit of a support group is that they can put you in touch with other resources that could help to

relieve some of the pressures you are undoubtedly feeling as the primary person responsible for someone's health and well-being.

2. *Recognize your limits.* You cannot be the perfect aide. If you try to provide everything, all the time, you will eventually break down yourself. Find ways to give yourself breaks from constant care, even if that means that someone else comes over for just a few minutes a day or a couple times a week. Take full advantage of that time away. Don't use it to grocery shop or do other chores for the person you're caring for. Take the time for yourself and engage in a mind-body practice.

3. *Set goals for yourself.* Break tasks into small steps and establish a daily routine. Don't take on added burdens. Say no to people who ask for your help with something outside of your caregiving duties. Limit your commitments and focus on caring for yourself.

4. *Accept help.* The only way for you to reduce your own burden is to allow other people to help you, even if they don't know the ways of the person you're caring for or they don't do things exactly the way you would. Learn to let go whenever you can. It will help to keep you strong and avoid disease.

5. *See a doctor.* Don't help keep someone else alive at the expense of your own health and well-being. It's better for both of you if you are putting yourself first.

6. *Engage in healthy behaviors daily.* One of the biggest problems faced by caregivers is that they tend to not take care of themselves, mentally or physically. Find a way to maintain your own health, even if that means playing an exercise DVD in your home or eating cut-up vegetables instead of cookies as a snack. Little things add up. Stay on the right side of your own health by making healthy choices every day and engage in healthy eating, exercise, stress management, and good sleep habits.

Stress and the Body

When looking at the dangers of stress on our health, it is important to understand the difference between chronic and acute stress. When we feel stressed—which means when we feel like we are in the presence of imminent or perceived danger—a cascade of chemical processes is triggered that courses throughout the entire body. We all know what happens when

we are startled: We're flooded with the stress hormones cortisol, epinephrine, and norepinephrine, our heart rate spikes, our breathing quickens,
then we may begin to sweat. These are biological signals that we are ready
to act! What primes us for action is the release of stress hormones, like cortisol, which, thanks to the efficient delivery system of our bloodstream,
highjacks our regulatory systems until the danger has passed.

But what happens when we can't turn off that fight-or-flee response and
we're awash in cortisol for an inordinate amount of time? This is when our
body starts to suffer from the interruption in regular service it's used to
getting from those key regulatory systems that have been instructed to shift
into "idle." Here's an analogy that may help. Think about what it's like when
you're driving to work and you hear a siren approaching from behind. You
glance into your rearview mirror and see that an ambulance, its lights
ablaze, is barreling toward you. What do you do? You slow down and pull
over to the side of the road. Once the emergency—the ambulance—has
passed, you get back on the road and continue your journey.

This is what acute, short bursts of stress look like, and these are inevitable and quite harmless to the overall healthy functioning of our key biological systems. But what if, when you try to get back on the road, you find
that you have a flat tire. Now the emergency continues (though it may look
a bit different). When you get out of the car to change your tire, a hailstorm
begins. You get the picture. What was just a moment of stress has become
a stress that, at least for now, sees no end in sight (you have to wait for AAA,
you are late for an important meeting at work, etc.). The longer the stress
hormones like cortisol, epinephrine, and norepinephrine, which were released to get you to pay attention, are still coursing through your veins, your
digestive, immune, and other regulatory systems will be put on a kind of
hold, or worse, will begin to falter. This is what being under chronic stress
does. It weakens us from head to toe.

Have you ever wondered why you finally get sick on the first day of vacation after a stressful period at work or why, after you finished your finals at
college, you immediately collapsed afterward? At Ohio State University the
husband-wife team of psychologist Janice Keicolt-Glaser and immunologist-
virologist Ron Glaser wanted to see if their hunch was right that this kind
of stress contributes to weakening the immune system enough to bring on
the post-exam colds and sore throats and coughs that OSU medical students seemed to suffer from every academic year, like clockwork.[56] So they

enlisted medical students who would let them track them and they did this for several decades. What they observed was a predictable uptick in stress hormone levels and a disruption to the immune system that made students more vulnerable to viruses and infections.

In another fascinating 2013 study, Ohio State University researchers measured whether dwelling on negative events, in this case a bad job interview, increased inflammation in the bodies of healthy young women.[57] The experiment was designed as a faux job interview. While each young woman (they were all in their thirties) did her best to pitch her talents, members of the "hiring" lab team sat in their starched white lab coats with their arms folded staring back at the young women and remaining expressionless and nonresponsive. (I get tense just thinking about it!) After the "interview," half of the "job applicants" were asked to think about what had just happened and an hour later, their blood was drawn. The other "job seekers" (the control half) were asked to think about more neutral things before their blood was taken. The test samples revealed that the women asked to marinate in their stress had increased levels of C-reactive protein (which promotes inflammation and is associated with injury, illness, increased mortality, and poorer cancer outcomes),[58-60] while the women who did not dwell on the stressful job interview showed no elevation of this inflammation-promoting, immunity-suppressing protein.

In terms of the effects of stress on cancer outcomes, in my own research I have found that kidney cancer patients who were more depressed and experienced more stress at the time of their diagnosis had a dysregulation of the stress hormone cortisol, as well as increased activation of key inflammatory gene pathways.[61] Notably, these stressed kidney cancer patients did not survive as long as their less-stressed, less-depressed counterparts.

The Interplay Between Stress and Gene Expression

Earlier in the book I mentioned the groundbreaking discoveries in the new field of human social genomics, which studies connections between social and psychological factors and the way our genes function. So many facets of the great research that's been done about how lifestyle affects disease progression comes together in this discipline in which we are now able to visualize the way gene expression—which controls the behavior of all cells and biological processes—is either positively or negatively influenced by lifestyle.

Steve Cole at UCLA is at the forefront of studying how long-term stressors, such as poverty, loneliness, grief, exposure to crime, or a diagnosis of a serious disease like cancer negatively impact our health in ways that go much deeper into our cells than most biologists (and oncologists) ever realized.[62,63] What Cole has pioneered is an understanding of how poor health behaviors and psychological processes like stress and loneliness, while not so bad on any given day, can cause serious health issues to develop over time.[64]

Researchers working in this space know that long-term social behaviors contribute to illness and disease, but we also know that these negative influences can be changed and the damage they cause may be reversed or even stopped. I believe that this kind of reversal of fortune, if you will, is what we see in long-term survivors like the late David Servan-Schreiber or Molly M., Meg Hirshberg, Gabe Canales, and so many others. To help us make this known to the rest of the medical world, Cole has been mapping the function of genes, examining them against stress, loneliness, and other health behaviors.[65] Cole notes that being able to do this is only possible because of the recent completion of the mapping of the human genome. Now researchers can pinpoint how specific genes react under the influence of specific external stressors. Now we can literally see how the outer world and inner world "dance" together to the beat of stress. This is a remarkable advancement in anticancer medicine. What Cole and others have now clearly documented is that chronic stress literally gets into our cells and increases aspects of gene expression making us more vulnerable to disease, while decreasing key gene pathways that help maintain our health and well-being.[65] These genetic analyses have given new scientific legitimacy to studies that look at the biological impact of mind-body practices like yoga, tai chi, and qigong. In a 2014 study by UCLA researchers (including Steve Cole), a twelve-week yoga intervention was found to reduce inflammation-related gene expression in breast cancer survivors who suffered from persistent fatigue.[66] Another UCLA study (also involving Cole) found that women with breast cancer who practiced tai chi for three months reduced their expression of genes related to inflammation.[67] Similar beneficial gene expression profile changes have now been documented with other yoga interventions as well as with qigong, meditation, and behavioral therapy programs.[31,66,68]

Resolving the Unresolved

What happens to us during childhood has an impact on our health later in life, particularly if our childhood experiences include high levels of stress and adversity. Research into the impact of adverse childhood experiences, or ACEs, shows a direct relationship between high levels of childhood adversity and multiple diseases, behavioral problems, substance abuse and addiction, and obesity later in life.[69-71]

Here are the categories of ACEs as defined by the U.S. Centers for Disease Control and Prevention:[72]

1. Abuse
   a. Emotional abuse
   b. Physical abuse
   c. Sexual abuse

2. Household Challenges
   a. Mother treated violently
   b. Household substance use
   c. Mental illness in household
   d. Parental separation or divorce
   e. Criminal household member

3. Neglect
   a. Emotional neglect
   b. Physical neglect

If you have experienced one or more of these, you are not alone. The Centers for Disease Control and Prevention teamed up with Kaiser Permanente to conduct one of the largest investigations of the long-term effects of childhood abuse and neglect ever undertaken. The CDC-Kaiser ACE study found that almost two-thirds of the more than seventeen thousand people surveyed reported that they had experienced at least one ACE.[73,74] One in five reported three or more ACEs, with physical abuse and substance abuse being the highest. Meanwhile, an extensive health-related phone survey, also under the purview of the CDC, contacted more than fifty-five thousand people from thirty-two states and found similar incidence, with one in five people experiencing three or more ACEs.[75]

The latest research shows that exposure to toxic levels of stress, especially in young children, affects not only brain structure and function but also the developing immune system, hormonal systems, even the way our DNA is read and transcribed.[76,77] Mounting evidence suggests a dose-response relationship between the number of ACEs we experience early in life and our risk of developing cancer, heart attacks and strokes, diabetes, and liver disease, as well as addiction, mental health problems, and behavioral problems as adults.[78]

Nadine Burke Harris, MD, has been at the forefront of the movement to educate the public about ACEs. She and her team at the Center of Youth Wellness in San Francisco screen every patient for childhood adversity and give them an ACE score to help assess their health in a more holistic way. In a study she conducted in 2011, Burke Harris found that, of the seven hundred patients she evaluated at her clinic, two-thirds had experienced at least one of the ACE categories. Children with an ACE score of four or more were thirty times as likely to have learning and behavior problems (compared with children with an ACE score of zero), and twice as likely to be obese.[79]

"One of the things I tell my patients, because of what's happened to you, your body makes more stress hormones than the average patient," Burke Harris explains. "We're helping people control their stress response."

In the same way an alcoholic reacts differently to alcohol, someone with a high ACE score reacts differently to stress and provocation, including a cancer diagnosis. In fact, numerous studies have found that breast cancer patients who had experienced childhood trauma reported higher levels of fatigue, depression, and stress and worse quality of life during treatment.[80-83] What's more, women with early trauma had decreased immune function, increased inflammatory markers, and heighted expression of genes linked with inflammation. What that means in terms of cancer prevention and survival is that for those who have a lot of childhood stress, adopting and sustaining a mind-body practice and creating a safe and supportive network could be the most important component of their anticancer lifestyle.

"There's no pill," Burke Harris explains. "If you had an ACE childhood, your stress response will fire faster and harder. There's never a time when someone is like, 'Oh, that's completely over and done with.'" In her recently released book, *The Deepest Well: Healing the Long-Term Effects of Childhood Adversity*, Burke Harris provides a prescription for dealing with toxic stress. It's not over, but it can be managed and mitigated.

Michelene H., whom you met in the last chapter, is one of the one in five people who have experienced three or more ACEs. As a child, Michelene experienced emotional and physical abuse, emotional and physical neglect, and the divorce of her parents. After leaving home at sixteen, and taking many turns in the road, Michelene realized she needed to address these past issues if she was going to be successful in maximizing her health. It was a long journey for her to get to where she is today: the only child in her family to have graduated both high school and college, and feeling healthier than before she had breast cancer. As she put it: "I ultimately came to terms and realized that although I was abused that didn't mean I had to live like I was abused, and I definitely wasn't going to abuse my children." Coming to terms with these early life experiences took time, but she had to address the issues head-on to achieve the health she feels today.

Bad experiences, like bad habits, have a way of catching up with us if they aren't addressed. While our tendency can be to ignore or deny things that are too hard or painful, moving toward an understanding of what has happened to us as children is important work for our health.

Cultivating a Positive Frame of Mind

Having a positive mind-set is uniquely and intimately tied to our ability to build a healthier community, but doing so requires a complete 180 from our evolutionary past. In early humans, being aware of and avoiding danger was a critical survival skill. But research shows dwelling on the negative is bad for our health and works against our efforts to build a sustainable and sustaining anticancer lifestyle.[84,85] Our natural tendency is to make decisions to avoid negative consequences. We are more influenced by negative news than by positive events, and we see people who say negative things as smarter than those who are positive. Research also shows that when we are not engaged in a task, our idle mind tends to focus on the negative, either past or future, and be in a state of "worry."[86] An excess focus on the negative can stimulate the stress response and trigger physiological inflammatory processes.[87] In addition to affecting our health, our mind-set and outlook impact our ability to utilize social support and build friendships and relationships based on trust and compassion. Being empathetic starts with recognizing and believing in your own self-worth. Believing in yourself means seeing and appreciating the good all around you, which in turn makes you happier, easier to be with, and more likely to form stronger, deeper connections with others. Growing your anticancer team begins with the attitude you are projecting knowingly and unknowingly to others.

When she left the hospital after her second brain surgery, our friend Molly M. began a year-and-a-half course of the first new brain cancer medication to be approved in North America in more than twenty years. She told her doctor she would stay on the drug until either she or the cancer died. She used an electronic stimulation treatment called AccuTherapy to boost her white blood cell count so the doctor would allow her to continue receiving chemotherapy, and she worked hard through all of this to cultivate a positive frame of mind. Her father made positive affirmation index cards for her to flip through, and Molly put sticky notes around her house—on drawers, mirrors, cupboards, the fridge. They weren't platitudes like "Keep smiling" or things like that. Instead, they conveyed positive, meaningful messages to remember, like, "You are healthy" or "This illness is not you" or "Be positive," which were direct challenges to the cancer and to the awful side effects of treatment Molly was trying to manage. As she explains, "I didn't have any illusions—nor did I want them. I wanted to stay grounded in reality, in life. I wanted to get my balance back (it's really knocked out of you when you have brain surgery) and figure out how to stay balanced. I had to figure out how to build up a sense of hope so I could do the hard work of educating myself and finding ways to get out from under the awful stress of the disease. So I just started eliminating all the external stress I could, which included things like watching, listening to or reading the news, which just made me feel lousier than I already felt." The notes were a way of redirecting her thinking and keeping her mind away from the kinds of thinking loops that can lead to anxiety, depression, or despair. In addition, she developed and religiously maintains a daily mind-body practice that centers her and enables her to feel sure of her path.

Cultivating Gratitude

One of the ways we can move from negative to positive thinking in our daily lives is to focus on what we are grateful for. Research shows that gratitude, like a lot of what we traditionally think of as "just in our heads," actually has a measurable impact on our physical and mental well-being.[88] In one 2003 study, researchers at the University of California in Davis had subjects write a few sentences each week. One group focused on things they were grateful for, a second group focused on things that irritated them, and a final group focused their writings on experiences that had neither a positive nor negative impact.[89] After ten weeks, the group that focused on gratitude reported increased optimism and self-confidence. Members of the group also reported that they exercised more and made fewer trips to the doctor.

I tried a variation of this experiment myself a few years ago. I have to admit that I initially found this exercise both difficult and frustrating. I realized that as an academic and scientist, I had actively trained my brain to focus on the negative. I spend my days searching for problems that need to be solved, either in studies, grants, or papers or some bad outcome that needs to be addressed and researched. It took real effort on my part to tune in to another side of things, which was in fact happening all around me. And the struggle paid off in ways I had not anticipated. As I continued, day after day, to recognize and record positive exchanges—strangers helping each other on the street, my colleagues laughing in the hallways, my kids being nice to each other—I found I was able to tune in to the good all around me, and my own behavior and outlook started to change.

One of the lead researchers in the ten-week gratitude study, Robert Emmons of the University of California in Davis, has gone on to compile a list of health data points from his own study and from other research related to gratitude. Research has found that actively practicing gratitude lowers the level of the stress hormone cortisol and reduces inflammation, two biomarkers linked to a variety of diseases, including cancer.[90,91] Studies also show that gratitude reduces depression and improves sleep quality.[89,92,93]

How Managing Stress Allows Healing to Begin

Like Jon Kabat-Zinn, psychoneuroimmunologist Mike Antoni, PhD, is at the forefront of finding ways to not only study how stress impacts our health but to come up with stress-management plans that can help us stay healthy and calm, even in the face of trauma and disease. For decades Antoni has led a research team that conducted a series of randomized trials that assessed how well breast cancer patients who engaged in CBSM (cognitive behavioral stress management) training in the early stages of their treatment fared over the long term.[94] The training included teaching relaxation skills (such as muscle relaxation and deep breathing) and techniques to reduce negative thinking. These were taught in weekly group sessions for a ten-week period. Antoni wanted to test whether this stress-management program could improve quality of life, impact biological processes, and decrease the risk of disease progression and mortality over the long term. And indeed, patients who participated showed increased survival rates and longer periods of remission at an eleven-year median follow-up.[95] This research shows that learning to effectively manage stress improves stress hormone regulation, immune function, and, more recently, gene expression, showing a down regulation in genes controlling inflammation and up regulation in immune function genes—all of which help to keep the metastatic process in check.[96]

Additionally, the CBSM participants reported improved quality of life and lower levels of depression and anxiety than those in the untreated control group, and these positive benefits held over the long term as well.[97]

What is so thrilling about this research, in terms of its application to anticancer living, is how long lasting the impact of early stress intervention is on the long-term survival and quality of life of these cancer patients, and ongoing studies suggest that this will be the case for everyone who engages in stress management.

Anticancer Living Begins When Stress Ends

The presence of stress undermines our good intentions and efforts to eat properly, rest well, exercise adequately, or make other health-enhancing changes, the most important being to improve our overall sense of satisfaction with life. Not only does stress inhibit our ability to do the right thing, it tends to trigger us to do the opposite, such as drink too much, or smoke, or lose our temper, or turn away from those we love.[98,99]

Stress will literally sabotage all our healthy intentions. If you come home from work stressed and exhausted, you are less inclined to spend the time chopping vegetables. Stress puts you in the position to say, I'm not going to exercise today, or let's go out for pizza. It can also keep you up at night, further jeopardizing your health by reducing your sleep.

Newsflash: Stress Cancels Dietary Benefits!

Here is an example of how stress can sabotage our good intentions around healthy eating. A team at Ohio State University found that prior-day stress eliminated the differences in biological response to eating a meal with high versus low saturated fat.[100] In other words, if stress was not managed, it didn't matter what people ate—the effects of healthy and unhealthy food was the same. All the women in the study, thirty-eight breast cancer survivors and twenty noncancer participants, ate a meal high in saturated fats and on a separate day ate a meal low in saturated fats. From blood samples drawn multiple times during the study, researchers examined two inflammatory markers (C-reactive protein and serum amyloid) of cell adhesion that are linked with plaque forming in the arteries, fat and carbohydrate oxidation, insulin, glucose, and triglycerides as well as an interesting measure assessing resting energy expenditure (how many calories you burn just resting).

Their first finding was that having experienced more stressors on the previous day resulted in lower post-meal resting energy expenditure, lower fat oxidation, and higher insulin levels.[100] For women who did not experience any stressors the day before their meals, the high-saturated-fat meal led to increases in the inflammatory and cell adhesion markers, while the low-fat meal did not. But for the women experiencing stressors the day before, there were no differences in their body's reaction to the meals. They had the same heightened inflammatory and cell adhesion markers after both meals. In other words, their body's response to the healthier meal was the same as if they had eaten the unhealthy meal.[100] The link between stress and diet in this study suggests that stress modifies metabolism in ways that may promote obesity and increases inflammatory responses, no matter what we eat. That is why stress management comes before diet and other healthy changes. If you don't control your stress, your other lifestyle improvements may be in vain.

Yet we also see that lifestyle factors can reduce the harms of stress. A 2014 study found that women who maintained a healthy lifestyle were protected from the effects of stress on their telomere length.[101] The study, which Epel and Blackburn participated in, looked at telomere attrition in 239 postmenopausal women over a one-year period and found that stress-induced telomere shortening was reduced if women engaged in healthy behaviors,

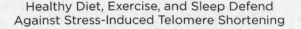

Healthy Diet, Exercise, and Sleep Defend Against Stress-Induced Telomere Shortening

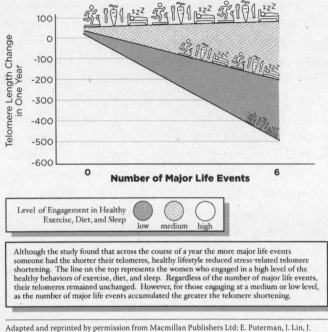

Level of Engagement in Healthy Exercise, Diet, and Sleep — low, medium, high

Although the study found that across the course of a year the more major life events someone had the shorter their telomeres, healthy lifestyle reduced stress-related telomere shortening. The line on the top represents the women who engaged in a high level of the healthy behaviors of exercise, diet, and sleep. Regardless of the number of major life events, their telomeres remained unchanged. However, for those engaging at a medium or low level, as the number of major life events accumulated the greater the telomere shortening.

Adapted and reprinted by permission from Macmillan Publishers Ltd: E. Puterman, J. Lin, J. Krauss, E. H. Blackburn, E. S. Epel, "Determinants of telomere attrition over one year in healthy older women: Stress and health behaviors matter," *Molecular Psychiatry* 20, no. 4 (July 2015): 529–35.
     Adapted in collaboration with Laura Beckman.

including a plant-based diet, regular exercise, and adequate sleep. This study replicated previous studies showing that healthy lifestyle buffered stress and was associated with longer telomeres.[102–104]

We are beginning to see how important it is to control stress, both in terms of its direct impact on our health and in terms of its indirect impact on everything from sleep to diet and exercise. The research points to a critical need for all of us to take time every day to relax and separate from the demands and responsibilities of our lives. Being in the moment, even for just a few minutes a day, can change your outlook and dramatically impact your health. Reducing and managing stress is key to your success in changing your life in other areas and maintaining those changes over time.

How you choose to reduce the chronic stress in your life is, like all aspects of anticancer living, largely up to you. When you tune in to your intuition and listen to what your body needs, you may surprise yourself by realizing that you no longer care to be triggered and stressed-out by follow-ing the news or by seeing pictures of the charmed lives of your friends on Facebook. You may realize it's finally time to quit the job that's draining your energy, give up the low-quality diet that makes you feel so uncomfort-able you can't sleep at night, or you may decide it's time to end an unhappy marriage or relationship. Or, if you are like most of us, you just need to learn how to unwind and experience a kind of peaceful easiness that eludes too many of us in this go-go world we live in.

I know for myself, I used to equate being under massive amounts of work stress with somehow being more committed or more successful than the next guy (yes, I realize this makes no sense at all), but I was wired with a fear that if I stopped, I'd somehow not be able to do my job as well or I'd somehow get left behind in the highly competitive world of cancer research. It took me a long time to make a commitment to be less motivated by stress (and fear) and more by the health benefits I'd reap if I slowed down. Little did I know that taking care of myself would not only relieve me of work anxiety but also make me more productive and focused despite my putting in fewer hours at the lab.

The Joy Protocol

Diana Lindsay is someone who has grown uniquely attuned to her mind, body, and spirit. But she tells me it was not always this way. "When I was first diagnosed with cancer, I had no idea how to heal myself and neither did my doctor," she explains. "One night, right after I got the news that I had stage IV cancer, I had a dream, and the next morning I invited all my friends to come over to our place. On a practical level, I didn't want to have to call each one and tell them I was sick—that just seemed too difficult. So my friends came over and we sang and danced and laughed and just had so much fun. It certainly wasn't a wake or anything like that. It was just a bunch of people I love getting together and getting really joyful. The next day, when I went in to find out my treatment options, I asked, 'What about the joy part?' I wanted to know because despite being so sick, I still clearly had a capacity for joy. I became determined to follow what I think of as my joy protocol. I researched what happens to your body when you feel intense happiness and I found out you get a great hit of endorphins, oxytocin, and dopamine—all are natural chemicals in the brain that make you feel good when you can let go of your worries and just be joyful. Then I found out that these substances all stimulate the immune system. So I got really serious about seeking out joy wherever I could find it. I'm certain this has been a major component of why I've defied the odds for so long. It's hard to keep someone who is enjoying life down."

Lindsay's embrace of her situation and her determination to find joy in the face of cancer exemplifies the goals of anticancer living. This is why it is so important for all of us who work in integrative oncology to address the psychological and emotional realities of cancer diseases and help patients develop the kind of mental and emotional resilience that will foster their healing. When we focus on reducing stress, then worry and fear are replaced by a sense of *calm* and often a renewed sense of appreciation for the beauty and joy of life.

THE ANTICANCER LIVING GUIDE
TO STRESS REDUCTION

Thoughts, both positive and negative, play a key role in our health, before or after a cancer diagnosis. Managing our negative thoughts, adopting a positive mind-set, cultivating hope and joy, and living in the moment—all these require practice. In the same way we train our bodies to swim farther or run faster, we must take the time to train our mind.

The Goal: Thirty Minutes a Day

Starting a mind-body practice is similar to starting an exercise routine—at first it can feel challenging, even painful, but over time you will come to enjoy the stillness and to crave this very special time to be with yourself and relax. The key is to get over that initial hump. If you try some of these practices once or twice, you will not see any results and you might think, "This is not for me." During the initial phase, keep your larger goal in mind. You will find that after a week or two of daily practice, you will feel more grounded and the little things will not get under your skin the way they once did. Remember that each time you engage in your stress-management practices you are boosting your immune system, slowing the aging process, and improving your mental outlook.

Goals of Your Mind-Body Practice

- To feel more in control, less bothered by the little things, and better able to handle the big stuff.
- To move away from that feeling of constantly being overwhelmed.
- To feel unencumbered, free, and light for a few minutes each day.
- To start living a more active, less reactive life.

Anticancer Stress-Reduction Techniques

In our work with cancer patients at MD Anderson, we use an array of techniques such as CBT (cognitive behavioral therapy), meditation, yoga, massage, tai chi, qigong, and other stress-reducing modalities to give patients the tools for general stress relief they will need to make healthy lifestyle changes in the other areas of their lives. As I mentioned, the mind-body practice is often what CompLife participants say had the biggest impact on their lives and their ability to sustain their anticancer lifestyle after the program ended.

HERE IS A BRIEF BREAKDOWN OF EACH TYPE OF STRESS-REDUCTION TECHNIQUE

> **CBT (cognitive behavioral therapy):** This short-term therapy teaches patients how to consciously change their thinking by replacing negative with positive thoughts and "rewiring" the default settings of their cognition. The positive long-term effects of this show up on Steve Cole's heat maps and in longitudinal studies of long-time survivors.[1,2]

> **Meditation:** For more than a decade, our friend Molly M. has started her day with her own self-designed mind-body practice based on the Canadian Healing Journey Program. Her daily practice helps to cleanse any stress she may have carried over from the day before and gives her a "clean" slate. She practices a combination of relaxation, imagery, and meditation. Molly is quick to point out, though, that her personally tailored visual imagery doesn't work for everyone.[3] What's important is to find a form of relaxation that feels right for you and that you are able to sustain on a daily basis.

> **Deep Diaphragmatic Breathing:** This can be practiced very formally or it can be practiced on the fly when we need to replace the buzz of stress hormones with the calming effect of oxygenating our bodies. Taking just a couple of deep, cleansing belly breaths can ground us and keep us present, especially when we're in the midst of an unavoidably stressful situation.[4]

Tai Chi and Qigong (and other formal movement practices): Combine movement with meditation and breathing practices that center and calm both the body and mind. I conducted a clinical study on the effect of qigong on nearly a hundred Chinese women who were undergoing radiation therapy for breast cancer.[5] Those who practiced qigong reported less depression, fatigue, and higher overall quality of life than the control group. These results, as with CBT and other stress-reducing techniques, had long-lasting benefits.[6]

Yoga: My grandmother, Vanda Scaravelli, was a legendary yogini. She started her yoga practice later in life. I lived with her for a year in order to learn yoga, so I know firsthand its healing power. It even formed the basis of my early research, which along with research from others showed that yoga imparts body awareness, flexibility, helps cancer patients sleep, improves mood, reduces fatigue, increases physical functioning, and helps to regulate stress hormones in the blood, among other benefits.[7-10] At a deeper level, yoga can increase our ability to find meaning in the illness experience and help transform our lives.[11,12] Vanda used to tell me, *"Stai attento."* This can be translated in two ways: (1) be careful or (2) be attentive. Many would think that as an Italian grandmother, she meant the former, doting on her grandson, but of course she meant the latter. Today, we use the term *mindful*, as in "Be mindful," but what Vanda meant was to be deeply engaged in all aspects of life. Yoga is a vehicle to help us become more attentive. As she wrote in her book *Awakening the Spine: Yoga for Health, Vitality, and Energy*: "It [yoga] is a living process that changes moment by moment, watching when we eat, how we eat, when we walk, how we walk, what we say and how we say it. All these things must be present in us and we must be passionately interested in them all."[13]

Be in Nature: Go outside and feel the sun on your skin. Nature is the greatest healer, the most gentle companion. Give yourself the healing gift of spending time outside being mindful as you walk and explore the outdoors. Even short doses of the natural world do wondrous things for our health and well-being.[14]

Three Steps to Optimal Anticancer De-stress

1. Develop a daily meditation practice that moves you through the stages of thoughtful introspection and sharing.
2. Integrate calmness into your life using meditation moments throughout the day.
3. Reflect on your mental state through reflective writing in a daily journal.

1. DEVELOP A DAILY MEDITATION PRACTICE

When practiced daily, meditation reduces stress, cuts the risk of illness, improves well-being, and helps to rewire our brain. This effect is not limited to adults. Many recent studies have found that meditation improved thinking and learning skills in children as young as nine.[15] After eight weeks of meditation, elementary school children in Korea reduced their aggression, lowered their social anxiety, and experienced less stress.[16]

For cancer patients, meditation has been shown to lessen the side effects of chemotherapy, lower cortisol levels, and reduce inflammation. By calming your mind through meditation, research shows significant downstream effects on your body and overall health.

Diaphragmatic Breathing

Although we all breathe, most of us hardly notice our breathing in everyday life. This exercise will help you practice deep abdominal breathing to make you more relaxed and calm at any point in the day, especially at times when you are feeling stressed, anxious, or angry. When you breathe from your chest, your breathing usually becomes shallow and rapid. When you breathe from your abdomen, you breathe more fully, deeply, and slowly.

A central component across different meditation practices is a focus on the breath. All practices encourage slow, diaphragmatic breathing, also known as belly breathing.

Directions: Sit in a chair or lie on the floor or a mat. At first, it may be best to practice deep breathing lying down, since this position allows you to better determine whether you are breathing from your chest or from your belly.

- To better monitor your breathing, place one hand on your abdomen directly below your rib cage.

- Inhale deeply through your nose and feel that you are able to reach the bottom of your lungs; in other words, send the air down as deeply as you can.
- If you are breathing from your abdomen, your hand should rise as you inhale, while your chest remains still.
- Take a full breath and pause before exhaling slowly through your nose. If exhaling through your nose is challenging, you can exhale through your mouth, but slightly purse your lips to slow the release of air. Exhale fully to create more room in your lungs for the next full breath.
- Inhale for a count of five seconds and then exhale slowly and deeply for a count of six seconds. Your exhalation can be slightly longer than your inhalation.

This is a wonderful practice to use when you wake up each morning and before going to bed each night. Spend a few minutes taking deep and cleansing breaths. Try to practice this for at least five minutes. When faced with a difficult task at work or at home during the day, pause and take three belly breaths to center and calm yourself before you begin. If you have children, encourage them to adopt this practice before bed or when they get frustrated. This is a great way to incorporate your own deep breathing into your day, spend quiet time with your children, and start to fill their anticancer toolbox with the lifelong skill of effectively and easily managing their stress.

Start with Focused Meditation: Now that you understand diaphragmatic breathing, the next step is to start a focused meditation practice. Focused meditation is maintaining an individual focus on one object, whether literal or figurative.

Directions:

- Sit on the floor or in a chair, or find another comfortable position that allows you to focus on your chosen object.
- Engage in your diaphragmatic breathing and spend up to five minutes getting focused on your breath.
- Even if you inadvertently shift your attention from your breath to the object of your choosing, continue your diaphragmatic breathing.

We recommend starting with breath-focused meditation. However, you could also focus on the flame of a candle or on a sound (e.g., chanting the syllable *om*, reciting a powerful word such as "calm," "joy," or "healthy," or a powerful phrase such as "I am strong . . . , I am worthy . . . , I am whole"). During the meditation, each time your mind drifts away or becomes wrapped up in thoughts or life issues, gently pull your focus back to your breath and then to the object of your focus.

Build to Mindfulness Meditation: Once your focused meditation practice is on solid ground and you have built up twenty minutes a day, try moving into mindfulness meditation. This guided sitting meditation will help you learn to quiet the mind and to look at yourself and others with equanimity. Studies show that practicing mindfulness meditation improves immune function, reduces depression, and improves overall well-being.

Directions:

- Start with five minutes of your diaphragmatic breathing focused meditation practice.
- Keep your focus on your breath, focused on the sensations of the air coming into your body and then gently leaving your body.
- Every time you find your mind wandering from your breathing, gently bring it back to the present, back to the moment, and continue to observe and notice the flow of your breathing.
- As you observe your breathing, you may find from time to time that you are becoming aware of sensations in your body. As you maintain awareness of your breathing, see if it is possible to expand the field of your awareness so that it includes a sense of your body as a whole, becoming aware of all the sensations you are experiencing.
- Be aware of these feelings and sensations without judging or reacting to them.
- Rather than following individual thoughts, let the thoughts come and go as you sit still, witnessing the thoughts and simply observing them. Let them float by like clouds in the sky or like birds flying by above you.
- As the meditation ends, slowly become aware of your surroundings. Try to carry the feelings of calm and peace you experience meditating into the rest of your day.

Expand to Compassion/Loving-Kindness Meditation: The ideal anticancer meditation practice begins with focused meditation, moves to mindfulness meditation, and ends with compassion, or loving-kindness, meditation. Loving-kindness meditation is essentially about cultivating and sharing love. If that sounds too touchy-feely for you, consider this: Research has shown that compassion meditation has both short-term and long-term effects on our health, well-being, outlook, self-confidence, and connection to others.[17–19] Loving-kindness meditation has been used to reduce depression and other symptoms in veterans diagnosed with PTSD, ease migraine and back pain, and improve vagal tone, a physiological marker of well-being.[20]

Directions:

- Start with a few minutes of diaphragmatic breathing.
- Shift to mindfulness meditation for an additional five minutes.
- Now bring to mind someone for whom you have deep feelings of love. Visualize this person and notice your feelings for them in your body.
- Let go of this person in your imagination, but retain an awareness of the feelings that thinking of them has brought to you. Think of yourself with these same loving thoughts. While directing these feelings toward yourself, repeat this phrase (or a statement you come up with on your own) either aloud or silently:

  May I be happy and joyful.
  May I be healthy.
  May I engage in my life with calm and focus.
  May I live in peace.

- Notice the sensations and feelings within you. Allow those sensations to arise and do not judge them one way or another.
- Next, try offering loving-kindness to someone who supports you, who has always "been on your side." Bringing this person to mind, imagining them perhaps in front of you, and repeat these lines directed to them, either out loud or to yourself:

  May you be happy and joyful.
  May you be healthy.
  May you engage in your life with calm and focus.
  May you live in peace.

- Then shift your focus to friends and acquaintances.
- Bring to mind the larger community in which you live. You might imagine your friends, your colleagues, or your neighbors. Say or think these phrases, directed at your community:

  May you all be happy and joyful.

  May you all be healthy.

  May you all engage in your life with calm and focus.

  May you all live in peace.
- As you close this meditation, bring to mind the larger world in which you live. Expand out from your family, friends, and colleagues to include all people and creatures on the planet, without exception, including yourself, and repeat:

  May we be happy and joyful.

  May we be healthy.

  May we engage in our lives with calm and focus.

  May we live in peace.
- Take a moment to feel that sharing from your heart. Feel the openness of your inner space, your awareness as light, the warmth of your loving-kindness, compassion, and inner joy.
- As you move back into the room, slowly become aware of your surroundings. Allow the benefits of this practice to expand into every aspect of your life.

The Ideal: Most studies examining the effects of meditation include at least a twenty-minute daily practice. Yet some studies have found benefits from even a twelve-minute daily meditation, including affecting your telomeres. If you begin with a shorter practice it is hard to settle in and feel or measure the benefits. Once you establish your twenty-minute routine, shorter periods of meditation will have a greater impact.

If You Need More Guidance: You may find it easier to engage in the meditation if it is guided. You can find the guided meditations we recommend in this chapter on our website.

2. MEDITATION MOMENTS

As you begin to build your daily meditation practice, it is important that you begin to work this new sense of calm and peace into your day, to reconnect with your breath and increase your awareness. Our close friend and colleague Alejandro Chaoul, PhD, introduced us to meditation moments, brief interludes that allow you to take a time-out from your life and reconnect to your breathing to center and ground yourself as you go through your day:

- **In Your Home or Office:** Stretch your arms upward. As you lengthen your back, breathe deeply through your nose into your belly and back out through your nose. Lower your arms and place your hands together, palms up on your lap. Close your eyes and take a few deep, long calming breaths.
- **Wash Your Hands, Wash Your Mind:** Put a sticky note on your bathroom mirror to remind yourself to focus on your breath and cleanse your mind each time you wash your hands. As you focus on washing your hands, breathe and feel that you are also clearing your mind.
- **Finding Peace on the Road:** We spend so much time in our vehicles that finding meditative moments on the road is essential. An American Automobile Association report found that Americans spend more than one hundred minutes a day driving, and across the course of a year the equivalent of seven forty-hour workweeks.[21] Whether that means taking our children to appointments, practice, or lessons or taking ourselves to work or school, we all need to find calm behind the wheel.

  When the traffic light turns red, take a moment to connect with yourself; put away your smartphone, turn off the radio, and pause to breathe in peace. When you exhale, release your thoughts and anxiety. For as long as the light stays red, breathe in calming, peaceful thoughts and exhale irritants, annoyances, and negative feelings.
- **Walking Meditation:** When you walk, do some mindful walking for one to two minutes—focus solely on everything to do with your walking: body movement, feeling of feet meeting with the ground, etc.

3. REFLECTIVE WRITING

Write for ten to fifteen minutes on the prompts listed below. Don't worry about spelling, grammar, or sentence structure. Use this time for yourself to reflect as deeply as possible on your life.

Meditation Reflection: At the end of your meditation, reflect on your meditation practice. What did you notice? Was it easier to keep your mind focused than it was last time? Where did your mind wander? Did your mind wander to positive thoughts and emotions or to negative feelings and anxieties? Explore some of the thoughts and emotions you experienced in the meditation practice.

Core Values Refection: Reflect on your core values from chapter 7. How are you staying aligned with your core values? What are the areas that lead you off course? How can your mind-body practice help you to stay aligned with what you believe in and value? What do you need to change to keep yourself aligned?

Triggers and Solutions Reflection: Explore what triggers your stress. Write down ideas for managing each trigger. Explore strategies you found successful for managing stress. How can you prioritize your stress-management practice?

THE ANTICANCER LIVING GUIDE
STRESS REDUCTION SUMMARY

1. **Meditate daily.** Build toward at least a twenty-minute practice that moves through all three types of meditation: focused, mindfulness, and loving-kindness.
2. **Engage in reflective writing.** Write about your meditation practice, core values, and triggers and ways to manage them.
3. **Find meditation moments throughout your day.** Stretch your arms upward for a few minutes and breathe from your belly. Take a mindful moment—washing your hands, brushing your teeth, at a stoplight, or try a few minutes of mindful walking.

Stress may be the most challenging area to get a handle on, but also the most rewarding when you do. Our recommendations are supported by research involving both healthy individuals and cancer patients and survivors. It has been said before, but deserves repeating: the best mind-body practice is the one you do every day.

CHAPTER NINE

The Need for Rest and Recovery

Just as there is a natural rhythm to life, there is a natural rhythm to health and healing. The human body is designed to run like clockwork. In fact, the body contains several internal regulatory systems that ensure our organs (such as the liver, pancreas, kidneys, lungs, and intestines) and immune, hormonal, and gene regulatory systems function smoothly and rhythmically by balancing periods of biological activity with rest. Governing these complex processes is an actual structure that we refer to as the "body clock," or the master system that regulates and interacts with the body's "secondary" timing systems, several of which I mentioned above.[1]

The body clock is actually two structures, located in the hypothalamus region of the forebrain in both brain hemispheres.[1] Within these structures, tiny clusters of neurons regulate our sleep-wake cycle in roughly the same twenty-four-hour cycle as the daily rotation of the earth's orbit around the sun. In fact, each individual neuron in a cluster also appears to operate on a roughly twenty-four-hour rhythm, so our body clocks are actually powered by thousands of tiny "clocks" working in harmony with the earth's natural phases of daylight and nighttime.[1] Tissues throughout the body also contain clocks.[2] In essence, the clock in the brain acts like an orchestral conductor, while clocks within tissue maintain rhythms locally, like a string or wind section, keeping time with the orchestra. These sub-clocks, working with the body clock, make up what we refer to as our circadian rhythm.[2]

We all know what happens when we don't get adequate nighttime rest: We feel pretty lousy the next day. And no wonder, because when we're tired from too little sleep, we become vulnerable to a cascading effect of negative biological consequences.[3] We may become both mentally and physically sluggish in ways that profoundly affect our quality of life and make us much more prone to accidents or illness, including chronic disease.[4–7]

Since our body clock regulates everything from sleeping and eating cues, core body temperature, hormone production, the regulation of insulin and glucose excretion, cell regeneration, brain wave activity—the list goes on and on—ignoring its cues costs us economically (in lost wages); socially (in poor communication and interpersonal stress); mentally (by prompting everything from depression to psychosis, depending on how "broken" our clock has become); and physically (in the suppression of the immune system and the weakening of the body's overall ability to fend off illness and re-generate health).[8]

So learning to identify and respect our unique circadian rhythm is es-sential to wellness and disease prevention. All it takes is a willingness to listen in to the subtle—and not so subtle—cues our biological clocks give us throughout the day and to adjust our lifestyle choices so that they acknowl-edge and support these natural signals. When you become attuned to the unique rhythms of your own body, you'll find that there is beauty to this synchrony. When you heed the cues to act or to rest, you have an opportu-nity to align your body and mind in profoundly healing ways. You will begin to experience a balanced state that will make you more present and more available to life by making your body more attuned to healing and disease prevention. This is the goal of anticancer living—to provide you the infor-mation you need to make choices that will synchronize your biology for maximum health.

Rest and rejuvenation are essential components of anticancer living and adjusting our lifestyles to include rest as an active part of our wellness ef-forts will fortify us to live better, healthier lives, whether we are living with cancer or not. As the Elizabethan dramatist Thomas Dekker wrote: *"Sleep is the golden chain that ties health and our bodies together."*[9]

Initially, I underestimated the importance of sleep when making my own anticancer lifestyle changes. I changed my diet and then looked into ramping up my exercise routine, but I just couldn't figure out how to fit that into my daily schedule. So I decided to wake up an hour earlier and get in an hour of working out before starting the rest of my morning routine. I thought that I'd try this for six days a week for a minimum of six months, in order to see if I'd enjoy the boost in well-being that I anticipated. So every day (except Sunday), I'd wake at 5:00 a.m., workout, shower, and leave the house feeling like I'd already accomplished some serious anticancer living. At first, I admit, I felt pretty self-satisfied with how easily I was able to make this adjustment, until . . . just a few months in I began to get some concerned feedback from my family and my colleagues. At work I was more irritable and less collegial and at home I was short tempered and crabby. Plus, my work started to suffer. I remembered that early morning was usually my most productive "brain" time, and now that prime problem-solving time had been replaced with an elliptical trainer. Finally, one evening after a particularly stressful day, Alison looked at me and said, "You look gray. You look unwell. I think you need to get more sleep." Of course, she was right. Instead of adjusting my schedule to accommodate the full seven-plus hours of sleep I need to function optimally, I had simply shaved an hour off my sleep time and given that hour to my waking life. Big mistake.

Sacrificing sleep to get more exercise turned out to be counterproductive for my overall well-being on several fronts: I was getting less done, so my stress levels increased. Because I was stressed, I was also more easily agitated and less fun to be around. In just a few short months, I went from feeling pretty good to feeling awful and totally out of whack. What I didn't know at the time was that getting one hour less of sleep a night was also negatively impacting me on a cellular level by increasing inflammation, decreasing immune function, and modifying how my genes were functioning. I decided that the 5:00 a.m. wake-up time had to go and that I'd have to fit exercise in during my waking hours, and I'll share more on that later. The point I want to make is that once I gave my body the sleep it truly needed, I immediately felt better and more available to my family, my work, and the rest of my life.

The Beauty of Our Circadian Rhythm

Our bodies are designed to function optimally and stave off disease when we are in a state of balance—even harmony—with the ebbing and flowing of so many of our internal systems. During the day, we're largely governed by the "circadian arousal system" that is marked by the release of the hormone cortisol at approximately 5:00 a.m. or at dawn.[10] As morning progresses and our cortisol level rises, our organs and cells begin to consume fuel, our hormones flow, and our brains become alert. Daytime is when, biologically, we are at our most energized, and, ideally, our most mentally and physically active. As the day progresses and the sun begins to wane, this system gives way to the "homeostatic sleep process," and as our cortisol levels begin to dip, we naturally feel an early afternoon desire to nap or rest (roughly between 1:00 p.m. and 3:00 p.m.). This is when many of us turn to coffee or candy or some other stimulant to keep us going—at least here in the United States. (In Mediterranean cultures like my native Italy, this biological slowdown was at one time acknowledged, and everyone stopped and stepped away from their workday activities for siesta.) As the day moves into evening, we begin to shift decisively out of the cycle of stimulation and light and into one of rest and darkness, as our bodies ease away from cortisol production and begin to produce the natural relaxant, the hormone melatonin. As darkness falls, our metabolic systems begin to slow, our minds begin to quiet, and our bodies begin to relax. Our body temperature drops, our breathing slows, and when we allow ourselves to, we drift off to sleep. During the time that we are actually asleep with eyes closed and minds not focused on tasks at hand, a tremendous amount of healing and repair takes place. We're no longer expending energy externally—now it's all being spent internally.

Our Broken Biological Clocks

When was the last time you went to bed when you felt the first signs of being "tired"? When was the last time you woke up feeling truly refreshed? Many of us would be hard-pressed to remember.

There are myriad reasons why our behavior has evolved in ways that work at such cross-purposes with our circadian rhythms. We live an electrified life, rarely experiencing the deep, enveloping darkness that can now only be found in the remotest parts of the world. Electricity shatters not just the darkness our bodies crave for optimal sleep, but it's allowed us to engage in behaviors that further chip away at needed downtime. These include the ability to work day and night (we see serious health problems among shift workers, including higher rates of some cancers); the intrusion of electronic devices into environments that were once blue-light free, such as our bedrooms, which are now outfitted with television sets, computers, reading tablets, and the ubiquitous cell-phone charger. In fact, light emitted by electronic devices can suppress melatonin and interfere with our ability to fall and stay asleep.[11] With electricity comes technology, and with easy access to information and a move to desk jobs, we've become sedentary in ways that measurably shorten our life span. This lack of movement, somewhat ironically, also interferes with our ability to sleep adequately.[12] It's hard to get enough rest when you're prone on the couch binge-watching your favorite programs, which stream twenty-four hours a day, or to get uninterrupted sleep when your cell phone rests on the bedside table, vibrating or pinging throughout the night with incoming texts and alerts.

Adding to the disruption of living in a brightly lit world, our eating habits (which are, ideally, regulated by our circadian rhythms) suffer, too, and this in turn adversely affects our sleep, which in turn affects our ability to concentrate at work or be physically agile, which in turn affects our weight and our overall health. You get the picture.[13-15] Our biological clocks are at the mercy of our ambition and invention. Now, research is showing that when we honor our circadian rhythms and rest when we need to rest and move when we need to move, optimal health is achieved.[16-20]

The Healing Power of Sleep

We spend about *one-third of our lives* sleeping, which means that should we live to age seventy-five (roughly the average life span for most Americans) we'll spend at least twenty-five years asleep.

Throughout the ages, poets and philosophers have been intrigued by the mystical, even romantic, aspects of sleep, but it's only in the past fifty years or so that understanding the phenomenon of sleep has become validated as a medical specialty. Now there is a growing body of compelling research and data that confirm what our bodies have always known: adequate, sound sleep is absolutely crucial to overall health and wellness.[21]

But let's face it, most of us are terrible sleepers.[22,23] Four out of five people say they wake up exhausted after a poor night of sleep at least once a week.[24] Fully 35 percent of the U.S. adult population characterizes their sleep as "fair" or "poor."[24] Worldwide, more than 20 percent of the population report some kind of sleep problem.[25] In short, most of us aren't getting nearly the quantity or quality of truly restorative rest our bodies and minds need to function optimally.

Daily living is hard on us physically as well as mentally. At night, our bodies should be able to step back from the stressors of the world and deal with the effects of those stresses on our organs and cells. Most of us know that sleep itself follows a regular rhythm, with various stages of sleep depth and activity occurring regularly throughout the night. What few of us realize is that we go through several sleep cycles during each night of sleep. At the height of nocturnal healing, human growth hormone (HGH) is released (interestingly, the bones of a child grow mostly during sleep), proteins are synthesized, and fat is broken down for tissue repair.[26-28] HGH, which is released during the deepest stage of sleep, stimulates cell division and repair.[29] Chronobiologists and other scientists can even pinpoint the maximum time of healing as being between 11:00 p.m. and 1:00 a.m.—which is likely where the old adage "Early to bed and early to rise makes a man healthy, wealthy, and wise" comes from, since, if we are to reap the benefits of this golden window of nighttime healing, we need to be already asleep long before 11:00 p.m., in order to reach this very desired, very deep phase of the sleep cycle.

While our body is repairing itself, our immune system is being rebalanced after working hard during the day to keep us healthy. Our immune system is the body's natural self-defense system, and it only functions optimally when we are well-rested. When we aren't well-rested, there are negative effects on key cancer hallmarks, including *increased inflammation* and *decreased immune function* making us vulnerable to infection and some research shows, exacerbation of tumor growth.[3,30,31] Emerging research also finds some associations between sleep disturbances and modulation of key circadian rhythm genes and other cancer hallmarks (including *activating proliferative signaling, enabling replicative immortality*, and *activating invasion and metastases*).[32-38] There is also evidence from my laboratory and others that a dysregulated twenty-four-hour cortisol rhythm, that should be high upon awaking and drop throughout the day and into the evening and not rise again until near the time of awaking, is linked with increased mortality in a number of cancers, including breast, kidney, and lung.[39-41]

Adequate sleep also promotes longevity by lowering our risk of daytime accidents; protecting us from the onset or exacerbation of mental health issues, such as depression and anxiety; allowing us to better cope and respond to our daily stressors; keeping our body weight in check, which minimizes our risk of the many health problems associated with being overweight, including the onset of some cancers; and keeping organ and cell degradation in check.[7,26,42-48]

It's not just our organs and cells that are given a rest while we sleep. Our entire musculoskeletal system is able to relax and rejuvenate. During the dreaming phases of our sleep (what we call REM, or rapid eye movement, sleep), we become somewhat paralyzed and our muscles relax.[49] This state of atonia, some sleep experts hypothesize, is designed to keep us in place while our brains replenish. On a more practical level, being so still quiets the production of nonessential hormones and lowers the energy being directed into non-repair-related metabolic processes.

So while you are sleeping, you are undergoing a profound round of comprehensive restoration and healing. Free radicals are vacuumed up and kept from bonding with oxygen and causing cellular damage.[50] Because this process happens most intensively while we're at rest, some scientists even refer to sleep as a natural antioxidant.[51] In fact, sleep is now being viewed by the medical world as being so essential to the successful blocking of free radical damage and for cellular repair that some scientists have even begun classifying sleep disruption, especially long-term shift work, as a "probable" carcinogen, as it is linked to increased inflammation and impaired immune function, both of which we know are tied to cancer development and growth.[3,52–56]

This all leads to one important and irrefutable fact: chronic sleep restriction (sleep time that is on average less than 6.5 hours per night for adults) is associated with increased mortality[6] and is now being studied as a possible cancer risk factor.

In one particularly revealing 2013 study, researchers at the University of Surrey in Great Britain took whole-blood RNA samples to examine gene expression profiles from more than two dozen people after they spent a week getting 8.5 hours of sleep per night.[38] They compared those samples with blood from the same participants after limiting their sleep to 5.7 hours a night for a week. They found that inadequate sleep affects hundreds of genes related to metabolism, inflammation, and immune response—all key cancer hallmarks.

Other research has also found that chronic sleep restriction is associated with shorter telomeres, which, as we've already discussed, is a known risk factor for cancer. A 2012 study by researchers in the United Kingdom found that telomeres were on average 6 percent shorter in men sleeping five hours or less per night compared with those sleeping more than seven hours per night.[57] The study looked at the sleep habits and corresponding telomere length of more than two hundred healthy middle-age and older men (with an average age of sixty-three) and found the effect held even when taking into account differences in age, weight, smoking habits, education levels, employment status, and whether the subjects reported being depressed. With all these other factors accounted for, their biological age appeared to be directly affected by how much they slept.

In addition, sleep is now the subject of several studies that are looking at the causal links between short or excessive sleep on tumor growth.[58,59]

Sleep and Peak Performance

An evolving focus in cancer medicine is on efforts to prepare people ahead of time for the steep challenges of treatments. This new "prehabilitation" model is in line with the philosophy of *prevention* versus the traditional rehabilitation or *treatment* model—wait for something bad to happen before we intervene. Prehabilitation aims to prevent something bad from happening, and, in the case of cancer treatment, to improve outcomes with fewer side effects.

Elite athletes know something about preparing for emotionally and physically demanding events. The mainstay of training has a focus on diet, exercise, and emotional balance. Many great athletes from across the sporting world also take their sleep very seriously. A great example is the American swimmer Michael Phelps, the world's most decorated Olympian and arguably one of the greatest athletes of all time. When Phelps is in active training, he swims seven days a week, logging between seventy thousand and one hundred thousand yards in the pool.[60] This means being in the water between three to five hours a day—which is nearly a full-time-job's worth of time—training at the highest level. In order to have the strength and endurance to do this, Phelps consumes a nutrient-dense, high-calorie diet. (Nutritionists have estimated that he needs roughly a thousand calories of food fuel for each hour of training, or six thousand calories per day).[61] But most important—he sleeps. A lot. When he's training, he sleeps eight hours a night and naps for two to three hours every afternoon.[60] That means that Phelps is clocking ten to twelve hours of sleep a day when he's training. "I really can't say it enough. I don't think people really pay enough attention to how important sleep is," Phelps has said.[60] And he is not alone. Basketball great LeBron James, it is reported, averages twelve hours of sleep at night during the NBA season. Tennis star Roger Federer also gets about a dozen hours of sleep a night, and the fastest human alive, Usain Bolt, swears by a minimum of ten hours a night, as does tennis star Venus Williams.[62]

Recent studies have shown that getting adequate sleep for these high performers improves their response time, their agility and accuracy, reduces the likelihood of injury and illness, extends their longevity as competitors, and improves their mental game, too.[63,64] Sleep, research shows, is vital to athletic success.

"If you told an athlete you had a treatment that would reduce the chemicals associated with stress, naturally increase human growth hormone, enhance recovery rate, and improve performance, they would all do it. Sleep does all those things," said Casey Smith, head athletic trainer, of the Dallas Mavericks.[65] So just as athletes harness the health-supporting powers of sleep for peak performance, we, too, need to foster high-quality sleep to keep our bodies in peak condition to maintain our health and prevent cancer or prepare ourselves for the challenges of cancer treatment and recovery.

The Side Effects of Sleep Loss

If we use athletics as evidence that sleep is a predictor of performance, most American adults are struggling. A 2013 Gallup poll found that the average American adult sleeps just 6.8 hours per night—which is down more than an hour over the last seventy years.[66] Back in 1942, the benchmark year Gallup used for their analysis, 84 percent of Americans slept for seven to nine hours per night—the recommended amount for optimal health and well-being that sleep experts still agree upon.[67,68] Yet today, only 59 percent of us are hitting this mark, which means that over 40 percent of us just aren't sleeping enough.[66]

And it's an even greater challenge among children—especially adolescents. This is because the teenage brain is undergoing a massive process of neural sculpting and development, and while this is going on, the adolescent brain operates in sync with a unique circadian rhythm that shifts a teen's day so that prompts for sleep (driven by hormonal and other cues) come most naturally later than for most of us, at roughly 11:00 p.m.[69,70] This means that a teenager who naturally falls asleep around 11:00 p.m. or midnight would need to sleep until at least 7:00 a.m. to 9:00 a.m., at minimum, in order to reach the recommended eight to ten hours of sleep for optimal health and well-being. But sleeping during this time frame, this 11:00 p.m. to 8:00 a.m. window, is, unfortunately, unrealistic for most teens given that school schedules tend to conflict with this natural biological rhythm. Studies show that only 15 percent of American teens are meeting the eight-to-ten-hour goal, and for the 85 percent who are not, the costs, in terms of physical, psychological, emotional, and academic performance are high.[71] In fact, one 2014 survey declared that more than 90 percent of all American high school students are sleep deprived.[72] Knowing that so many diseases are gestating years and years before they appear—especially cancers, which can be "seeded in the body" up to forty years before they ever become detectable— makes this fact particularly difficult for me to bear, not just as a professional in the cancer care and prevention world, but as the father of teenagers. Mary Carskadon, a sleep researcher and professor of psychiatry and human behavior at the Warren Alpert Medical School of Brown University, has described the conflict between the adolescent biological drive to stay up late and the need to wake up early for school as a "perfect storm."[69] Simply put, societal norms about school start times clash with adolescents' circadian biology.

A study published in February 2015 in the *Journal of Youth and Adolescence* surveyed a diverse sample of almost twenty-eight thousand high school students in Virginia.[73] Only 3 percent of this group of teens reported getting the mean goal of nine hours of sleep a night, and 20 percent indicated that they sleep less than five hours per night. The average reported was 6.5 hours per night. From the questions asked, the researchers deduced that with each hour of lost sleep, feelings of sadness or despair increased by 38 percent, feelings of being suicidal increased by 42 percent, and substance abuse increased by 23 percent. There is no way, of course, in this kind of survey to conclude that sleep deprivation was the sole cause of an increase in mental health complaints, but given that we know that teens are already at risk for high rates of depression, insomnia, and other mental health issues, these findings are notable.

So if inadequate sleep is causing such a huge raft of psychological and physical problems for all of us, what are we doing about it?

When we don't get sufficient sleep, we're sluggish, and in an effort to prop ourselves up, we turn to stimulants such as coffee, cigarettes, food, alcohol, or drugs—all of which offer us some short-term benefits, but at tremendous cost to our long-term health. When we don't get enough sleep, we enter a chronic state of stress that can cause a domino effect of poor

THE HIGH COST OF SLEEP LOSS

Sleep medicine as a specialty arose in the 1970s when scientists began to understand that not getting enough sleep was a leading cause of death by accident in this country. The majority of traffic fatalities are related to driver drowsiness, and sleep restriction and working at a time that humans are biologically driven to be asleep have been connected by investigators to a series of high-profile catastrophic accidents, including nuclear melt-downs at Three Mile Island and Chernobyl, the grounding of the Exxon Valdez oil tanker, and the explosion of the space shuttle *Challenger*.[74] More recently, train crashes in New York and New Jersey, including a 2013 crash that killed four people, have been tied to sleep-restricted engineers.[75] Today, it is estimated that 47 million Americans—well over 10 percent of the population—suffer from disordered sleep.[76] And nearly 9 million of us are taking prescription sleep aids in an effort to remedy this.[77]

In 2016, it was estimated that sleep loss was costing the U.S. economy $411 billion due to lost productivity and workplace accidents.[78] This is vastly higher than any other country on earth.

lifestyle choices, such as overeating, moving too little, experiencing depression and anxiety, and, most notably, making our bodies vulnerable to infection, inflammation and illness.

Lack of sleep also changes how we metabolize food and contributes to the current worldwide epidemic of obesity and type 2 diabetes, by changing the way our bodies regulate insulin and other key hormones.[79] Research also shows that across the life span, people who get less than six hours of sleep per night are more likely to become obese, even if they exercised regularly.[80] Research also shows that not getting enough sleep affects hormone levels that increase hunger the next day.[81] In a 2013 study of almost fourteen hundred teenagers from suburban high schools in Philadelphia, researchers found that each additional hour of sleep was associated with a reduction in body mass index, with the highest reduction shown for teenagers who were the most obese.[82] In adults, inadequate sleep has been associated with ailments ranging from diabetes to stroke and heart disease.[83,84]

The best remedy for inadequate sleep is . . . sleep. But there is a way to sleep well, and it's not by shortchanging yourself on sleep during the week

---

THE ANTICANCER LIVING BENEFITS OF SLEEP

- Sleep regulates our appetite, and so when we sleep well, we eat well and are more able to sustain a healthy weight.[81]
- Sleep regulates key biological processes linked to obesity.[79]
- Sleep is essential to being physically at our best. Our muscles and cells need sleep to regenerate, detox, and heal.[26]
- Sleep is essential to positive mood.[85] Being well-rested allows us to effectively respond to stressors throughout our day and have healthy relationships.[86,87]
- Sleep is essential for mental performance.[88,89] We need to be well-rested to be responsive and avoid accidents and injury.[4,90]
- Sleep is the timekeeper of our health: if we sleep well, we are more likely to prevent disease and have better outcomes, including with cancer.[23]

---

and then oversleeping on the weekend. Sleeping in on the weekends can actually cause a "social jet lag," not unlike traveling across time zones.[91] Sleep rhythms are regular and somewhat fixed, though they are unique to each individual. Learn to listen in, and when your body and mind give you the cues that it's time to sleep, heed them.

How Much Sleep Is Enough?

Since so many of us are conditioned to believe that sleep is not a meaningful activity, we're always trying to find ways to cut back on it, but as those of us who've dragged ourselves through our days know, this never works. Sleep is a complex process. It's a series of physiological events that need adequate time to unfold and progress to completion. The idea that we can somehow hack this process and take a shortcut just isn't plausible. As sleep researchers learn more about the physiological processes at work while we sleep, they've been able to hone and adjust their understanding of what constitutes optimal sleep time.

We included the following recommendations to show that our understanding of why sleep duration is important is evolving. Scientists are becoming more aware of the peak hours of rest and are increasingly able to understand the specific biological processes of sleep. Our lives are fluid

In 2015, the National Sleep Foundation (NSF) issued new recommendations for goals for sleep duration per age group.[67] The new recommendations are as follows:

Age	Recommended amount of sleep
Newborn (0–3 months):	14–17 hours per day (narrowed from 12–18 hours)
Infants (4–11 months):	12–15 hours per day (widened from 14–15 hours)
Toddlers (1–2 years):	11–14 hours per day (widened from 12–14 hours)
Preschoolers (3–5 years):	10–13 hours (widened from 11–13 hours)
School-age Children (6–13):	9–11 hours (widened from 10–11 hours)
Teenagers (14–17):	8–10 hours (widened from 8.5–9.5 hours)
Younger Adults (18–25):	7–9 hours* (*this is a new category)
Adults (26–64):	7–9 hours (unchanged)
Older Adults (65+):	7–8 hours* (*this is a new category)

and so our biological rhythms are somewhat fluid, too. This explains why optimal sleep time is framed as a range—but it's not for the reasons most people think: It is actually possible to oversleep as well as undersleep, and it is estimated that up to 30 percent of the U.S. population sleeps too much.[92] If we look then at healthy sleep duration as a curve, with 40 percent falling below the target range and another 30 percent sleeping beyond the target range, only a sliver of us—roughly 30 percent—are getting sleep right.[92,93]

Too Much of a Good Thing

Michael Irwin, MD, at the Semel Institute for Neuroscience, UCLA, is one of the world's leading researchers on the intersection of sleep and disease and is keenly aware of how vital it is that we really aim for that eight-hour-a-night sweet spot.

The population that engages in more than eight hours of sleep typically isn't enjoying quality sleep, according to Irwin. Long sleepers are particularly prone to disease. For example, oversleeping can raise one's risk of developing heart disease by nearly 35 percent.[94] There is also compelling scientific evidence that oversleeping plays into other conditions that affect mortality, such as obesity, depression, and chronic illnesses like diabetes and cancers.[6] What we don't know is which comes first: the health problem or the poor sleep, but the question of which causes which isn't as important as changing the dynamic, according to Irwin. "Poor sleep, whether it's too much or too little, is linked to increases in inflammation, which is a known pathway that has been implicated in a whole host of health problems, including the onset or exacerbation of serious diseases such as cancers." Later in this chapter, we'll discuss how to make the lifestyle adjustments you need to reach the sweet spot of sleep.

The Wild Nightlife of the Brain

When we think of sleep and the brain, we think of dreams and Carl Jung and the mind as an ethereal, untethered abstraction, and until very recently, we really didn't give much thought to what was happening to the literal mass of cells and neurons and vessels that make up this amazing organ when we're asleep.

Even though the brain only takes up approximately 2.5 percent of the body's total mass, it uses 25 percent of the energy we generate and 25 percent of the oxygen we breathe.[95,96] The brain is made up of nervous tissue that relies on the glucose supplies produced by the rest of the body to function. As the command center for the entire body, it can be argued that the rest of the body processes energy primarily to fuel the brain.

What happens then, when we go to sleep? We know that deep sleep refreshes us, clears our mind, and gives our body the rest it needs, but what about the brain?

In 2013, a team of researchers at the University of Rochester in New York explored a seemingly simple question: What happens to the brain at night? What this team, led by Maiken Nedergaard, MD, discovered is that the brain actually undergoes a vital cleansing process while we sleep.[97]

Nedergaard and her team looked at the brains of mice while they slept. What they saw astounded them. The brain cells of the mice literally contracted so that glia cells could expand and wrap around neural blood vessels and transport cellular waste via cerebrospinal fluid out of the brain. Nedergaard named this network of glia cells and this extraordinary removal of neurological toxins and waste the "glymphatic system," as it mirrors the essential cleansing properties of the body's lymphatic system. What her team saw was that the sleeping brains of the mice were anything but at rest; they lit up while this unique network of vessels flowed with fast-moving cerebrospinal fluid as it bathed the quiet cerebral cells and neurons.[97]

Most startlingly, Nedergaard's team noted that during the day the glymphatic system was not active. This flushing away of neural toxins, which only occurs at night, begs the ultimate question: is this extraordinary process of brain cleansing actually one of the key reasons we sleep?

We certainly know how much critical thinking, judgment, reflexes, and other processes are harmed by inadequate sleep, and perhaps it is because we interrupt this natural cleansing process. Researchers are now actively investigating the link between the work of the glymphatic system and the presence of protein plaques (beta-amyloid) known to be associated with diseases such as dementia and Alzheimer's.[98–100] This would help to explain the research showing a direct link between sleep and cognitive functioning and that sleep loss is a risk factor for early-onset dementia and Alzheimer's.[101–103] In fact, recent research shows that even in individuals not suffering from a sleep disorder or any form of dementia, those who experienced the worst sleep had the highest concentration of beta-amyloid in their brains, and another study found that if study participants had their deep sleep disrupted by the experimenters, this resulted in increased beta-amyloid even after just one night of disrupted sleep.[104] Could conditions like Alzheimer's be a by-product of a faulty neural cleaning system, which might be the result of poor sleep? And if so, are there other diseases, including some cancers, that are affected by a lack of adequate nightly brain cleansing?

What this research highlights, more than anything else, is that the brain is more than just a computer, a set of neurons that fire on and off. It is a fragile organ that needs to be cared for and maintained, and the best way to do that is by creating habits that support its health, the chief one being getting the appropriate amount of restful sleep.

Sleep and the Body

Just forty minutes. That's all it takes for us to miss per night for our bodies to become vulnerable to a whole host of illness-related conditions.[105] It's been well studied that getting under seven hours of sleep (the low end of the recommended healthy range for adults) results in conditions that increase mortality. These include higher rates of diabetes, measurable weight gain, and, most noticeably, heart disease.[106,107]

Cancer and Sleep

In addition to being linked with weight gain, diabetes, cardiovascular disease, and Alzheimer's disease, poor sleep has been linked in many studies to increased cancer risk and poorer outcomes for cancer survivors. A 2012 study by researchers at Case Western Reserve University in Cleveland found that postmenopausal women who have a chronic lack of sleep were more likely to develop more aggressive forms of breast cancer and had increased risk of recurrence.[108] The study looked at the pre-diagnosis sleeping habits of more than one hundred recently diagnosed breast cancer patients and found an association between a chronic lack of sleep and the recurrence of early-stage hormone receptor positive breast cancer. The fewer hours the study subjects slept, the more likely their cancer was to return. This correlation remained significant when adjusting for age, a history of smoking, physical activity, and whether participants were overweight or obese.

In terms of colon cancer, some of the same researchers at Case Western found that patients who reported sleeping less than six hours a night had a 50 percent greater risk of colorectal adenomas, a precursor to colon cancer, compared with those who reported sleeping only an hour more, at least seven hours a night.[109] That 2011 study involved more than twelve hundred study participants who completed sleep surveys before undergoing colonoscopies.

While a lack of sleep has not been directly identified as a cause of cancer, it is now universally accepted that poor sleep after a cancer diagnosis leads to worse outcomes. So, much of the focus in the medical field is on helping those who have cancer get adequate rest to improve their chances of survival and lower their risk of recurrence.

In one of the more compelling studies to date, researchers in Europe found that patients with advanced colorectal cancer died sooner if their circadian rhythm was disrupted during chemotherapy (a common side effect).[110] Researchers tracked the circadian rhythms of seventy-seven patients who were receiving chemotherapy and found that those who were able to maintain normal sleep patterns survived significantly longer than those who had disrupted sleep during treatment. The researchers speculated that preventing circadian disruption during chemotherapy could reduce the toxicity of the treatment and improve its effectiveness as well as improve mortality rates.

While the science in this area continues to develop, we already understand the most important outcome—good sleep and rest are essential to high quality of life and overall health, whether or not one is living with cancer.

Less Stress, More Sleep

Arguably, the number one reason most of us don't get enough sleep is due to psychological stress. When we slow down and the lights go out, we tend to ruminate on our problems, be they social, financial, work related—you name it. But for those who are also contending with cancer, the stress can be multiplied by the combining of psychological or existential stress with physical stress and symptoms such as pain.

I talk to many cancer patients who tell me that the problem that is most vexing for them—and it is one that can last long term—is being able to relax and get high-quality sleep.

The reasons for this are both psychological and practical. Certainly, the existential stress of knowing that one's body is harboring something potentially lethal can be overwhelming. At night, a cancer patient has no choice but to make a certain kind of peace with his or her body, despite knowing that the cancer itself isn't resting.

Medical stress often prompts us to come face-to-face with our mortality, which is, arguably, one of the most potent causes of insomnia. When we're at rest, our psychological and emotional defenses are down, and we become vulnerable in ways that put us in touch with the fact of our natural biological fragility.

Martica Hall, PhD, has been studying the connection between stress and sleep for the past twenty years at the University of Pittsburgh. Her research has pointed to a link between stressful events, such as a cancer diagnosis or the loss of a loved one, and disrupted sleep.[47,111,112] Hall and her colleagues have demonstrated that sleep is the link between stress and poor health.[113-115] Moreover, it seems that poor sleep is what allows stress to literally get under our skin and into our cells, making us more vulnerable to illnesses and, possibly, poor outcomes. We cannot remove all the stressors in our lives (though we can certainly make valiant efforts at cutting them down), but perhaps improving our sleep will counteract the harms that stress can otherwise cause our bodies to incur.

I have seen firsthand how improving sleep in the breast cancer patients in our CompLife Study helps these women experience less stress and regain their vitality. When Brucett, whose story we shared in chapter 8, joined the study, she slept, on average, only four to five hours a night. She attributed this to being a "natural worrier," and she was concerned that, now that she was diagnosed with cancer, she wouldn't get any sleep at all. But we worked closely with her on learning how to manage her stress and we watched as her sleep improved. Now four years post-treatment, she continues to sleep well and feels sleep has been an important part of her healing. "Honestly, I just don't stress like I used to," she recently told me. "I don't just lie down in bed and stare at the ceiling. Now I go right to sleep."

When we relax and let go as best we can, our minds and bodies are better able to do what they do best—to heal and strengthen us. Sleep then becomes an act of faith: we learn to trust the processes that occur when we sleep, and we begin to gain an appreciation for the diurnal nature of healing and disease prevention.

Taking Pills versus Changing Habits

I am a strong proponent of cancer survivors and others avoiding sleeping pills. There are of course times when taking sleeping pills may be appropriate, under the guidance of a physician, to help break a bad cycle or for a limited period to help with jet lag. But it is vital to understand that sleeping pills do not tackle the root problem leading to sleep disturbances. Also, pill-assisted sleep is not truly restorative sleep. While sleeping pills do put you to sleep, benzodiazepines and other drugs do not move you through all stages of sleep. In fact, no drug on the market increases the deepest stages of sleep, the restorative part of sleep, critical for maintaining health. So, you may feel like you have gotten a good night's sleep, but the true restoration needed to improve your health will still be missing. As Michael Irwin put it: "There are significant changes in sleep architecture associated with the use of benzodiazepines, including the loss of slow wave sleep. Such findings raise very real questions about the impact of benzodiazepine as an insomnia treatment, on mitigating insomnia-related inflammatory responses, or helping the person who has insomnia return to normal physiologic homeostatic state." Older adults who use sleeping pills can also wake up in the middle of the night and have coordination problems leading to dangerous falls.[116] There are also concerns for daytime function with the use of sleeping pills. As Irwin explains, "We know from a number of studies that sedative-hypnotics have daytime consequences such as problems with cognition, memory, and visual spatial abilities that impact their functioning."

Methods for Improving Sleep

There are several anticancer living approaches to addressing the stressors that inhibit healthy sleep, and these include the following:

COGNITIVE BEHAVIORAL THERAPY-INSOMNIA (CBT-I)

This short, focused talk therapy is extremely effective in treating insomnia. In just a few weeks, patients learn to change their sleep habits and research shows that it is much more effective than prescription drugs in providing long-term results.[117–119] CBT-I can be delivered in person, in group formats, by telephone, or via internet-based treatment and has been shown to have long-term benefits for improving sleep in cancer patients.[120–124]

TAI CHI

In his work at UCLA, Michael Irwin has done remarkable research that looks at the efficacy of tai chi for helping breast cancer survivors who suffer from insomnia. The results show that tai chi promotes "robust" improvements in sleep duration and quality, which are comparable to CBT-I, or talk therapy, and provides additional benefits of reduction of depression and daytime fatigue.[125] This is a remarkable finding in that CBT-I has been the gold standard nonpharmaceutical treatment for insomnia—but it can be expensive. Tai chi, on the other hand, is often offered at community or senior centers, public libraries, or in outdoor parks, for little or no cost. Plus, there is the added benefit of doing it as part of a group, which bestows additional health benefits associated with being connected to a social group or network. Irwin notes that the subtle, rhythmic movements of tai chi relax the body, slow breathing, and reduce inflammation, which is associated with cancer recurrence.

Irwin's study recruited ninety breast cancer survivors ranging in age from forty-two to eighty-three. Half the women were in a group that engaged in weekly CBT-I and the other group did weekly tai chi for three months. Both groups were closely monitored monthly, and fifteen months later both groups reported continued improved sleep and less fatigue. Not only was tai chi as effective as CBT-I at improving sleep outcomes, Irwin found that tai chi led to greater reduction in inflammatory markers than CBT-I. They also demonstrated that this practice reduced inflammatory gene expression profiles—a key factor in preventing disease onset or progression, including cancer.[126]

This study, Irwin believes, points to the importance of sleep in terms of overall health and homeostasis (internal balance). "We know that quality sleep is important to the regulation of our endocrine system, the sympathetic nervous system, and the immune system—three systems that need to be well balanced in order to stave off serious diseases, including cancers. Making lifestyle changes such as engaging in tai chi, for example, can rebalance one's circadian rhythm and restore and reinforce healthy sleep architecture, which are thought to be important in promoting health and even possibly in preventing cancer recurrence."

MEDITATION

Meditation has also been shown to promote restful sleep. Irwin and his team taught meditation to a small group of people over fifty-five years of age who complained of moderate sleep disruption.[127] These meditators were compared to another control group of the same age that was given basic sleep education. The meditators not only slept better but also reported less depression and daytime fatigue. Also important, in study after study we see that participating in meditation also leads to higher melatonin levels, the hormone that is necessary to help us initiate and maintain our sleep.

YOGA

In a study conducted at the University of Rochester, four hundred cancer survivors who were experiencing sleep disturbances reported that both their subjective and objective sleep quality improved after attending two yoga sessions a week for just four weeks.[128] In addition, research we conducted at MD Anderson in women with breast cancer undergoing radiotherapy found that those who practiced yoga up to three times a week during radiotherapy had better cortisol regulation than a light stretching control group at the end of treatment and one month later.[129] In fact, cortisol levels for the women in the yoga group dropped more on a daily basis than that of the control group, allowing the body to relax and prepare itself for sleep. We have also found that women undergoing chemotherapy who practice yoga at least two times a week or more also report improved sleep outcomes.[130] Though more research is needed to show if tai chi, meditation, yoga, or other mind-body practices have a long-term impact on sleep quality and health outcomes, the data we've gathered is promising.

Cancer and Fatigue

For cancer patients—even for those who are years out from treatment and "cured"—the fatigue that accompanies the disease can be pernicious. So much so that it has its own name: cancer-related fatigue (CRF). CRF is a complex syndrome that is a result of cancer treatment and the high levels of stress both the illness and the treatments put on our bodies. CRF is defined by the National Comprehensive Cancer Network as "a distressing, persistent, subjective sense of physical, emotional and/or cognitive tiredness or exhaustion related to cancer or cancer treatment that is not proportional to recent activity and interferes with usual functioning."[131]

The powerful medical treatments, especially chemo and drug therapies, not to mention surgery (particularly the anesthetics and sedatives used) are known to disrupt our circadian cycle and to interfere with cellular repair processes, endocrine modulation, and nerve function.[132-134] These disrupted biological systems can cause pain, insomnia, and physical symptoms such as hot flashes—all of which can make sleeping soundly nearly impos-

---

CRF FACTS[135]

- CRF affects between 25 and 99 percent of cancer patients.
- CRF can persist for up to five years—or longer—after completion of treatment.
- CRF is not relieved by a rest (a particularly cruel aspect of the syndrome).
- CRF is associated with impairment of quality of life both during and after treatment.
- CRF is linked to recurrence of cancer and to decreased rates of overall survival.

---

sible. In fact, patients with CRF have heightened levels of inflammatory markers that lead to worse levels of fatigue and sleep quality. So when sleep becomes physically uncomfortable, what can one do?

Let There Be Light

In addition to behavioral therapy designed specifically to improve sleep health, light therapy (using a light box with full-spectrum or high-lux LED lights or exposure to natural sunlight) is a promising technique that is being studied as a way to improve sleep during chemotherapy and to reduce CRF. And light therapy is even less expensive than tai chi. In fact, all you have to do is step outside and enjoy the sun (without wearing sunglasses).

One of the leading researchers in this area is Sonia Ancoli-Israel, a professor of psychiatry at the University of California San Diego School of Medicine and director of the Gillin Sleep and Chronobiology Research Center. In her research, Ancoli-Israel has found that breast cancer patients who are exposed to short doses of bright light before and during chemotherapy report lower levels of fatigue.[136] "My hypothesis was that patients undergoing chemotherapy are so fatigued that they never go outside. They just get into this cycle of being fatigued, having disruptive sleeping rhythms, and just sitting around the house. The lack of light makes all those things worse."

Ancoli-Israel and her colleagues conducted a study where they exposed women to bright light for thirty minutes every morning and studied the effects on their fatigue during chemotherapy.[136] Those who were exposed to bright light did not suffer additional fatigue, while those who were exposed to less-intense red light for the same period every morning saw their fatigue significantly increase. Patients in the bright light group also recovered better and more quickly from the disruptive effects of chemotherapy.

Ancoli-Israel and her team have now completed a similar study on cancer survivors and found that exposure to bright light reduces daytime sleepiness, decreases depressive symptoms, and improves quality of life.[137] Most recently, she has turned her attention to the impact of light therapy on chemo brain (decreased cognitive function that can result from chemotherapy treatment); we look forward to the results of this important study.

After two decades focused on the impact of sleep and circadian rhythms on disease progression, Ancoli-Israel has no doubt about the vital importance of sleep, for those with cancer and those who hope to avoid a cancer diagnosis: "Just like you have to eat and just like you have to drink liquids, you have to sleep. Without good sleep, all the rest is impossible. Everything falls apart if you don't have a good night's sleep."

Listening to Our Bodies

Overcoming CRF takes a willingness to give up our expectations about what we can do for the short term and to really listen in to the body, perhaps for the first time. Cancer is, above all else, exhausting, but learning how to modulate your energy after cancer treatment can put you on a path to true anticancer living. Fatigue is a powerful messenger and learning to listen to it is part of learning to listen to what the body needs to heal. We all know that when we're sick, rest is the best medicine. But for all of us—including cancer patients—it's important to rest but not too much. Being conscientious and deliberate about your sleep-and-wake cycle will help you recover more quickly and efficiently.

Staying physically active during the day is crucial to being able to rest well at night, and it also helps alleviate CRF.[138] Of course going to the gym or rejoining your softball team after going through treatment for cancer (or any illness or disease) isn't well advised, as your body has been under tremendous pressure. But engaging in activities like walking or stretching or gentle yoga are ideal. In fact, multiple studies have found that patients experiencing CRF benefit tremendously from participating in yoga, tai chi, and MBSR (mindfulness-based stress reduction).[139–141] The goal is to reignite muscle memory and to reactivate your respiration and circulatory system— to begin to gently reengage with the world. As your strength increases, you'll know when it's time to get back into the game more fully. Speaking of strength, one of the major shifts cancer patients often need to adjust to is learning how to take care of themselves instead of others. It can be very difficult to make this shift, but when energy levels are low, it's important to use limited energy supplies wisely and learn to put your own health and healing first. This redirection of energies is a game changer for many.

Experts like Michael Irwin at UCLA and Sonia Ancoli-Israel at UCSD have dedicated their careers to studying and finding antidotes for sleep disturbances and CRF because they know that healing cannot occur when the body is in a state of constant sleep restriction. Researchers in the Netherlands tracked the white blood cell count of fifteen healthy young men who got eight hours of sleep and then compared those numbers with white blood cell counts during twenty-nine hours of sleep deprivation.[142] They found the effect of sleep deprivation mirrored what the body goes through during the acute stress response, triggering the production of a type of white blood cell that helps the immune system fight off viruses and bacteria. Although having increased immune cells might sound like a good thing, this is not ideal in the absence of a pathogen against which you want this type of response. In fact, researchers found that, after responding to these repeated phantom attacks, the immune cells lost their typical day-night rhythmicity—their natural circadian rhythm. In other words, much as the functioning of a person who is sleep deprived declines, their white blood cells are similarly affected, and, over time, sleep loss leads to immune suppression and increased inflammation.

The goal is to break this cycle and get our chronobiology back and our sleep-wake cycle into sync so that our bodies do what they do best, which is to generate health and wellness.

I think it's most useful to reframe how we view sleep and to see it as a vital, health-promoting activity rather than a passive timeout. Without sleep we become low functioning, miserable, and sick. I'd like to see us begin to value sleep the way we do athletic, academic, or work success and put that much thought and consideration into sleep health. Once you make sleeping well a high priority, the quality of all your other endeavors will improve, including your ability to adopt healthy lifestyle changes in all the other areas of the Mix of Six. Your life will just get better all the way around.

THE ANTICANCER LIVING GUIDE
TO BETTER SLEEP

ANTICANCER ACTION STEPS

1. Evaluate your sleep health.
2. Identify your sleep patterns and challenges.
3. Understand if you need to consult a health-care professional.
4. Improve your day to improve your night.
5. Use your "senses" for optimal sleep health.

1. Evaluate Your Sleep Health

Sleep disturbances fall into six main categories:

- Trouble falling asleep
- Trouble staying asleep
- Waking up too early
- Not sleeping long enough
- Irregular sleep schedule
- Overall poor sleep quality

Take a moment to assess what your sleep health looks like. Do you face multiple sleep challenges, or do you have a specific area that needs attention? Do you have problems every night, or are your sleep disturbances intermittent?

If you want a clearer picture of your sleep issues, consider keeping a sleep diary to understand your sleep patterns or use an activity monitor that you wear on your wrist when you go to sleep. This information is then downloaded and provides an organized view of your sleep patterns. Track the following with honesty:

- Time you went to sleep
- Time you woke up (did you wake up before it was necessary?)

- Total hours of sleep
- Amount of time it took to fall asleep
- How many times you woke during the night
- How long you were awake overall during the night
- Rate your overall quality of sleep on a scale of 0 to 10

TRACK YOUR SLEEP PATTERNS FOR SEVEN TO THIRTY DAYS

It may take time for your specific sleep picture to emerge, including how regular or irregular your sleep patterns are. Record your sleep patterns until you have a clear picture of your sleep health.

2. Identifying Your Sleep Patterns and Challenges

Consult the box on page 174 to view the sleep recommendations for your age. How does your nightly sleep line up with the recommended amount of sleep for your age group?

Your first goal is to get at least 6.5 hours of sleep and preferably between 7 and 8 hours a night. Once you are getting enough sleep, the question to ask is whether your sleep quality is good. In other words, are you sleeping well? Judging whether your sleep is good is a subjective measurement, but it is also simple to assess. Do you feel tired during the day? If so, it is likely that you are either not getting enough sleep or your sleep quality is poor. Common problems, along with too little sleep, include taking a long time to fall asleep, waking up too early, and repeatedly waking up during the night. Do you follow a regular sleep pattern? If you are getting enough sleep, but still feel tired during the day, it is likely that you are encountering one or more of these issues. While your sleep time is good, your sleep efficiency is not.

If you find you're having trouble falling asleep or if you wake up in the middle of the night and can't get back to sleep, try meditative breathing. Breathe in deeply through your nose and feel your stomach rise on the inhale. Pause for a few seconds and then breathe out slowly through your mouth. Repeat this technique for as long as it takes you to settle down and relax. Meditative breathing slows the heart rate and blood pressure simultaneously and helps you let go of any stress or anxiety that might be keeping you awake. Do your best to maintain a regular sleep pattern that does not deviate by more than an hour—you don't want to induce jet lag on a regular basis.

3. Understanding If You Need to Consult a Health-Care Professional

Your sleep issue may require a doctor to evaluate your symptoms and make recommendations. Consider if you need professional help. One sleep expert described a more formal sleep disorder in the following way: If a sleeping problem occurs three times a week for three months, it qualifies as a clinically significant sleep issue. If this applies to you, consider seeing a professional to get advice about how to proceed. Cognitive behavioral therapy for insomnia is now recommended as a first-line treatment for sleep disorders. CBT-I has lasting effects because it teaches you how to optimize your sleep. Ask your doctor about that option before they write you a prescription for sleeping pills. Treat the problem, not just the symptoms. Other nonpharmacological approaches such as tai chi, yoga, or stress-management techniques are also effective.

4. Improve Your Day to Improve Your Night

- **Light Therapy:** Without wearing sunglasses, go outside for half an hour every morning when you first wake up. This could involve an outdoor breakfast, or even better, a walk. If you don't have the energy for that, just sit outside on your balcony or in your backyard (or sit close to a light box). By exposing yourself to bright light early in the morning, you can reduce your fatigue and improve your energy throughout the day.
- **Bedroom:** If you are having trouble sleeping at night, make sure your bedroom is for sleeping and intimacy only. If you want to use your laptop, curl up on the couch, but be sure to limit your light exposure. If you want to watch television or listen to the news, do that in the living room. If you find yourself drifting off, get up and go to bed. Once you start to associate the bedroom exclusively with sleep, your body and mind will become more receptive to sleeping when you enter your room of rest.

- **Routine:** Go to sleep at the same time every night. Hitting the sack at or near the same time will help you improve your sleep quality and circadian rhythms—you'll feel like a perfectly tuned orchestra!
- **Napping:** If you must nap, limit your naps to thirty minutes or less, and don't nap after 5:00 p.m. Longer naps can disrupt your circadian rhythm and prevent you from falling asleep and staying asleep during the night.
- **Work Your Body:** Aerobic activity for as little as ten minutes a day can dramatically improve your sleep quality. Yoga and tai chi have also been shown to improve sleep quality and duration. But avoid strenuous activities and workouts close to bedtime.

5. Use Your "Senses" for Optimal Sleep Health

The first thing to look at when trying to improve either sleep duration or sleep quality is to make an honest assessment of your sleep environment and sleep habits. In thinking about sleep quality and how to improve our sleep, Alison and I like to consider our five senses—smell, sight, sound, taste, and touch. This is a straightforward way for us to remember all the things that influence sleep and home in on things we can do to improve our own sleep health and the chances of our three teenagers getting deep, restorative sleep every night.

YOUR *NOSE* KNOWS

- Breathe deeply. It is important to engage throughout the day in your deep diaphragmatic breathing that you learned about in the last chapter and to do so especially before bed.
- Meditation can be used across the Mix of Six. Before bed, meditation can be very effective at switching off the monkey mind, rewiring, and disengaging. It is also an effective tool to help you get back to sleep after waking during the night.
- Use essential oils like lavender to help with sleep initiation. Consider an organic lavender essential oil spray on your pillows at night—it feels fresh and helps with sleep initiation. You can also get a diffuser to fill the room with the relaxing smell.

SEE THE PROBLEM

- Decrease exposure to ambient light in the bedroom—LED lights, outside lights, etc.
- Limit exposure to TV and all electronic devices thirty minutes before bed. They emit a blue light that makes it difficult for your pineal gland to start releasing the necessary melatonin to start your sleep cycle.
- Your phone doesn't belong in your bedroom. With your phone by your bed you are more tempted to look at it in the middle of the night, especially if you are having trouble sleeping or want to knock a task off your list that has just come to mind. Banishing your phone to another room is tricky in this day and age. With elderly parents or with teenagers out for the night we want to be available and reachable. Until someone develops an app that allows for a Do Not Disturb Except in the Case of Emergency setting, we are going to find this challenging. Consider placing your phone far enough away that you will hear it ring but not hear any bothersome texts at two in the morning. Also consider establishing a cut-off time with texting and emails. At nine or ten o'clock Alison and I stop looking at our phones and computers. Admittedly, it has been a challenge to get our children to abide by this rule, but we are always encouraging them to turn off, shut down, and disengage when it gets close to bedtime.
- I swear by my eye mask. I wear the kind of mask that has recessed spots for the eyes so that the mask does not push on your eyeball and obstruct eye movement during REM sleep. Blackout curtains are good, but they are also surprisingly expensive. As a cheap alternative, a friend of ours bought thick foam and cut it to her window shape and size.
- Travel with electrical tape to cover LED lights in hotel rooms. It is shocking how much light the TV red LED emits. That light hitting your retina in the middle of the night if you open your eyes can disturb your sleep pattern.

HEARING SOLUTIONS

- Sound—neighbors talking, partner snoring, outside noises, etc. An easy solution is earplugs. The use of a light pillow over your head may also do the trick.

- Sound machine—using a sound machine that makes white noise is a popular option. It masks the background noise by imposing a steady white noise sound.
- Snoring is a challenge in a partnership—encourage sleeping on the side or stomach, as this often helps. Consider sleeping in a separate room or raising the snorer's side of the bed with pillows.

TASTE BARRIERS

- Watch your alcohol consumption. While alcohol does have that sedative effect people enjoy and can help with sleep initiation, when alcohol is metabolized in the second part of the night, it becomes a stimulant and can cause you to wake up or sleep less deeply.[1]
- Watch your daytime caffeine intake. Don't drink coffee or caffeinated drinks after noon. Chocolate, while delicious, can have the same effect due to its caffeine content, especially the dark chocolate that we know is also healthy for us.
- Eating close to bedtime means your body is busy digesting when it is supposed to be sleeping. If you mix in rich food, alcohol, and sugar, it will likely cause you to have difficulty getting to sleep. Heartburn is a common reason people can't get to sleep or stay asleep. An easy solution: don't eat rich food, citrus fruit, or carbonated beverages close to bedtime.

FEELING SLEEPY

Temperature matters for sleep initiation and sleep maintenance.

Are your pj's too warm or cool? Surprisingly, this makes a real difference in Houston—given the large swings in temperature, one needs to go from light cotton to warm flannel, sometimes from one night to the next. The amount and type of covers you have (and if your partner pulls off your covers in the middle of the night) can lead to the same effect.

Do you need to adjust the thermostat before bed? We sleep better in a cool room. One degree of temperature change can be the difference between a good night's sleep and a poor one. A fan is an inexpensive solution.

Your body temperature naturally fluctuates during the night.[2] When you sink into deep sleep, your body temperature drops. You do not want bedding, like an electric blanket, that interferes with this natural process. Down covers or the like are ideal as they cool down as your body cools and hold heat as your body heats up.

Are your bed and pillow comfortable or do they need to be replaced? Signs you need a better pillow or mattress—neck gets cricks, you sink to the middle of the bed, or you've had your mattress for over ten years.

Until you optimize your sleep health, you can't know why you struggle in certain situations or in other areas of your life. Only when you adopt a steady sleep schedule and are getting a good night's rest can you move on to address other more obvious lifestyle choices, like what you eat and how much you exercise.

THE ANTICANCER LIVING GUIDE
SLEEP SOLUTION SUMMARY

For those experiencing sleep problems, below is a summary of the possible approaches to get your sleep on track.

During the Day

- Light Exposure: without wearing sunglasses, go outside for half an hour every morning when you first wake up.
- Bedroom Ambience: the bedroom should be for sleeping and intimacy only.
- Bedtime Routine: go to sleep at the same time every night.
- Nap Time: if you must nap, limit naps to thirty minutes early in the afternoon.
- Body Work: exercise for at least ten minutes a day.

USE YOUR SENSES AS YOUR SLEEP GUIDE

1. Smell

- Deep diaphragmatic breathing
- Meditation before bed
- Aroma therapy—lavender

2. Vision

- Create a dark bedroom free of all types of light. Consider a padded eye mask.
- Limit exposure to blue light (laptops and tablets) thirty minutes before bed.
- Establish a spot outside of your bedroom for your phone at night.
- Travel with electrical tape to cover LED lights.

3. Hearing

- Earplugs or light pillow
- Sound machine
- Snoring—encourage sleeping on the side or stomach, sleeping in a separate room, or elevating the snorer's side of the bed.

4. Taste

- Control and watch your alcohol intake, especially right before bedtime.
- Don't drink caffeinated beverages in the afternoon or evening.
- Limit chocolate and sugar consumption, especially at night.

5. Feeling

- Temperature matters for sleep initiation and sleep maintenance—dress for bed with temperature in mind.
- Control your bedroom temperature—cool is best.
- Body temperature fluctuates at night—down covers work well at helping to regulate body temperature.
- Consider replacing your mattress and/or your pillow.

CHAPTER TEN

Moving for Wellness

As you're reading this, I bet most of you are sitting, a few may be pedaling along on a stationary bike, walking on a treadmill or an elliptical trainer, and some are even, possibly lying down. Reading used to be one of the very few activities that could only be accomplished if we were sitting still. Due to the wonders of technology, we can now listen to an audiobook while we jog or prop a portable reading device in front of us while we count our calories and log our steps in the gym. But in large part, most of the hours of our lives are spent sitting.[1] This is where, I think, technology has, at least temporarily, stranded us. We sit to work, we sit to eat (of course), we sit to binge-watch TV (for more hours per day than at any other time in history). We sit in our cars and on planes and trains. This is why scientists and researchers have discovered that sitting is becoming a major health liability, and it is as detrimental to our health as smoking or eating poorly or any other number of less-than-healthy lifestyle choices that make us vulnerable to disease.[2]

The human body, which is an evolutionary masterpiece of biological engineering, is designed to be in motion. Think about it: We're a brilliantly put-together vessel of muscle, bone, sinew, organs, and fluids, capable of moving fluidly and swiftly at a thought's notice. We can bend, stretch, reach, or lift with exquisite precision and range. Most of us can also run, swim, and throw things, and throw them pretty hard with surprising accuracy, especially if we practice. No wonder, then, that we enjoy things like watching a young Olympic gymnast defy gravity with elegance, strength, and, not surprisingly, a level of joy and confidence that we rarely observe in our day-to-day lives. But what if I were to tell you that you can tap into this sense of personal satisfaction simply by getting up and taking a step? That's literally all it takes.

Move More for More Synergy

Movement can be the ultimate synergizer when it comes to the Mix of Six.

Physical activity can encompass more than just exercise. *Physical activity is defined as any skeletal muscle movement that increases energy expenditure above what is used while at rest. Exercise, on the other hand, is defined as physical activity performed in a structured, repetitive, organized manner with the objective of changing physical or psychological fitness or health-related outcomes.*[3] With this in mind, we see that just moving is considered physical activity. When we're in motion, we often cross paths with others, and when we do we're enriching ourselves not just in mind and body but socially, too, and this keeps us healthy. Being active allows us to participate with others on a somatic level, which lets us experience mutual joy and satisfaction in nonverbal ways.

Reduce Stress and Promote Mental Health: Exercise has been shown to measurably increase the output of specific neurotransmitters that are associated with mental and visual acuity, heart rate regulation, emotional regulation, and other cognitive functions.[4-8] These are the very neurotransmitters (the chemical messengers that facilitate communication between the body and the brain) that also protect us from mental health issues such as depression and anxiety. Richard Maddock, MD, a professor of psychiatry and behavioral sciences at University of California–Irvine, recently authored a study that found that vigorous exercise releases the neurotransmitters that promote physical and mental health:[4] "From a metabolic standpoint, vigorous exercise is the most demanding activity the brain encounters, much more intense than calculus or chess, but nobody knows what happens with all that energy," Maddock said. "Apparently, one of the things it's doing is making more neurotransmitters."[9] And more neurotransmitters mean greater brain-body health. Jennifer Carter, PhD, a lead sport psychologist and assistant professor in the Ohio State University Sports Medicine Program, views incorporating regular, balanced exercise into one's daily lifestyle as essential to treating mental health issues: "If clients are depressed, I educate them that the two best self-help strategies are exercise and social support.

For anxious clients, I teach them how exercise helps reduce worry, panic, and other symptoms."[10,11]

Sleep Better: In 2011, a team led by researchers at Oregon State University looked at a national sample of twenty-six hundred men and women aged eighteen to eighty-five who engage in 150 minutes (the amount recommended by the U.S. Department of Health and Human Services) of moderate to vigorous activity per week and they found that they reported less daytime sleepiness than those not exercising.[12] Physical activity resets our circadian rhythms that help us sleep better at night and be more alert and refreshed during the day.[13] Brad Cardinal, a professor of exercise science at OSU and one of the study authors, says, "Increasingly, the scientific evidence is encouraging as regular physical activity may serve as a nonpharmaceutical alternative to improve sleep."[14] The study participants, it is important to note, are not among the approximately 40 percent of the U.S. population that reports difficulty getting adequate deep sleep and staying alert during the day. For this population, studies show that regular physical activity also improves their sleep—though it may take longer (several weeks or more) for the positive effects to take hold.

Have Lower Obesity Rates: Researchers at Stanford University examined national survey results from 1988 through 2010 and found that rising rates of obesity kept pace with rising rates of inactivity—while calorie consumption remained constant.[15] Though careful to frame this as a correlative, rather than causative link (correlation is not necessarily an indicator of causation), they were struck by how dramatically rates in inactivity had risen. In women, this had spiked from 19 percent to more than 50 percent during this twenty-two-year period (while obesity rates rose from 25 percent to 35 percent); while in men, rates of inactivity climbed from 11 percent to 43 percent (with obesity rates rising from 20 percent to 35 percent). The fact is that we burn more calories when we're active than when we are *sedentary*. So if our diet remains constant, when we up our calorie burn rate, owing to physical activity, we are likely to burn the energy that is stored in fat. Additionally, research done at Brigham Young University suggests that daily exercise may act as a natural appetite suppressant, as it releases hormones that promote a sensation of "perceived fullness."[16] But, as rigorous physical activity may also cause one to overeat, it's important to maintain a sensible eating plan when engaging in physical activity so that body fat might be replaced with leaner and more energy-efficient muscle mass.

Get to Spend Time Outdoors: Working out in a gym is great, but for most of us, nothing beats being outdoors in the sunshine and fresh air. Studies of the health benefits of a "green environment" on exercise efficacy are new, but observational studies show that people who spend time outdoors—in any capacity—report greater feelings of revitalization and positive engagement.[17,18] These studies show that mood and sense of self-esteem also rise (especially in the first few minutes of engagement). Unfortunately, whether indoors or outdoors, worldwide nearly 31.1 percent of adults are physically inactive.[19] This is largely due, of course, to advances in technology, particularly in computers and digital connectivity. With work moving so decisively indoors, exercise seems to have followed suit, though this shift in location isn't necessarily a good thing. These studies revealed that not just mood, or affect, is improved when we spend time in natural, green surroundings; there are also beneficial physiological responses. Japanese studies monitoring the physiological effect of walking within real forest environments (*shinrin-yoku*, or forest bathing) reported similar findings.[20] Significantly lower systolic and diastolic blood pressure occurred following both viewing alone and walking in the forest environment when compared to the same activity in an urban environment. In nature we're able to relax, let our minds wander, and simply be. Additionally, research suggests that exercise may feel easier when performed in an outdoor versus a laboratory setting and people may tend to exert themselves more.[21] Being in nature, which is where we spent our waking hours prior to urbanization and industrialization, calms, relaxes, and yet invigorates us, awakening the body's impulse to move.

Move Your Body, Improve Your Health

Along with being linked to obesity, being sedentary causes a whole host of serious yet highly preventable health problems including the following:

- Increased insulin resistance, which is a precursor to the onset of type 2 diabetes, which in the United States, India, China, Mexico, Brazil, and many other countries is at epidemic proportions.[22] It's estimated by the CDC that more than one-third of all Americans suffer from unidentified insulin resistance.[23]
- Higher rates of heart attacks and other cardiovascular-related diseases.[24] The Nurses' Health Study found that women who are physically

active for three or more hours a week cut their risk of heart attack and stroke by 50 percent.[25] Active men cut their risk for stroke by two-thirds and their risk of heart attack by one-third.[26]

- Immune-deficiency issues and difficulty with keeping airborne illnesses, such as colds and flus, at bay.[27]
- Greater risk for depression and other mental health issues.[28]
- Bone health diminishes without the regular exercise needed to maintain adequate mineral content and strength.[29] The same is true for muscle health.[30,31] Both degrade more rapidly among the sedentary than among those who are active.[32]
- Cognitive decline and the onset of diseases such as dementia and Alzheimer's.[33]
- General physiological aging on all levels, from cellular and vascular, to increased organ deterioration.[34]

There is something almost paralyzing that happens when we get used to being so inactive. The laws of physics, particularly the one about inertia, take hold and we begin to feel as though not moving is what our bodies are designed to do. Not true! We need to put our focus on moving to aid the body in fulfilling its true purpose, which is to be actively nourished to control disease and function optimally.

For myself, once I had tried and failed to add exercise as another task to my already overbooked day and prioritized my sleep, I decided to try a new approach. Instead of looking at physical activity as a burdensome add-on, I began to view it in the context of what I was already doing.

I started to notice moments where I could cut out the "convenience" factor (there it is again: the word that tips us off to where we may be undermining our anticancer living goals) and incorporate more movement into my daily routine. When I got to work in the morning, instead of looking for the parking space closest to the elevator, I parked farther and farther out (where there were, of course, more available spaces) until I was walking across the whole garage. I also began parking on the upper decks and walking the seven flights of stairs down. Once inside, I began to skip the elevator, and take the stairs another handful of flights up to my office. I decided I'd take the elevator only if I was traveling with colleagues, or better yet coax them to join me, and I've stuck to this commitment long enough that stepping onto an elevator now feels really strange and unnatural to me.

At one point, I began tracking this kind of everyday activity on a fitness-tracking device, and I was surprised to see that by simply walking instead of riding during my workday, I was logging ten thousand steps without even thinking about it. I also realized that I was climbing, on average, fifty flights of stairs a day—which is a lot of steps. And which, frankly, is not something I'd be doing if I were standing in an overly lit gym on a stair machine.

This data inspired me to do more. So I began to view every parking lot as a place to walk and, whenever time allows, make it a game to park as far from my destination as I can. At our kids' soccer games, Alison and I began walking around the grassy perimeter of the field instead of sitting motionless for two hours, and soon other parents joined us and it became a great way for the grown-ups to catch up while the kids played.

And the bonus? I didn't need to give up an hour of sleep, sneak out of work, or give up time with family. And the benefits I reaped began showing up in surprising ways. I felt calmer, more balanced, and alert. I noticed, too, that even though I was spending a lot less time actually sitting at my desk, I was getting better quality work done in less time. My sleep and diet were also benefiting as my own natural circadian rhythm was fortified.

I realized this was a start, but what about the fact that my job is primarily sedentary except when walking from meeting to meeting? I bought a standing desk to use for work and laptop desks for the family at home. Although we know that standing is better than sitting, was there a way I could stand and move, too? I looked into treadmill desks. When I spoke to the powers that be at MD Anderson about possibly getting one, they voiced concern about the potential risk and liability. I understood their concerns, so I asked for a stationary bike instead—but was turned down. (The reason: "If we allow you to get one, we'd have to allow everyone to get one," which, come to think of it, might not be such a bad thing.) So I stopped looking for corporate approval and instead went rogue.

I found a $150 semirecumbent bike that fit nicely under my new standing desk and set that up so I could work and pedal at the same time. On average, I now pedal for an hour or two every day while working on my homemade "bike desk." I pedal with just enough tension so that I feel some resistance without getting too winded or working up too much of a sweat, with the goal being that I feel more energized, rather than tiring myself out. When I'm not pedaling away, I ask my colleagues, especially if we're meeting one-on-one, if we can have a walking meeting and, if so, preferably outside.

I've found that we connect more easily when we're side by side rather than across a desk from one another, and it seems like our creative brains just fire better when we're moving. I've found solutions to work problems during these walks that I doubt I'd find if I were just sitting alone and "thinking hard" about them. Getting some natural vitamin D and other nutrients from sunshine refreshes me in ways I cannot find anywhere else, and I know that by incorporating outdoor time into my workday, I'm working better and I'm a better colleague as well.

Now, I'm both talking the talk and walking the walk when it comes to understanding how to include more movement and activity into my day without the inconvenience and expense (in both time and money) that carving out a whole new category of work—as in "working out"—brings with it. This isn't to say that going to the gym is a bad or unhealthy thing (unless, again, it's costing you money or sleep or time in a way that just adds more stress to your life). If that works for you, great! Just make sure that when you're not in the gym that you're also getting out of your chair, moving as much as you possibly can and sitting as little as possible. A 2016 study published in *Medicine & Science in Sports & Exercise* found that even for people who already exercise, swapping a few minutes on the couch or in an office chair with some kind of movement was associated with reduced mortality.[35] The study charted data from three thousand people between the ages of fifty and seventy-nine. Lead author Ezra Fishman, part of the University of Pennsylvania's Population Studies Center, said that even getting up and washing the dishes or sweeping the floor seemed to have an impact on mortality. Over the course of eight years, the least active people were five times as likely to die compared to those who were the most active.

After a cancer diagnosis, physical activity is equally if not more important. Researchers in Canada followed more than eight hundred prostate cancer patients for seventeen years and measured their daily exercise.[36] Men who were the most active reduced their mortality by as much as 40 percent. You do not need to be an elite athlete to garner the benefits of exercise after a cancer diagnosis. In the Canadian study, researchers found benefits for prostate cancer survivors, even if they just took a daily thirty-minute walk. A study published in the *Journal of the American Medical Association* found that breast cancer survivors who exercised at a moderate level had a 50 percent reduced risk of recurrence, even somewhat better than those who exercised more.[37] Researchers have found that getting regular physical activity creates a more inhospitable environment for tumor development in both breast and prostate cancer survivors, and that aerobic activity makes tumors more vulnerable to the effects of chemotherapy.[38-42]

Does a Lack of Exercise Cause Cancer?

Certainly one of the Holy Grails of cancer prevention research is to determine, with enough scientific evidence, whether or not exercise can actually prevent the onset of cancer diseases. As with diet, the research, at this point, is largely epidemiological and observational and so, per the standards that must be met to establish scientific proof, they're not yet there. Nonetheless, there is enough evidence, gathered by the meta-analyses and cohort studies of vast quantities of data that have been summarized by the National Cancer Institute (NCI), to suggest that engaging in physical activity is associated with lowering one's risk of developing certain kinds of cancers.[43,44] Exercising, even moderately, has a positive impact on risk:

Colon Cancer: A 2009 analysis of fifty-two epidemiological studies found that very physically active people had a 24 percent lower risk of developing colon cancer than those who ranked among the least physically active.[45] In an analysis of another set of studies that looked at those who engage in "leisure" activities, the data showed a 16 percent reduction in risk of onset. Physical activity is also associated with lower occurrence of colon polyps, which are believed to be the precursor to full-blown colon cancer. According to the American Institute of Cancer Research, forty-three thousand cases of colon cancer each year in the United States are linked to a lack of physical activity.[46]

Breast Cancer: A 2013 analysis of thirty-one studies showed that women who engaged in physical activity lowered their risk of onset by 12 percent.[47] Interestingly, this is most evident in post-menopausal women, indicating that exercise is as important to older women as it is to younger women where cancer prevention is concerned.[48-50]

Endometrial Cancer: In an analysis of the data from thirty-three studies, those with high physical activity lowered their risk of onset by 20 percent compared to those with low physical activity.[51] The possible low physical activity–obesity link is of interest here as endometrial cancer is also highly associated with obesity.[52,53]

Additionally, in a study that tracked over one million people, "leisure" activities were linked to a reduced risk for onset of many more types of cancer, including liver, kidney, esophageal, and bladder, and these results are supported by other large studies and meta-analyses of internationally sourced data sets.[43]

So though we can't say with scientific precision that a sedentary lifestyle increases one's risk for the potential for developing cancer diseases, the overwhelming evidence we've gathered to date certainly points in this direction.

The Value of Adding Physical Activity to a Cancer Treatment Protocol

Kerry Courneya, PhD, a professor and Canada Research Chair at the University of Alberta in Edmonton, is one of the world's leading experts on the positive impact exercise has on cancer diseases. When Courneya began his research more than twenty years ago, exercise was barely on the radar, in terms of looking at its effect on the general quality of life for most cancer patients. Courneya looked at charts tracking the exercise patterns of cancer patients before, during, and after treatment, and he noticed that most patients fell into a period of marked inactivity after diagnosis and during active treatment.[54,55] This was true even when patients were physically active before diagnosis. He noted that, when treatment is completed, physical activity resumes, but rarely reaches the same precancer levels.[56] In other words, cancer seemed to have a very negative impact on a person's physical activity.

Courneya became interested in looking at the flat zone on a patient's physical activity graph, and he wondered, "What would happen if a patient engaged in a structured exercise program right after diagnosis and while undergoing treatment? Would this have any effect on the efficacy of the treatment? Would it have any effect on a patient's general quality of life going forward?" What he discovered not only surprised him but also fundamentally changed our view of how movement and activity might augment traditional cancer treatment protocols. "For many years, the accepted wisdom was that you should take it easy and rest up during treatment for cancer, but the research is showing that resting makes the side effects of cancer treatments (from surgery and chemo through radiation and immunotherapies), including things like neuropathy (nerve pain), cancer-related fatigue (CRF), generalized pain, brain fog, and so many others, worse." *Adding to this, a recent review of multiple studies showed that the best treatment for CRF was physical activity, with the evidence showing that physical activity was better than any pharmacological treatment.*[57]

When Courneya and his colleagues studied the impact of exercise on the efficacy of treatment within the context of formal clinical trials, the results, though counterintuitive, were consistent. Patients who exercised while undergoing chemo or radiation were more likely to have received all their treatments on time; experienced increased self-esteem and physical functioning; reported less brain fog and more mental clarity; experienced less fatigue and improved sleep; reported less nausea and improved appetite; experienced less nerve pain and numbness in extremities; had improved mood and less depression and anxiety; experienced shorter hospital stays and fewer trips to the doctor; and, most important, experienced a higher general quality of life.[40,58,59]

Courneya was also part of a meta-analysis in 2016 that looked at more than two dozen studies and found that cancer deaths were cut by more than a third when breast, colorectal, and prostate cancer patients engaged in physical activity.[59] Those findings, published in *Clinical Cancer Research*, also found a reduction in recurrence rates when comparing study subjects who exercised the most with those who exercised the least.

One of the most interesting findings of Courneya's research is that physical activity seems to prime the efficacy of the actual cancer treatments, and this finding got the attention of oncologists the world over. It brought this question to the fore: if being physically active helps the treatments we're using to cure or control cancer, then should we make sure that our patients are educated about the benefits of exercise and incorporate some kind of tracking of their physical activity into our work?

Over time, as more data have been gathered, exercise has also been shown to be associated with a lower rate of recurrence and with a lower risk of death from a number of different cancers, including breast, prostate, colorectal, endometrial, and others.[37,60-63]

But it's important to realize that inasmuch as we know the benefits of exercise, the evidence suggests that cancer survivors need to work on reducing their sedentary behavior. A study published in the *Journal of Clinical Oncology* reinforces both the positive benefits of exercise and negative effects of sitting. First the good news: Adults diagnosed with nonmetastatic colon cancer who engaged in about 2.5 hours of brisk walking per week reduced their mortality over a fifteen-year period by more than 40 percent.[63] The bad news: Colon cancer patients who sat more than six hours a day had an almost 30 percent increase in mortality over the same period, *even after controlling for physical activity*. In other words, even if they were physically active, sitting for extended periods of time was still harmful. In short, our bodies are not made for extended periods of sitting. "The lesson in all of this is don't take cancer lying down," Courneya explains. "The level of benefit in terms of recurrence and death can be as much as 30 or 40 percent lower when comparing the least active to the most. It's fairly profound."[64]

Finding the Next Gear

For Glenn Sabin, whose story we shared in chapter 5, "movement" is a foundational part of his prescription. More than twenty years ago, when he was diagnosed with an incurable cancer, little was known of the link between exercise and cancer. He, like others, was often told to not exert himself; Glenn intuitively knew that exercise was going to be critical for his success in controlling his disease. Before his diagnosis with chronic lymphocytic leukemia at age twenty-eight, Glenn was an on-again, off-again exerciser. He regularly lifted weights, but cardio was inconsistent at best. That all changed after his diagnosis. After reading about the health benefits of physical activity, Glenn made a commitment to exercise daily, a commitment he has stuck to now for twenty years. He incorporates at least an hour and a half of exercise into his day, everything from Pilates and weight lifting to yoga and swimming. But at the heart of his routine is walking. Glenn walks more than twenty miles a week, a practice he maintains whether he is home, on the road, attending conferences, or working with clients. No matter where he is or what he's doing, Glenn makes time to walk. "I'm not on an exercise program, per se," he explains, "it's just become part of my lifestyle and it makes me feel good."

EXERCISE AND CHEMOTHERAPY

Oncologists at the University of North Carolina (UNC) have directly measured the impact of chemotherapy treatment on biological aging. Hanna Sanoff, MD, MPH, assistant professor with the UNC School of Medicine and member of UNC Lineberger Comprehensive Cancer Center, and colleagues measured the level of p16, a protein that causes cellular aging, in the blood of thirty-three women over the age of fifty who had undergone chemotherapy for curable breast cancer.[65] Samples were taken for analysis of molecular age from patients before chemotherapy, immediately following chemotherapy, and a year after therapy finished. *The results showed that curative chemotherapy caused an increase in molecular age that was equivalent to fifteen years of chronological aging.*

Exercise and physical activity effectively counteract the accelerated aging caused by chemotherapy and the benefits persist over time. Research by Lee Jones, PhD, a pioneer in exercise research in cancer, found that exercise could counteract the negative cardiovascular and biological effects of chemotherapy that they documented in the control group, with exercise even decreasing inflammatory gene expression.[66-68] Jones, who was working at Duke Cancer Institute, Duke University Medical Center when this research was conducted and now works at Memorial Sloan Kettering Cancer Center, found that by just exercising, survivors slowed the biological clock to where it was supposed to be, neutralizing the aging effects of chemotherapy.

How Exercise Impacts Your Biology

The research of Courneya and others suggests that making time for more physical activity in our lives, the way Glenn has, should be part of the standard treatment for cancer patients and survivors (as well as part of everyone's daily routine). But what does exercise do to us that makes it so beneficial? Does it change our bodies and affect us at a cellular level?

An extensive body of research says yes. In fact, exercise impacts *ALL* the cancer hallmarks and especially *sustaining proliferative signaling, metabolism, immune function,* and *inflammation.*[67,69-76] As part of a brilliant Swedish study published in 2014, researchers basically made each study participant, both the intervention and control arm (or more accurately "leg"), work out one leg and not the other.[77] After three months, researchers found that gene expression was changed in the exercised leg in ways that influence metabolism, insulin response, and inflammation. More than five thousand positive changes were discovered in the genes on the exercised leg that remained unchanged in the leg that was not exercised.

This same genetic impact has been found in multiple studies looking at the effects of exercise on men with prostate cancer and women with breast cancer. Physical activity down regulates, or turns off, genes that promote tumor growth and up regulates, or turns on, genes that help prevent tumor growth.[67,76,78] Meanwhile, evidence is mounting that exercise can have effects within the tumor microenvironment, modifying key regulatory pathways.[79-81] Tumors thrive in a low-oxygen environment. Exercise pumps oxygen into tissues, which could reduce tumor growth.[79] The latest research shows that different tumors react differently to exercise, which may mean that, at some point soon, we will have different recommended exercise interventions specifically designed for a particular type and stage of cancer.[81]

While more research is needed to draw a direct causal relationship between exercise and tumor development, the early indications suggest that exercise could help cancer survivors live longer, enjoy life more, and avoid a recurrence. Notably, no studies have found adverse reactions in cancer survivors who exercised. So, while the extent of benefits is still being debated, there is little or no downside to engaging in daily exercise, even, and perhaps especially, if you are a cancer survivor.

What Kind of Exercise Is Best When It Comes to Cancer?

Karen Mustian, PhD, a leader in the field of exercise oncology at the Wilmot Cancer Institute at the University of Rochester, New York, knows how hard it is to enlist cancer patients to exercise. "Nearly fifteen years ago, when we started this work, a lot of people believed it wasn't even safe for most cancer patients to exercise," she recently reported. Fully 80 percent of the patients who enroll in her studies are sedentary, and she finds that the overwhelming nature of cancer and cancer treatment makes it hard for patients to hear and take in information about the benefits of exercise.[82] So Mustian (like Courneya and others) is careful about how she presents her findings to patients. She wants them to know that:

- exercise does not have to be expensive. There is no need to buy fancy equipment or join an expensive gym;
- walking is as effective as any other form of exercise in terms of reducing inflammation and protecting against cognitive side effects like chemo brain (cognitive impairment that can follow chemotherapy) and memory loss;[83]
- exercise works better than medications to reduce cancer-related fatigue, the most common side effect of cancer treatment;[57]
- yoga and tai chi are gentle yet effective forms of physical activity that reduce stress, fatigue, anxiety, insomnia, pain, and cognitive symptoms;[84-89] and
- patients see improvement in their overall quality of life after only four weeks of regular walking or using resistance-band strength training that they can do at home.[90]

What Works Best Is What Works for You

An important takeaway from all this exciting research is that there is no one-size-fits-all exercise program for cancer patients—or even just one plan for an individual cancer patient. As with all of the anticancer living Mix of Six lifestyle factors, an individual must listen to her body to determine what is most beneficial at any given point in time. Postsurgically, a patient who played tennis regularly may need to scale back and focus on regaining flexibility and strength and regaining her ability to get a full, restful night of sleep before she goes back out on the court. Practicing yoga may be the right choice for her at this stage in her treatment. Later, when her treatment is completed and she's feeling stronger, she may find that the stress-reducing benefits she got from yoga improved her tennis game (especially her serve), despite a six-month hiatus from the sport. Experts are referring to this as a "precision medicine" approach to using exercise for therapeutic purposes in cancer treatment, as physical activity needs to be tailored to the very unique and individual needs of each patient.[91,92]

Additionally, many things count as physical activity that we tend to overlook, especially among the older population, which is the demographic that is the hardest hit by cancer diseases. Gardening is a wonderful form of activity, as it keeps the body moving and limber while it also provides an opportunity to be out in the sunshine and fresh air. Walking a dog is another great way to get up and get out, and even doing household chores counts as physical activity, too. It's even been shown that we benefit simply from standing rather than sitting, so making a point of standing up when you take a phone call or attend a meeting or watch TV is also beneficial.

Dancing through Fear

Deborah Cohan, MD, is an obstetrician and gynecologist and professor at the University of California San Francisco School of Medicine. She is also the mother of two young kids. And she knows firsthand how profoundly healing movement can be.

In September 2013, at the age of forty-four, she was diagnosed with stage IIB breast cancer. She got the news just after dropping her daughter off at school, and so she called her boss and took the day off. That evening, she went to a Soul Motion class, a form of conscious dance, which she refers to as her "weekly sacred ritual." She walked into class that evening filled with nearly overwhelming fear: Would she leave her children motherless? Would she be disfigured? Would she be unlovable? Would she die alone? But she didn't go to distract herself from these fears; instead, she let her body, through this deeply transformative practice, draw her deep into and ultimately through those fears.

Cohan allowed her body to feel all the emotions that her diagnosis brought and to express those emotions through dance. While she initially felt numb and detached from her body, by the end of the class, she had come to a new place, remarkably to a place of joy. "In effect, my body was teaching my mind that I could feel joy," Cohan explains, "even within just a few hours of getting diagnosed with cancer."

Cohan took this cathartic experience as a sign that dance would be her medicine. Her cancer became a wake-up call to prioritize self-care and pay attention to her physical, emotional, mental, and spiritual health. She started dancing every day to help her work through the complex emotions that came with her diagnosis that she couldn't express with words alone. Her friends, who were helping her with her kids and driving her to her appointments, kept asking, "What else can I do?" Cohan realized that what she wanted more than anything was to be surrounded by joy and love, so she asked her friends to dance for and with her. She discovered a Beyoncé song she found inspirational called "Get Me Bodied," and she asked all her friends to record themselves dancing to it, so she could watch them dancing while she was recovering from surgery. She created a social media page and invited all her friends to join her virtual dance party. Then Cohan took it a step further. She asked her anesthesiologist if she could come into the operating room dancing to "Get Me Bodied." He agreed. The day before her surgery, Cohan rented a studio and with a close friend danced to the Beyoncé song until, as she puts it, "the joy I experienced was imprinted on my body."

The next day, she walked into the operating room totally unmedicated and calm. When "Get Me Bodied" started playing, the imprinted joy filled her body and she danced with the entire operating room team, filled with feelings of joy and freedom. The anesthesiologist videotaped the operating room flash mob, and one of Cohan's friends posted it to YouTube while she was undergoing surgery. "When I woke up, it had gone viral," Cohan explains. To date, Cohan's video of an entire operating team dancing to Beyoncé before her surgery has been viewed more than eight million times.

Cohan became something of an instant celebrity, and she used this newfound platform to talk about the multidimensional nature of healing and how finding peace and joy through movement can actually be very powerful medicine. She continued to dance during her four rounds of chemotherapy that followed her surgery. In 2014, she created the Foundation for Embodied Medicine, a nonprofit program affiliated with Commonweal (Michael Lerner's program), to offer dance and movement practices for patients, caregivers, and medical professionals so that they can experience the body's innate wisdom and healing guidance.[93]

Negative Comparisons

In a 2017 study published in the journal *Health Psychology*, Stanford University School of Business PhD candidate Octavia Zahrt and psychologist Alia Crum looked at data from the National Health Interview Survey and the National Health and Nutrition Examination Survey, and they found that "individuals who thought they were less active than other people their age were more likely to die, regardless of health status, body mass index, and so on," Crum reported.[94] What they found is that there is a kind of negative placebo effect that happens when people compare themselves to others—even when their perceptions are all in their head. How much you think you exercise is not as consequential to your long-term health as your actual level of physical activity, but the fact that it can have measurable negative consequences is worth noting. Part of what may be "psyching people out" is the pressure they feel if someone tells them they need to work out. If we feel pressured, even bullied, it just makes us feel lousy and it undermines our efforts to make anticancer living lifestyle changes. What is most important is that you engage in activities that bring you pleasure and make you feel good. These are strong indicators that you're giving your body exactly what it needs, whether it's a leisurely walk, a 100-mile bike ride, or a mind-blowing hour of HIIT (high-intensity interval training).

In Blue Zone areas, where residents routinely live to be more than one hundred years old, Dan Buettner notes that they don't differentiate between life and activity—it's all one and the same.[95] In these small pockets of health, moving freely and naturally is the name of the game.

How Much Is Enough?

The American Cancer Society recommends that cancer patients aim for 150 minutes, or 2.5 hours, of physical activity a week.[96] Broken down over seven days, this amount of time averages out to about twenty-two minutes a day. If you think about it this way, this is an incredibly doable goal. What's even better is that even those twenty-two minutes don't have to be done at once. In fact, research suggests that shorter bouts of exercise may have greater health benefits than longer endurance workouts.[97] A 2016 study by Martin Gibala and his colleagues at McMaster University found that in previously sedentary individuals brief, but strenuous (ten minutes total, with only three twenty-second episodes of flat-out exertion) exercise bouts three times a week for twelve weeks resulted in similar improvements in physiological and biological measures of fitness compared to those who exercised forty-five minutes a week for twelve weeks.[98] Previous research found the same effect for three ten-minute walks compared to a thirty-minute walk in adults with borderline hypertension.[99] The shorter walks had the same effect on blood pressure, but unlike the thirty-minute walk, they also reduced spikes in blood pressure, and so they had greater implications for overall health. We also know that simply sitting less and moving more is the ideal approach, as research suggests that: walking more and sitting less is even healthier for you than exercising an hour a day if you are then sedentary for fourteen hours; replacing thirty minutes of sedentary time with light activity will reduce mortality risk; and short bouts of activity will result in reduced inflammation.[63,100–104]

Alison and I believe that the best coach is our own body, so listen to your body and respond to its requests and needs. If you feel strong, balanced, flexible, and confident, you're likely on the right track. Getting aerobic exercise (elevating your heart rate) on a regular basis is important, as is keeping your muscle strength up.

Though the bulk of research on the effect of exercise on cancer outcomes has centered on breast cancer patients, Gabe Canales, whose story we shared in chapter 3, is actively working to change that. September is Prostate Cancer Awareness Month, and through his nonprofit Blue Cure, Gabe and his team are creating programs and events that are not only raising awareness around this type of cancer, which is the third leading cause of death in America (one in seven men will be diagnosed at some point in their lives), but also teaching people how to prevent prostate cancer through lifestyle changes.[105]

Gabe Canales's Bike

When we spoke recently, Gabe, who is now forty-two and who has PSA levels that are lower than they were before he was diagnosed at age thirty-five (and whose cancer has remained inactive), told me managing the stress that comes with knowing, every day, that he is living with cancer, has been his biggest challenge. It's also inspired him to reach out to men and boys in unique and highly effective ways by tapping into places where men come together—which means bringing the prevention and anticancer lifestyle message to sports fields, tracks, and stadiums across the country. Blue Cure has professional athletes on its board of directors, and the organization hosts night runs and basketball camps, and has partnered with professional soccer and the AAU (the Amateur Athletic Union) to spread the word about healthy lifestyle habits helping to prevent prostate onset and improve outcomes.

When Gabe started this work, he changed his life wholesale: He sold his big house in the Houston suburbs and bought a one-bedroom apartment in the city so he'd be closer to the Blue Cure offices. The early years of the organization were super lean. (He gave up an impressive salary as president of his own PR firm to not drawing a salary at all in the initial stages of founding a nonprofit.)

He remembers a pivotal moment when he was about to sign a lease for a new Chevy Tahoe. He had the pen in his hand and was getting ready to put his name on the contract, when he started to think about all the stress he had when he was driving, how he was always either texting or on the phone, always racing to the next meeting. As he thought about these things he could feel his stress increasing, his blood was pounding, and his breathing was shallow. With everything he was going through, Gabe realized in that moment that he had to find a way to get more grounded and reduce his stress, and buying a new Chevy Tahoe was not a step in that direction. He put the pen down and stood up, "You know what? I'm not going to do this." The dealer looked up at Gabe and said, "What are you going to do?" To which Gabe replied, "I'm going to buy a bicycle."

Three years later, Gabe bikes an average of fifteen miles a day. So far, the change has not only modified his mind-set and improved his health, it has also had a positive PR impact on his nonprofit, showing that, when it comes to anticancer living, Gabe is more than just talk. "If I walk into a meeting with my bike helmet under my arm and casual clothes on, people get it," he explains. "I'm promoting an anticancer lifestyle and I think it really helps people to get on board to see that I'm actually living it."

As Gabe's example illustrates, nothing makes us feel more at ease in our body than testing out its physical potential. I'm convinced that when we try any kind of new activity—but especially something that asks us to move— we're activating our senses in ways that positively impact all aspects of the anticancer living Mix of Six. It's all about achieving a state of healthy balance and disease-free longevity.

THE ANTICANCER LIVING GUIDE TO EXERCISE

Exercise as part of an anticancer lifestyle is all about putting movement back into your day—more time standing and moving, less time sitting and being idle. While this sounds simple enough, in our culture, being active requires you not only to move but also to move against the grain.

Monitor Your Daily Movement

Start by honestly assessing or evaluating your physical activity. We like this step because you have to know where you are to know where you want to go. Simply keep track of how many steps you take and how many hours you sit each day on average:

- Monitor your steps—most phones have a step program, or consider purchasing an activity monitor. It is truly the best way to know how many steps you take in a day.
- Along with your steps, keep track of your sitting time for a week.

After monitoring your activity for a week, answer the following questions:

- What can you do to simply increase your movement each day?
- If you already have an exercise routine, what can you do to make the rest of your day include more movement?
- By increasing movement, you increase steps taken in a day. There is no magic number of needed steps. The number is simply more than what you were doing before. Some aim for ten thousand steps—five miles—per day, but this practice is more about increasing your individual activity levels.

Break Up Your Sitting Time

Based on multiple studies, we encourage you to break up your sitting time by at least standing up:

- Don't do this once in a while, but hourly.
- Standing will feel strange at first, but stick with it. As with most habits, after your body gets used to standing up, you will start to prefer this to sitting down to do work.
- The ironing board is a great (and cheap) substitute for a stand-up desk at home and allows you to spread out your work.
- Try standing when you watch television or shows on your computer.
- Consider buying a laptop desk (which start at around forty dollars) and can be carried to and from work easily.
- Think about your children. School-age children need stand-up desks. They sit most of the day and then come home and sit for most of the evening—doing homework, playing video games, eating dinner, or watching TV.
- Get in the habit of standing when you are attending events or out on the town. Stand at the back of the lecture hall, stand during intermission of a performance, stand during meetings, encourage others to stand after meeting for an extended period, engage your friends and coworkers in standing and walking more.

Walk Instead of Sitting

- Don't do this occasionally, do this every day, at least once every one to two hours, even if you are merely walking around your house, around the block, or around the office.
- Take the stairs at work, at the movie theater, at the airport, at doctors' appointments—anytime you are going up or down, use the stairs.
- Conduct walking meetings. Carry a clipboard to take notes. If someone at work wants to discuss an idea, suggest that you walk outside as you talk.
- Park away from your destination and walk a few extra steps.
- Walk to work, if possible, or bike.

- Walk after dinner with those you care about—it allows you time to catch up and connect. Walking after a meal (especially a big meal) helps your body process food and could keep older people from developing diabetes.
- Listen to a book on tape while you walk.

Develop a Fitness Routine

- When you are ready for aerobic training and fitness, we suggest finding a friend to join you. For Alison, having a workout partner is an essential part of improving her fitness that helps keep her motivated and makes her responsible to someone other than herself.
- Start with something easily accessible that works with your schedule and temperament. Alison admires the runners who jog by our house every morning and evening, but she has no desire to be one of them. Be honest with yourself about what you want to do and what you can sustain. You don't have to run a marathon. You just have to find a way to move more that works for you. Establish a short exercise routine you can follow with a friend, online or via DVD.
- Work on your flexibility and range of motion. Our joints thrive on being used and lubricated. Engage in activities that encourage lots of full range-of-motion movements, such as swimming or yoga.
- Build your strength and your stamina. Resistance work is great for building muscle mass and protecting bone health. And your own body is your best source of resistance. A near perfect exercise is the simple plank. This activates your large muscle groups and builds arm strength. You can include free weights or resistance bands to create more tension on the muscles.

Break Up Your Day with Exercise Bursts

- Use short workouts to break up your day instead of long, endurance-style workouts at the gym. Three brisk ten-minute walks help to break up a long day of sitting.
- If you like to run, a series of short sprints burns more calories than a long jog.

- Consider adopting an intense seven-to-ten-minute workout that you can return to and repeat on a consistent basis. This helps not only your muscles but also your heart. The most popular models require only a chair to complete and involve a series of exercises performed in a row, with thirty seconds of rest between each.

Model an Active Lifestyle

- Incorporate movement as a part of your family plans.
- When you are taking a break from the routine or celebrating an individual achievement, involve physical movement, whether it's a trip to the park or a day at the beach.
- Have fun. Running around with your kids or kicking a soccer ball with a group of old friends on the weekend count. Being active is synonymous with being social, and both combined will up your anticancer living quotient.

Active Travel

For many of us, life on the road is part of the job. Finding ways to stay active when your normal routine is disrupted can be a challenge, but if you take a few small steps, you can ensure that you don't fall out of your healthy habits even when you're away from home.

Keep Moving on the Road

- Bring workout clothes and tennis or running shoes. I realize this sounds obvious, but I can't tell you how many times I've arrived somewhere that had the potential for a great hike or a hotel with a surprisingly good gym only to find that I did not pack an appropriate outfit. Don't let your clothes or lack of proper shoes hinder your ability to stay fit while you travel.
- Stand up periodically on long flights. I'm that guy who gets up and waits in line for the bathroom even if I don't really have to go, because it's often the only way to stand up during a flight without appearing to be a threat to passenger safety.

- Bring your routine with you. We recently had a visitor stay with us in Houston who had a sheet of paper with the 7-Minute Workout. He brought a chair out to the living room and, in less than ten minutes, went through his routine and worked every muscle group in his body while also increasing his heart rate.
- Resistance bands pack easily and can be used anywhere.
- Travel with a yoga mat to continue your morning practice.

You don't have to be an endurance athlete to see the benefits of physical exertion. In fact, being more active—sitting less, and taking regular breaks from sitting—is more important than pushing yourself to run farther or faster. Take small steps. Start today. The research shows that continuing our sedentary routines is killing us slowly. Form a habit that is good for you and will keep you getting up for years to come.

THE ANTICANCER LIVING GUIDE
EXERCISE SUMMARY

1. Keep a daily log of your physical activity for a week.
2. Find ways throughout your day to walk when you would normally be sitting.
3. Break up your sitting time by standing up every hour. Break up your day with short bursts of exercise.
4. Develop a fitness routine.
5. Incorporate physical activity into family events, time with friends, and trips.
6. Plan for exercise and find ways to stay physically active when you travel.

CHAPTER ELEVEN

Food as Medicine

W hy do we eat the way we do, in our particular place and time? How does the way we feed ourselves relate to our health and wellness? Food is the fuel that powers the human body. That, right there, is the basic biological fact. But at this juncture, a complex web of factors, from cultural traditions to convenience, affects our daily choices. Many of these are far from conscious awareness and have instead become automatic habits, aided and abetted by the food and advertising industries. Yet our bodies—and current scientific research—tell us something else, that it's time to become much more aware about what and how we are feeding ourselves. Whether you are a gourmet, a gardener, or a fast-food grabber, it's time to tune in to a growing body of research and thinking about food and healing and collectively turn the page on how we feed our bodies.

Recognizing Food's Healing Power

After Dorothy P. (who you met in chapter 7), was diagnosed with aggressive breast cancer in 1998, she underwent a year of intensive treatment that included taking corticosteroids, which are used during chemotherapy to help prevent nausea and vomiting. A common side effect of corticosteroids is weight gain. In the course of her treatment, Dorothy gained twenty-two pounds. When she was finished with her treatment and ready to lose that extra weight, Dorothy faced a realization—she couldn't go about this the way she once had. She couldn't simply starve herself to lose weight or eat only salads. This wasn't about fitting into a wedding dress or looking good in a bikini; this was something deeper. She needed food to help her recover—healthy food. As she puts it, "I had to start thinking about food as my friend." This fundamentally changed her relationship to eating.

At dinner every night, her kids, eleven and nine, made a game of counting how many different fruits and vegetables they could pack in a single meal. It became a challenge. On her own, Dorothy became a label reader. She avoided hydrogenated oils, sugars and chemicals, and processed foods of many types and started buying organic fruits and vegetables. Over time, it led to deep, sustainable change. She was no longer *dieting*, but eating to live.

As a by-product of her new dietary pattern, Dorothy lost weight, not quickly, but in a way that has allowed her to keep the weight off over the years since her initial diagnosis. More important, she has improved her health and given her body the nutrients it needs to stay healthy and strong. Another noteworthy side effect: Dorothy has passed on healthier eating habits to her children, who are now adults with families of their own, as well as to her ninety-year-old Texan father, who spent most of his life as a meat-and-potatoes guy. Her changes have had a cascading effect through her family.

Cancer as a Wake-Up Call

As with other areas of lifestyle, cancer has a way of sweeping aside cultural clutter and allowing us to see clearly how daily decisions impact our health. But all of us, whether or not we have cancer, need to reconnect with the true purpose of food, which is to nourish, heal, and sustain us. According to the most recent Dietary Guidelines published jointly by the U.S. Department of Health and Human Services and the U.S. Department of Agriculture, roughly half of U.S. adults have a chronic illness related to poor diet or lack of exercise, and more than two-thirds of adults are overweight or obese.[1] Only one in four Americans eats one fruit a day and only one in ten eats the recommended amount of vegetables.[1] In fact, Americans eat so few foods rich in antioxidants that beer represents the fifth-largest source of antioxidants in the standard American diet.[2,3] By contrast, the average amount of kale an American eats each week is half a teaspoon, even with the vegetable's newfound popularity in some circles.

Our CompLife Study participants face the temptation to eat unhealthy foods both within the halls of MD Anderson and at other hospitals where cafeterias offer fried chicken, french fries, and slices of restaurant-chain pizza. A few pioneering hospitals have come up with innovations such as planting organic vegetable gardens on-site, which has numerous benefits for the whole community.[4]

During the intensive six-week portion of our CompLife study, participants meet weekly with registered dietitian nutritionists and receive lessons on how to shop for healthy foods and how to cook those foods to maximize their nutritional value and make them taste delicious. When they return home, which for most means a small, close-knit town in Texas or Louisiana, participants often find their refrigerators and freezers stuffed full of the very foods we've been telling them not to eat. Here they are trying to make sustainable changes to the way they eat (for many the hardest component of the program), and they arrive back home to find an abundance of creamy casseroles, lasagna, and pies—"comfort food"—often prepared by caring, empathic friends. So we try to troubleshoot for this, too. Friends and family genuinely want to be helpful, and with a few simple guidelines, what's waiting in the fridge can be healthy and sustaining as well as delicious and comforting.

The idea that food that is bad for us will make us feel better is a strange idea but one that is thoroughly ingrained in our culture. And we are not only spreading the Western diet to each other but also exporting our unhealthy diet to the world. It is no coincidence that cancer and other chronic diseases are taking hold in the very places where the Western diet is most readily adopted.[5] In fact, cancer rates are on the rise in countries that once had the lowest rates in the world (breast cancer in China and India and colon cancer in Japan).[6] What's more, the increasing incidence is concentrated in urban centers, where people are most exposed to fast food and highly processed food.[7,8]

The dangers of exporting American eating habits were illustrated dramatically in a 2015 study that had African Americans and a rural tribe in South Africa switch diets.[9] Stephen O'Keefe, a professor at the University of Pittsburgh School of Medicine, wanted to know why South Africans have such healthy colons and such a low risk of colon cancer, whereas African Americans have the greatest risk of colon cancer of any race in the United States. O'Keefe and his colleagues had twenty people in each country switch diets for two weeks. The South Africans ate a high-fat, low-fiber, high-animal-protein diet that included things like pancakes and sausage for breakfast, burgers and fries for lunch, and meatloaf and rice for dinner. Meanwhile, African Americans in the study ate the typical low-fat, high-fiber diet of South Africans—foods such as hi-maize corn fritters and salmon croquettes for breakfast; fish tacos, homemade Tater Tots, and mango slices for lunch; and okra, tomatoes, black-eyed peas, and pineapple for dinner. After only fourteen days on the new diet, researchers noted profound changes in each group. The African American participants experienced rapid changes in their intestinal biology and microbiome (the bacterial balance in their gut). Risk factors associated with colon cancer, like inflammation, decreased. Meanwhile, the South Africans had changes in their intestines associated with increased colon cancer risk. In support of these findings, a recent study summarizing the findings of research that included more than 800,000 people found that those eating a diet characterized as causing inflammation had an increased risk of colorectal cancer (51 percent for men and 25 percent for women).[10]

The extent to which an unhealthy diet is a part of our Western culture is disconcerting, but it does not have to be permanent. As is graphically illustrated in the South African study, changing to healthier foods that nourish the body can have a dramatic impact, and the effect can take hold quickly. As O'Keefe explains, "In just two weeks, a change in diet from a Westernized composition to a traditional African high-fiber, low-fat diet reduced these biomarkers of cancer risk, indicating that it is likely never too late to modify the risk of colon cancer."

Managing Your Microbiome

One of the most noteworthy results from the South African diet study is how quickly nutritional shifts (both good and bad) could impact the ecosystem of bacteria, fungi, and viruses—living on and inside our bodies—known as the microbiome. Even if you take baths daily, brush your teeth, and wash your hands, you are walking around accompanied by your own unique ecosphere of microbes, roughly a hundred trillion bacteria, some good, some bad. In fact, our human cells are outnumbered ten to one by these nonhuman cells along for the ride. Mapping the microbiome, like the genome-mapping project, is an ongoing global effort.[11–13]

An unhealthy microbiome has now been linked with multiple diseases and conditions, including clostridium difficile infection, psoriasis, reflux esophagitis, obesity, childhood-onset asthma, gastrointestinal disorders, neuropsychiatric illness like depression and anxiety, multi-drug-resistant organisms, cardiovascular disease, and cancer. Research also points to a link between gut bacterium and the key hormones ghrelin and leptin, which regulate appetite.[14,15]

Study after study shows the greater the diversity of our microbiome, the better the health outcomes.[16–18] Increased diversity is also linked with lower overall body fat, decreased insulin resistance, and a decreased inflammatory profile, one of the cancer hallmarks and a profile linked with lower cancer risk.[16–18] Research shows a clear connection between the microbiome and a number of different cancers, including colon, liver, pancreatic, lung, and breast, as well as emerging data in melanoma.[19–21]

While human studies haven't conclusively shown a causal link between the microbiome and cancer, studies involving animals have been able to draw a more direct link. Multiple mechanisms link the microbiome and cancer,[22,23] one of which is increased inflammatory processes.[22] The immune system is closely connected to the microbiome. In fact, scientists now believe important aspects of our immune system and immune response reside in our gut.[24,25] Gut-based microbiota play an essential role in activating, training, and modulating the immune response.[25,26] The microbiome likely influences carcinogenesis through additional mechanisms that remain to be discovered. In the meantime, immunologic dysregulation is likely to provide important insights into how our microbiome influences cancer development and cancer therapies.

It may sound obvious, but it is important to note that what we eat has a direct impact on our microbiome, and evidence is mounting that creating and maintaining a healthy microbiome could play a significant role in the effectiveness of cancer treatment. One of my colleagues at MD Anderson, Jennifer Wargo, is at the forefront of microbiome research. In a 2017 study of patients with advanced melanoma, Wargo found that the diversity and makeup of someone's gut bacteria affects how well they respond to immunotherapy.[27] Her findings suggest that the immune system is aided by certain microbes when responding to immunotherapy drugs. While more research is needed before people rush to the store to purchase probiotics in hopes of improving their response to cancer treatment, the research points to clear benefits from maintaining a healthy microbiome. The more diverse the microbiome, the lower the inflammation in the body and the healthier the immune system.

Adopting the Plant-Based Diet

The key to creating a healthy microbiome without going overboard with untested supplements and pills is to feed the good bacteria in your body and crowd out the bad by eating a plant-centered, high-fiber diet rich in whole grains and complex carbohydrates.[28,29] In fact, a landmark animal study published in *Science* in 2013 found that when mice were fed the standard American diet and then had a healthy microbiome transplanted into their gut, the microbiota would not colonize.[30] They recognized their new environment as an unsuitable place to live and grow.

The diet that has shown the greatest benefit in terms of health and cancer resistance is the Mediterranean diet, as was also noted by David Servan-Schreiber in *Anticancer*.[31] As the son of Italian and American parents who wrote two popular cookbooks on Mediterranean cooking in the 1980s, I hold a special place in my heart for a diet heavy in vegetables, olive oil, whole grains, and nuts. As a teenager, I was lucky enough to serve as a taste tester for an incredible variety of vegetarian soups, entrées, and side dishes. Research has long connected the Mediterranean diet with reduced risk of cardiovascular disease and diabetes. More recent studies point to potential impacts on cancer risk and connections to brain health.[32–37] A 2015 study analyzing the diets of more than five thousand Italian women found that those who followed the Mediterranean diet most closely had a 57 percent reduced risk of endometrial cancer.[38] They also reported a dose-response effect. Those who followed the diet most closely had a substantial cancer risk reduction, while those who followed the diet less stringently had only moderate risk reduction.

A 2017 study by researchers in the Netherlands found a clear association between the Mediterranean diet and the risk of postmenopausal breast cancer.[39] Researchers used data from the Netherlands Cohort Study involving more than sixty-two thousand women between the ages of fifty-five and sixty-nine and tracked their dietary and lifestyle habits over the course of twenty years. They found that, with estrogen receptor negative breast cancer, which generally has a poorer prognosis, adhering to a Mediterranean diet reduced risk by about 40 percent relative to those not adhering to a Mediterranean diet. Moreover, for both estrogen receptor positive and negative breast cancer, the higher the adherence to the Mediterranean diet, the lower the risk of breast cancer.

WHY FOOD IS BETTER THAN SUPPLEMENTS

I consciously decided to forgo adding supplements to the CompLife Study protocol, just as I'm suggesting now that you begin your anticancer diet without them. Food is designed specifically to deliver nutrients to the body in the most efficient and usable way. That's not to say that supplementation isn't often warranted (I encourage patients with low vitamin D, for instance, to take additional D, given that we know it is linked to the onset of certain cancers).[40] But we tend to put too much faith in pills and elixirs instead of trusting that food—our daily diet—will, over time, give us everything we need. I'm a true believer that most of us can get everything we need when we hone our skill for choosing the widest variety of nutrient-dense foods possible. For people undergoing cancer treatment, it is ideal to consult with a registered dietitian nutritionist certified as a specialist in oncology (CSO).

A key aspect of the Mediterranean diet is consumption of vegetables and fruits. When it comes to fruit and vegetable intake, the evidence suggests more might be better. A meta-analysis of ninety-five prospective cohort studies found that people who regularly eat ten portions of fruit and vegetables a day have significantly lower risk of chronic diseases, including heart disease and cancer.[41] Researchers found that for each additional 200 grams of fruit and vegetable intake (two portions) cancer risk went down by 3 percent. They concluded that 7.8 million early deaths from cancer, heart disease, stroke, and all causes could have been prevented by people eating ten portions a day of fruit and vegetables. Adding to this evidence is a startling 2017 study that shows diet quality in teen and early adult years predicts risk of breast cancer later in life.[42] The study, conducted by Karin Michels and her colleagues at UCLA, tracked more than forty-five thousand women enrolled in the Nurses' Health Study II over the course of twenty-two years. Researchers scored diets based on the degree to which they were *inflammatory*. Compared to the women with diets with a low inflammatory score, those with the most inflammatory diets during their teenage years had a 35 percent higher risk of breast cancer. Similarly, those in the highest inflammatory group during their early adult years had a 41 percent higher risk of developing breast cancer than women who reported eating more anti-inflammatory foods when they were younger.

These were observational studies. But a large randomized controlled study conducted in Spain published in 2013 examined the effects of a Mediterranean diet supplemented with extra virgin olive oil versus a Mediterranean diet supplemented with extra nuts compared to a moderately reduced fat diet in men and women at risk for heart disease to see if they could decrease the incidence of major cardiovascular events. The study worked, and they reported in the *New England Journal of Medicine* that both Mediterranean diet groups resulted in fewer strokes across a four-year follow-up period.[43]

From this same clinical trial, the authors have reported that the Mediterranean diet led to reduced weight, lower rates of diabetes, reversed metabolic syndrome, decreased oxidative stress, and lower levels of C-reactive protein (a general measure of systemic inflammation).[44–47] Most important for us in the cancer world, women who were randomly assigned to the Mediterranean diet high in extra virgin olive oil reduced their breast cancer risk by over 70 percent over the course of five years compared to the control group that ate the moderately reduced fat diet.[48] So it seems that what's good for the heart is likely also good for the prevention of cancer.[49]

Evidence is also mounting that a plant-based diet is important to adopt post-diagnosis for a number of different cancers. A 2015 study found that men diagnosed with prostate cancer were more than 50 percent less likely to die from the disease if they followed a "prudent diet," rich in fruit, vegetables, and whole grains and low in fat, sugar, cholesterol, and sodium.[50] On the flip side, the same study, which involved more than twenty-two thousand male physicians, found that those who stuck with a typical Western diet were over 2.5 times more likely to die from prostate cancer.

One of the reasons why the Mediterranean diet, or the very similar prudent diet, in study after study is consistently linked with good health may be in part attributable to modifications in key cancer hallmarks, including decreases in angiogenesis, improvements in immune function, and decreases in overall inflammatory load. Dark-green leafy vegetables, such as the cruciferous vegetables, whole grains, and other high-fiber foods are great sources of micronutrients and phytochemicals and are linked to lower levels of multiple inflammatory markers.[51–54] Vegetables and fruits are not only rich in vitamins and minerals but also contain antioxidants, which may play a role in preventing the early stages of cancer.[55–57] Importantly, cruciferous vegetables in particular have a high level of indole compounds such as sulforaphanes, phytonutrients found to be effective in fighting the growth and development of cancer through reduced cell proliferation, inflammation, and epigenetic biomarkers.[58-60] The other benefits of a high-vegetable diet are its low-calorie and carbohydrate content and low glycemic index, which are linked with decreased inflammation. In fact, dietary factors influence all the cancer hallmarks, either in a favorable way when eating for health and to decrease tumorigenic processes or eating in an unhealthy way that increases tumorigenic processes. [55,60-77]

The Mediterranean diet also reflects a more natural, relaxed interplay between humans and the immediate environment they live in. Historically, Mediterranean cultures eat what is readily available to them, which means they eat what is seasonally grown, what can be caught from the sea, what can be farmed or raised on a small plot (including chickens), or what can be harvested nearby. Of course, this has changed as industrial farming has spread to even remote corners of the globe, but fortunately for all of us, the key principles of the Mediterranean diet (and culture) remain intact.

The same can be said of most healthy diets across the globe—Mediterranean diet, Asian diet, or South African rural diet. There are similarities in all these largely plant-based diets: They include vegetables, fruits, nuts, seeds, whole grains, and other fiber-rich foods, and minimal servings of animal protein, processed foods, and added sugars. Eating in this manner helps to keep our microbiome well fed. While the names and details might differ, the basics of these diets are largely the same.

Healthy Diets, Different Names

A great example of this overarching pattern of healthy diets can be seen clearly in the Blue Zones,[78] communities scattered around the world where residents frequently live to a hundred years of age, with little or no incidence of disease. On the face of it, the diets of Blue Zone residents couldn't be more different: In Loma Linda, California, the community, which is centered around the Seventh Day Adventist Church, favors a vegan diet. In Sardinia, Italy, the standard diet is high in oils and fats, but the healthy oils and fats found in nuts and olives. Costa Ricans who live in Nicoya favor a diet that includes meats but is high in vegetables, especially the flourishing indigenous tuberous kinds. In Okinawa, Japan, the emphasis is on fresh fish and vegetables and starches, like rice, but low in fat. In Ikaria, Greece, the diet is the closest to the classic Mediterranean. While on the surface all five

Blue Zone diets seem remarkably different, what they have in common is an emphasis on local, fresh, whole foods and a near wholesale absence of processed foods. In other words, they share the same principles of the Mediterranean diet but with food choices that best exemplify what is available, based on their local culture, climate, and environment. Although we can't say with absolute certainty that these dietary patterns decrease one's risk for developing cancer or improving outcomes for those with cancer, the overwhelming evidence gathered to date certainly points in this direction.

I recently spoke to David Katz, MD, about the similarities between different healthy diets, and he shared a similar observation he had when he attended a recent gathering of experts at the Oldways Common Ground conference. There were breakout sessions on various diets, each touting the specific benefits of focusing in one area. The Paleo advocate talked about animal protein, while the vegan group discussed dairy-related inflammation, and those in the Mediterranean diet session heard about healthy fats. When everyone broke for lunch, Katz noticed that their plates looked nearly identical. Everyone had a lot of vegetables and salad, a small portion of protein, some fats and some grains. "In the end, we were all on the same page thematically and this struck me as the key takeaway," Katz explained. "There's so much noise in the nutrition diet arena but there just doesn't have to be. I realized that we create a lot of confusion when what we're all aiming for is simply this: we need to eat *wholesome foods in sensible combinations.*"

This healthier plant-centered dietary pattern, no matter how you label it, runs contrary to what the culture promotes and what is often the easiest choice in terms of what we eat and drink. For most of my life, I participated in an addictive food culture that feeds our cravings for sugar, salt, and fat. I was once questioned about eating this way during a cancer conference, and responded, "Those are the rules for cancer patients. We don't have cancer." But what I have come to realize is that we must take a more proactive approach to healthy eating if we hope to lower our cancer risk and improve our chances of surviving a cancer diagnosis. David Servan-Schreiber's mantra still rings true—cancer lives in all of us, but not all of us will get cancer. We can reduce the likelihood that those cells will activate and multiply by the lifestyle choices we make every day—and our nutritional choices are key.

Unplugging the Donut Machine

It was the summer of 2015 when a colleague emailed me a photo of the do-nut machine with the subject line: "Good for Business." When I realized this contraption was on MD Anderson's grounds, I went immediately to see for myself. The aroma of fresh donuts greeted me even before I caught a glimpse of a brightly colored cart on rollers, that said "Dough'Yo on the Go" on its side, surrounded by a throng of hospital workers in scrubs and patients with excited children. The cart was positioned on the sky bridge outside the parking garage that leads to the main hospital and the faculty/staff building. The location is directly outside a top-tier hotel, where patients stay with their families during cancer treatment.

It was a surreal moment for me. We face so many rules and regulations at MD Anderson. If you wanted to serve fresh vegetable juice on campus, I can't tell you how many committees there are from which you'd have to seek approval or how many details would have to be worked out (we tried, in fact, but in the end we were defeated by concerns about the risks of unpasteurized food). But if someone wants to roll a donut machine into the main thoroughfare where faculty, staff, patients, and their families pass on their way to and from their cars, apparently they could just plug it in, turn it on, and let the show begin.

The man operating the machine, the executive chef from the hotel chain next door, was beaming with pride. When I asked if this was to be a permanent fixture at the hospital, he said, "It's a very expensive machine. We'll have to sell a lot of donuts, if it's going to last." No doubt he was thinking I would rush back to my office and call an emergency staff meeting, "Hey, folks. This is important. We all need to eat more donuts!" From the look of things, this was, in fact, the response he was having so far on his opening day. And I have to admit that I felt overpowered. Everyone seemed so happy. The smiling face of the executive chef who was handing out pink bags of sugar-coated fried dough as fast as he could make them, the big eyes of the waiting hospital workers and patients, all spelled a big success for a daily dose of grease, carbs, and sugar.

After taking a few pictures, I did return to my office but, rather than urging on the pace of donut consumption, I fired off an email to Dr. Ron DePinho, who was president of MD Anderson at the time. For the record, I am not in the habit of dashing off emails to the hospital president. But I cannot stand idly by knowing what I know about the connection between diet and disease. We now know that obesity is linked to thirteen types of cancer and accounts for one in five cancers globally.[79,80] When you add a sedentary lifestyle to an unhealthy diet, cancer risk increases by more than 30 percent.[81] That means almost a third of all cancers could be prevented if people ate a healthy diet and stayed active. In fact, if every adult in the United States reduced his or her body mass index (BMI) by 1 percent (losing just over two pounds each), the National Cancer Institute estimates it would result in the avoidance of one hundred thousand new cancer cases (of the additional half million new cases predicted by 2030 in the United States).[6,82–85]

Despite these incredible statistics about how much cancer could be avoided if people ate more vegetables and fewer donuts, the prevailing tendency is to blame cancer on causes beyond our immediate control: our genes, genetically modified foods, hormone-injected meat, air pollution, and so on. The latest Cancer Risk Awareness Survey from the American Institute for Cancer Research shows that fewer than half of Americans are aware that diets low in vegetables and fruit increase cancer risk and only half know of the link between obesity and cancer.[86] Only one in three know that eating a diet high in red or processed meat has been repeatedly tied to colon cancer.

So, while the evidence continues to mount about the connection between diet and cancer, what gets through to the public is murky and fragmented. Hospital staff waiting in the "Dough'Yo" line could have been discussing their patients or talking about their daily rounds without the slightest sense of contradiction or irony. Patients might have been lamenting their next round of chemotherapy without any sense that what they were about to eat could counteract the intended effect of chemotherapy to reduce the size of their tumor before surgery.

But with those happy smiles looming before me, I composed my email without much hope of being heard.

Much to my amazement, when I returned from vacation, the donut machine was gone. The president had written, thanking me for "being such a great watchdog," but I imagine far more people considered me a buzzkill or party pooper. The truth is, I don't want to be either of those things, but in the current climate, I often find myself in such roles. When you're up against multibillion-dollar industries intent on addicting us to potentially lethal products, banishing the donut machine was for me more than just a symbolic victory.

Not So Sweet: The Dangers of Sugar

An example of powerful forces we are up against became clear in a 2016 study by researchers at the University of California, San Francisco, who examined internal sugar industry documents from the 1960s and '70s. The documents revealed a campaign of disinformation that looks eerily similar to the effort by the tobacco industry to downplay the dangers of smoking. Fifty years ago, the sugar industry sponsored a research program to cast doubt on the role of sugar in heart disease risk and to promote fat as the dietary culprit.[87] Studies linking sugar to cancer also did not see the light of day.[88] That campaign was largely successful and led to a series of recommendations based on the role of fat and cholesterol in heart disease while downplaying the role of sucrose.

But while fat consumption has gone down, the epidemic of heart disease and other chronic diseases, including cancer, has continued to grow,[89-92] along with our consumption of vast amounts of sugar that were added to foods to replace the fat. The average American now consumes around twenty-three teaspoons of sugar per day, more than twice the daily intake recommended by the World Health Organization and more than three times the amount recommended for women by the American Heart Association.[93]

While the idea that "sugar feeds cancer" is still disputed by many oncologists as an oversimplification, research in the past ten years suggests a clear connection between high blood-sugar levels and certain types of cancer.[94-100] In a 2011 study, researchers at the Albert Einstein College of Medicine in New York City analyzed health data from forty-five hundred postmenopausal women over a twelve-year period and found that those with the highest blood-sugar levels were twice as likely to develop colon cancer.[101] In a long-term study published in 2012, Swedish researchers showed that men who drank one twelve-ounce soda a day increased their risk of prostate cancer by 40 percent.[102] For that study, scientists tracked the health of more than eight thousand men between the ages of forty-three and seventy-five over the course of fifteen years. They also found the increased risk was connected with faster-growing forms of prostate cancer, which are more likely to be fatal.

While proving a direct link between cancer and sugar requires more research, the connection between sugar intake and the international explosion of type 2 diabetes is beyond question. Type 2 diabetes affects more than 420 million people, almost one in ten adults worldwide,[103,104] and people with diabetes are almost twice as likely to be diagnosed with pancreatic and colon cancer.[105] So, even if you remain unconvinced about the implicit dangers of sugar, it's hard to ignore or downplay the path to cancer through diabetes as a real and dangerous trend.[106]

THE ALCOHOL QUANDARY

Alcohol is listed by the National Toxicology Program as a known human carcinogen.[107] The more someone drinks, the higher their risk of developing certain types of cancers, including head and neck, esophageal, liver, stomach, breast, and colorectal.[108–112] In 2009, an estimated 3.5 percent of cancer deaths in the United States were alcohol related.[113] The latest research suggests that even moderate alcohol use increases cancer risk and the risk of death from cancer.[107,113,114] A study published in 2013 found that those who consume three or more drinks a day account for a majority of alcohol-related cancer deaths.[113] But the study, which involved researchers in the United States, Canada, and France, also concluded that those who drink 1.5 drinks a day or less account for more than a third of alcohol-related cancer deaths. So, when it comes to cancer, the less you drink, the better, and perhaps it is prudent to remove this risk factor altogether.

If your cancer is not on the list with identified ties to alcohol, something to consider is that alcohol is sugar, sugar causes inflammation, and we know cancer is an inflammatory disease. If you consume alcohol at all, the American Institute for Cancer Research (AICR) recommends no more than one drink a day for women and not more than two a day for men. And to decrease that sugar spike, make sure you do not drink on an empty stomach. If you drink alcohol, it's better to consume like Europeans do—with a meal.

Reducing Your Glycemic Load

Sugar isn't the only culprit behind blood-sugar spikes. Highly processed and refined foods like white bread, white rice, breakfast cereals, and crackers have what is called a high glycemic index.[115] That means the body can digest these foods and convert them into sugar quickly, literally within moments after they are consumed. So, just like eating candy or drinking soda, eating foods with a high glycemic index creates blood-sugar spikes, which lead to the release of insulin and the increase of ß-catenin, a protein known to be a major factor in the development of certain cancers.[116,117] A 2016 study headed by my colleague at MD Anderson Xifeng Wu, MD, PhD, found that patients eating foods with the highest glycemic index had an almost 50 percent greater chance of developing lung cancer compared to those with the lowest glycemic index.[118] For people who never smoked and had the highest glycemic index, their increase in lung cancer risk was more than 80 percent.[118]

SUGAR SUBSTITUTES

At every talk Alison and I give where we discuss the harms of excess sugar consumption, someone will invariably ask, "What about the calorie-free, zero glycemic-load sugars?" These noncaloric sweeteners fall into two main categories: (1) natural sugar substitutes such as stevia, xylitol, and some of the other sugar alcohols, also appearing in a processed form, for example, Erythritol, or (2) artificial sugar substitutes such as saccharin, acesulfame, aspartame, neotame, and sucralose. There is contradictory research linking the artificial sugar substitutes with increased cancer risk. To date, there have been no such studies linking the naturally derived sweeteners with cancer. Unfortunately, simply substituting a sweetener, either artificial or real, may not be as effective as we would like in terms of weight loss. (This is, after all, why most people turn to sweeteners, to get the sweet taste with no calories or weight gain.) In fact, these sugar substitutes might actually desensitize the brain's reward response, resulting in increased food consumption.[119-121] That means that tricking the brain with no-calorie sweeteners could actually backfire. Some sugar substitutes have been associated with weight gain, glucose intolerance, and even diabetes.[119-121] The ideal approach is to retrain your sweet tooth and tame your sugar addiction.

Similar data exist for a link between sugar, glycemic load, and the risk of prostate, breast, ovarian, colon, and endometrial cancers.[94–96,122,123]

Given the extent of research and the growing understanding of the role of highly processed carbohydrates and sugar in cancer risk and outcomes, why does it seem so normal, even comforting, to encounter free candy at a doctor's office, or, for that matter, donuts in the lunch room? Why is the message about sugar and refined carbs not getting through to the public, or even penetrating into the offices of our top cancer centers?

The Dangers of Red and Processed Meats

Although the messages coming at us daily about our diet and what is and is not healthy seems to be a moving target, it is clear at this point that red and processed meat are linked with cancer. In fact, excessive consumption of red meat has been related to more than a dozen cancers, including breast, prostate, colon, and liver.[124,125] Basically, if you're eating bacon every morning, burgers every night, and steak on the weekend, you could be creating an environment of chronic inflammation, and we know inflammation fuels cancer growth.

In 2015, the International Agency for Research on Cancer and the World Health Organization classified processed meat as a carcinogen and red meat as a probable carcinogen.[124,126] Researchers at Cambridge University concluded that if men cut their consumption of processed meat in half, it would result in a 12 percent reduction in colon cancer.[124,126,127] Other studies have connected red meat consumption with increased prostate, colorectal, and breast cancer risk.[127,128]

One factor linking red meat to cancer is through the carcinogens that are released in the cooking process. These compounds are formed when meat is cooked at high temperatures or is charred.[128–132] Unfortunately, they are also formed when meat is cooked at normal temperatures, including pan fried, broiled, or grilled.[128–131]

Another factor that increases the harm of red meat is a result of the food we feed animals to make them fat and bring in more profits for the farmers. Cows that graze all day in the fields eating grass up until the time they are killed for their meat have a nice balance of omega-6 and omega-3 essential fatty acids; approximately a four-to-one or two-to-one ratio. However, cows that are raised on a feedlot and fed corn and/or soy, even for the last part of their lives, are devoid of omega-3 fatty acid by the time they are slaughtered.[133] Feedlot-raised beef is essentially an omega-6 delivery vehicle. Omega-6 is an essential fatty acid, meaning we need it in our diet, but we also need it in the right balance alongside omega-3 fatty acids. Excess omega-6 fatty acid in our diet, which is the case for the majority of people eating conventionally raised meat, increases inflammation, which is connected to cancer.[134] There are also other theories emerging for the link between red meat consumption and cancer, but more research is needed to substantiate these in humans.[135,136] Less is known about whether the harms of red meat consumption are diminished if you eat pasture-raised, organic meat. In theory, this meat would have a better omega-6 to omega-3 ratio. Yet to date, no one has done the animal or human studies to determine the relative risks.

Let Them Have Choices

Despite the known dangers of sugar and red and processed meat, most hospital cafeterias serve excess amounts of all these foods—let them have choices, they say. Down the hall, patients and their families can finish their high-fat, carcinogenic meal with a heaping cup of soft-serve ice cream sprinkled with crunchy candy toppings. While the portable donut machine is no longer rolling down MD Anderson's walkways tempting survivors and hospital staff with the scent of deep-fried dough and powdered sugar, our hospital cafeterias, like our culture in general, is awash in diabetic, obesogenic, carcinogenic temptations.

The rationalization I have repeatedly encountered at MD Anderson and elsewhere is that as long as a healthy option (and often only one) is offered, it justifies an abundance of unhealthy items. As long as you have a salad or smoothie on the menu, you can check off the healthy category and then offer a plethora of burgers, fries, and sugary desserts. This strikes me as a false choice (not to mention an obvious imbalance between healthy and unhealthy options). Knowing what we know about the addictive qualities of foods high in sodium, sugar, and fat,[137–139] we should not be offering any health-depleting meals to our patients and staff. Or, as a compromise, why not offer one unhealthy option and the rest healthy choices? The argument that people want these foods and only these foods is also a specious one. As has been documented at New Milford Hospital, in Connecticut, when offered healthy choices, patients and workers appreciate them. "Often, patients will be discharged and will ask if they can stay for lunch," says Chef Kerry Gold.[4] How many hospitals can make that boast? We've all been held hostage too long by false arguments.

Interestingly, research shows that highly processed food has the same effect on the brain as drugs like cocaine and heroin. A 2015 study by scientists at the University of Michigan found that the propensity of people to binge on unhealthy foods was directly related to how much those foods were processed.[140] Highly processed foods such as pizza and ice cream have the capacity to override willpower and overwhelm biological signals that relate to hunger.[141] (In other words, you keep eating them even if you are full.) Healthy foods such as broccoli and salmon don't trigger this same response in the brain. No one is tempted to binge on brussels sprouts or carrots. This is not because brussels sprouts and carrots don't taste good. It's because those healthy foods are not inducing the same response from our neurochemical reward centers. I can tell you from my own experience when I was an undergraduate with a growing Doritos addiction, and more recently with my craving for movie popcorn flavored with artificial butter, food addictions are no joke. When you realize that certain foods are feeding addictions, and that many of us are either addicts or recovering addicts, the idea that hospital cafeterias serve pizza or that doctors' offices offer free candy becomes even more disturbing.

The Body Weight–Cancer Connection

Because studies that examine the link between weight and disease have been largely observational, for many years it was easy for the medical-scientific community to dismiss this data as lacking the kind of granular specificity (and, more important, reproducibility) that made it worth promoting. But over time, the consistency of the links and trends we were seeing simply became undeniable. For instance, we've been able to track how a change in diet affects one's vulnerability to disease by monitoring cancer onset rates of people from Asia or Africa who migrate to Western countries. It's been clearly shown—over decades of gathered data—that those who emigrate from these cultures experience an increase in obesity rates and a spike in diseases associated with a Western diet (which is high trans-fat, high sugar, highly processed), including increased incidence of many cancers at a rate much higher than in their home countries that (after a single generation) mirrors the rates in their newfound home.[142-144] In other words, people who move here assimilate in ways that aren't always very good for their health, and the Western diet of convenience is, quite clearly, one of these unhealthy adaptations. As noted earlier, we have also been quite successful at exporting our processed and fast-food diet to other nations, and their rates of obesity are increasing, as are the Western diseases. In a developing country like Brazil, in the not-too-distant past people were underweight and struggling to get enough calories due to poverty. But a 2011 study showed that 48 percent of the Brazilian population is now overweight, which is thought to be due to the increased consumption of fast and processed foods; foods that are low in nutrition. Brazilians, like millions around the world today, may be an overweight yet undernourished population due to the poor quality of food people are eating.[83]

There are many variables and factors at play when it comes to making a direct link between high body mass index (or BMI) and disease,[145,146] but research now clearly shows that being overweight or obese:

- increases levels of insulin and the production of insulin growth factor 1, which are believed to contribute to cancer proliferation;
- promotes chronic inflammation which is linked with cancer risk;
- increases estrogen production in fat tissue (estrogen is known to drive the proliferation of some cancers, such as breast and endometrial cancers); and
- multiplies fat cells that appear to affect the processes that regulate cancer cell growth.

You are at greater risk of these metabolic disturbances if you had a high birth weight, have gained weight as an adult, or have gained or lost weight repeatedly over time.[147-149] As you age, you are also at increased risk of metabolic dysregulation and special attention is needed in this area.

A patient rarely feels well supported when it's pointed out that she is overweight. But if we were to share with patients—especially our cancer patients—all the reasons why carrying excess fat imperils their health, we'd not only be doing our jobs better, but we'd see better outcomes as well. What if the patient is told that losing weight will, for example, bring down her high blood pressure, perhaps free her from her dependency on insulin (due to the type 2 diabetes she developed in her forties), and/or improve her cancer prognosis? If she learns this, she will likely not only sit up and listen but also likely become very interested in participating in her own care. If her doctor goes one step further and tells her that she can easily change her diet and that when she does, her body will respond in ways that will improve every aspect of her life, she may feel downright inspired. I know for myself that when I've provided the information that helps a patient step into action, really good things begin to happen.

I recently heard an inspiring story from my MD Anderson colleague Anil Sood about a patient named Verna G., who experienced a remarkable turnaround. When Sood first met Verna, she suffered from obesity, hypertension, adult-onset diabetes, and metastatic endometrial cancer that had moved to other areas of her body. Her condition was so compromised that immediate surgery was not an option. "My first reaction was: This person is not going to live for more than another year or so," Sood explains. Verna went through chemotherapy, then radiation for the cancer that had spread to her pelvis. Sood talked with her about lifestyle changes she could make to improve her quality of life and her health. "I don't know what clicked, but she actually took our recommendations to heart," Sood says. Verna lost weight and her blood pressure stabilized. She was able to go off her blood pressure medicine, and, significantly, she never relapsed. Eight years later, Verna is alive and well. "She's just defied all the odds," Sood explains. "Can I say it's all due to lifestyle factors? We'll never know, but certainly, losing weight and healing herself from the other health problems caused by being obese contributed to a fantastically positive outcome for her."

The Higher Your Weight, the Greater Your Cancer Risk

One of the leading pioneers in creating and analyzing the data gathered from large, longitudinal epidemiological studies of the human diet is Walter "the Father of Nutrition" Willett, MD, who is a professor of epidemiology and nutrition at Harvard's Chan School of Public Health and professor of medicine at Harvard Medical School. Willet revolutionized our understanding of the causal link between weight and health when his data revealed the connection between being overweight and the onset of diabetes,[150] a disease that now affects well over one hundred million American adults, according to a recent study released by the CDC (Centers for Disease Control and Prevention) in July 2017.[151] Willett says, "Getting Americans' diet right can mean the difference between being healthy or ill." This breakthrough in linking weight to diabetes put Willett and other Harvard researchers to work studying how high body mass may be influencing other diseases, including cancers. In fact, the combination of being sedentary combined with being overweight is now considered by many experts to be a more serious threat to one's health than smoking.[152–154] Conditions negatively impacted by obesity include heart disease, stroke, high blood pressure, type 2 diabetes, bone and joint problems, breathing and sleep disturbances, metabolic syndrome, social and emotional problems, and many types of cancer.[153,154]

Researchers have made reliable inferences from looking at massive amounts of data gathered from worldwide studies that have assessed millions of people who are overweight or obese. Where looking at the onset of cancers is concerned, the findings are startling with more than a dozen cancers linked with being overweight or obese. Here are just some examples of how excess weight increases your risk of developing certain cancers:[97]

- **Breast Cancer:** In postmenopausal women (the age most prone to this type of cancer), overweight women increase their risk of developing breast cancer by 20 to 40 percent.
- **Colorectal Cancer:** Overweight people have a 30 percent greater risk of developing colorectal cancer than their normal weight peers, with men being at slightly greater risk than women.
- **Endometrial Cancer:** Overweight women have a two to four times greater risk of developing this cancer, and extremely obese women have a seven times greater risk. The risk goes up even higher in overweight women who have used hormone therapy for menopausal symptom relief.
- **Liver Cancer:** Overweight people are twice as likely to get liver cancer than those of normal weight. As with colorectal cancers, obese men have a slightly higher risk than obese women.
- **Pancreatic Cancer:** There is a 1.5 times increase in onset of this cancer if you are overweight.
- **Multiple Myeloma:** There is a 10 to 20 percent increase in the risk of developing multiple myeloma if you are overweight.

Obesity is linked to increased mortality risk from the most common forms of cancer in men (prostate, kidney, colorectal, esophagus, stomach, pancreas, and liver) and women (colorectal, ovary, breast, cervical, kidney, endometrial).[155–157] Interestingly, this relationship holds true even for cancer sites where the link between obesity and cancer risk is less clear, including a 75 percent increase in mortality in premenopausal women diagnosed with breast cancer. Meanwhile, obese men are more likely to develop more aggressive prostate cancer and to have more advanced disease at the time of diagnosis.

According to the most current research, there are numerous mechanisms and pathways that are either triggered or suppressed in people who are overweight or obese and which create an opportunity for cancer to develop. These include the following:

- **Chronic Inflammation:** Obese people tend to suffer from chronic, low-grade inflammation, a condition that, over time, can damage DNA and prompt cancer cell growth.[158]
- **Excessive Estrogen Production:** Fat (adipose) tissue produces estrogen and raises a person's baseline estrogen levels in ways that have been associated with breast, ovarian, endometrial, and other cancers.[159]
- **Insulin Resistance:** Along with the increased risk of developing type 2 diabetes, obese people are more prone to having high insulin levels, which have been associated with colon, kidney, prostate, and endometrial cancers, among others.[159,160]
- **Hormone Interference:** Obese people are at greater risk for hormone disruptions that promote cancer cell proliferation by changing cell growth regulation and even cellular structure.[159]
- **Inference with Proliferative Signaling and Growth Suppressors:** Fat cells release adipokines, cell-signaling proteins secreted by fat that may stimulate or inhibit cell growth. Fat cells may also have direct and indirect effects on tumor growth regulators.[159]
- **Depressed Immune Response:** Obese people are known to produce more stress hormones, which, in turn, weaken our immune responses to disease.[159]
- **Increased Oxidative Stress:** Excess body fat can produce an imbalance between oxidants and antioxidants, which prevents the body from neutralizing the harmful effects of free radicals, or highly reactive oxygen by-products.[161] (Oxidative stress has been tied to a host of conditions, including Parkinson's, Alzheimer's, heart disease, chronic fatigue syndrome, and cancer.)[162]

Fortunately, being overweight is a reversible condition, and we've seen remarkable diminishment of all of these risk factors in our patients who understand that striving to reach or maintain a healthy body weight not only helps them fight their disease but also restores their quality of life. In fact, research shows it's worth it to lose those extra pounds. Data from the Women's Health Initiative suggests that weight loss over the course of three years is associated with reduced risk of endometrial cancer eleven years later.[163] Women who lost more than 5 percent of their body weight had a 29 percent reduced risk of endometrial cancer, and obese women with intentional weight loss had a 56 percent reduced risk of developing endometrial cancer. Unfortunately, the opposite was also true. Women who gained more than ten pounds during the three-year period had an increased risk of endometrial cancer. And we know that obesity will also interfere with physical activity goals and make us less likely to exercise.

Nella A., one of our CompLife participants, joined our study on her first day of radiation therapy in the spring of 2017. She'd recently been diagnosed with stage III hormone positive breast cancer and had had surgery to remove twenty-four lymph nodes (twelve of which were cancerous). Her oncologist here at MD Anderson encouraged her to work with us as her type of cancer tends to be slow growing, and if she focused on making healthy lifestyle changes—including lowering her BMI—it could slow even further. When she joined us, Nella didn't give much thought to how the things she ate could impact her health. "All I cared about were calories and that's how I'd tried to lose weight my whole life—which, by the way, never worked," she explains. As someone with a doctorate in education, Nella prides herself on being educated, but she was shocked to discover how little she knew about the effects of different foods on cancer. If she drank green tea it reduced the growth of new blood vessels needed for tumors to grow and spread. Broccoli and cabbage could prevent precancerous cells from developing into tumors. Berries and dark chocolate had the potential to slow tumor growth. Suddenly, her diet became less about calories and more about protecting herself and giving her body the substances it needed to heal and remain cancer-free. "Now I eat a ton of vegetables, some meats, but no fish, no cheese, no dairy, no sugar, no salt, no oil," Nella says. "And here's the crazy thing: My diet has expanded tremendously." In the process, Nella has lost pounds. But more important, her new diet has reconnected her to her body in a positive way. She now feels that she is feeding her body with the fuel it needs to heal. "I'm working in unison with my body now—not fighting against it—and I'm giving it food that's come from the earth, not a factory, because it knows what to do with real, whole food," she explains. Now that her body is supported by her diet, it has blossomed in ways Nella did not anticipate. "I've still got a ways to go, but my body is so different: The fat that I could never lose before, on my hips, no matter how few calories I ate, is gone. I have seen my percentage of body fat go down as my percentage of muscle has gone up! It's as though my body is reorganizing itself around healthier principles. It's pretty remarkable."

Like Dorothy P. and Gabe Canales and so many others (including Alison and me), Nella stopped eating for convenience and started eating for health. This is the basis of anticancer eating.

But What if My BMI Is Just Fine?

Unfortunately, just because you eat a healthy diet doesn't mean you won't get cancer. When Cynthia Thomson, who heads the Canyon Ranch Center for Prevention and Health Promotion at the University of Arizona Cancer Center, was diagnosed in 2003 with colorectal cancer at the age of forty-four, everyone in her family was shocked. Thomson was the one who did everything right—exercised, ate a healthy diet. How could she get cancer? Thomson, who had been researching the connection between nutrition and cancer for a decade, saw it differently. She realized that her own healthy living would give her a better prognosis and a greater chance of surviving her diagnosis, which she has succeeded in doing now for fifteen years.

Another thing she realized when she underwent surgery and woke up surrounded by flower arrangements is this—her friends and family thought she was going to die. The people who gave her flowers were concerned that a diagnosis of cancer inevitably meant she would die. Thomson had worked with enough cancer survivors and done enough research to know that she could survive, and it was vital to her survival that she resume physical activity as soon as possible and get back to her healthy diet.

Thomson's research shows that eating right lowers the risk of cancer recurrence. In 2011, she was the lead author on a follow-up study looking at more than three thousand breast cancer survivors involved in the Women's Healthy Eating and Living (or WHEL) Study.[164,165] The initial WHEL Study

Breast Cancer Recurrence with High Cruciferous Intake and Varying Overall Vegetable Intake

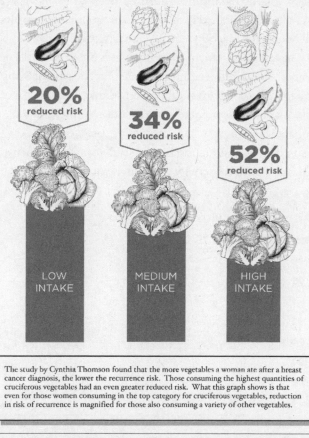

20% reduced risk

34% reduced risk

52% reduced risk

LOW INTAKE

MEDIUM INTAKE

HIGH INTAKE

The study by Cynthia Thomson found that the more vegetables a woman ate after a breast cancer diagnosis, the lower the recurrence risk. Those consuming the highest quantities of cruciferous vegetables had an even greater reduced risk. What this graph shows is that even for those women consuming in the top category for cruciferous vegetables, reduction in risk of recurrence is magnified for those also consuming a variety of other vegetables.

Adapted from: C. A. Thomson, C. L. Rock, B. J. Caan, et al., "Increase in cruciferous vegetable intake in women previously treated for breast cancer participating in a dietary intervention trial," *Nutrition and Cancer* 57, no. 1 (May 2007): 11–19.
     Adapted in collaboration with Laura Beckman.

results were viewed as disappointing because they did not show a clear link between vegetable intake and breast cancer recurrence risk.[165,166] But what Thomson and her team found in their follow-up analyses was that when they compared the women eating the lowest numbers of vegetables to those eating the most, the women eating the most had a 31 percent reduced risk of recurrence of disease.[167] And risk reduction was even greater for the women taking Tamoxifen who were eating a high variety of vegetables that also included cruciferous vegetables such as broccoli, kale, and brussels sprouts.[167] When a healthier diet (at least five fruits and vegetables a day) was combined with physical activity (thirty minutes of brisk walking, six times a week), the risk of dying of cancer during the up-to-eleven-year follow-up period was reduced by half relative to the women not eating fruits and vegetables and not exercising.[168] In fact, women who modified just diet or physical activity had survival outcomes similar to women who did not change either behavior. This reinforces our message that the Mix of Six is the most effective when applied synergistically and not taken as this particular diet or that particular exercise or mind-body practice. Lifestyle changes have the greatest impact when implemented simultaneously.

Thomson is now heading the largest study of its kind focusing on the effects of diet and physical activity on women with ovarian cancer.[169] She is

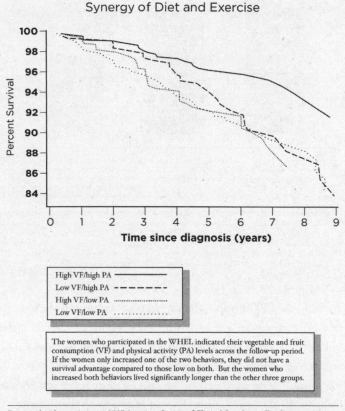

Synergy of Diet and Exercise

High VF/high PA ———————
Low VF/high PA — — — — — —
High VF/low PA ·····················
Low VF/low PA · · · · · · · · · · ·

The women who participated in the WHEL indicated their vegetable and fruit consumption (VF) and physical activity (PA) levels across the follow-up period. If the women only increased one of the two behaviors, they did not have a survival advantage compared to those low on both. But the women who increased both behaviors lived significantly longer than the other three groups.

Reprinted with permission. © 2007 American Society of Clinical Oncology. All rights reserved.
Pierce JP, et al. "Greater survival after breast cancer in physically active women with high vegetable-fruit intake regardless of obesity," *Journal of Clinical Oncology* 25, no. 17 (2007): 2345–51.
   Adapted in collaboration with Laura Beckman.

also examining the role of "energy dense foods" and cancer risk.[170,171] When it comes to research searching for the ideal cancer diet, she believes that the traditional reductionist approach is antithetical to how nutrition works. "Everyone is searching for the magic bullet, whether that's vitamin E, beta carotene, or curcumin [the active ingredient in turmeric]," she explains. "This approach is destined to fail because it doesn't take into account reactions and interactions with the other foods we eat as well as other health behaviors known to modify risk. Diet is like a low dose of twenty thousand compounds that, over the years, protects us from disease."

Nutritional Synergy

We have already noted in the previous chapters the way other areas of the Mix of Six affect diet and vice versa. Eating a big meal close to bedtime can disrupt your sleep because your body is still actively processing your late-night dinner. Recent evidence also suggests a meal too close to bedtime disrupts the sleep-wake cycle of your circadian clock and leads to weight gain.[172] Drinking caffeine can keep us up at night and add to our stress during the day. Sleep deprivation also modifies insulin, ghrelin, and leptin regulation, disrupting our body's signals that tell us when we need to eat and when we are full.[173,174] On the flip side, eating a healthy diet can help alleviate stress and is linked to sleep.[175–177] Leafy greens such as spinach are high in folate, which help the body produce serotonin and dopamine, hormones that relax us. Meanwhile, like sleep deprivation, excess stress and depression are also linked with obesity and dysregulation of ghrelin and leptin signaling, which leads to overeating.[178,179] Recent research also links the health of our microbiome to our mental health and stress levels, as the gut is rich in serotonin and the release of this serotonin is dependent on our gut health—the brain-gut axis.[180] This is perhaps one reason why stress can interfere with the health of our gastrointestinal tract and modulates how we process food, be it healthy or unhealthy food. In terms of exercise, eating the right foods helps keep energy levels up throughout the day and sustains us through physical activity.

What is more surprising in terms of diet synergy is the way foods interact with each other to boost disease prevention and to promote health. Research shows that nutrients in foods work better together than they do individually. A study of more than one thousand Chinese women found that the more mushrooms they ate, the lower their breast cancer risk.[181] The researchers found similar effects from green tea. But the effects of doing both, drinking green tea and eating mushrooms, reduced breast cancer risk even more. This synergy between healthy foods also occurs with vegetable variety. The ideal is to have a rainbow on your plate—vegetables of different colors—to achieve the healthiest meal possible. Vegetable variety has been associated with lower breast cancer risk, even when women carry the BRCA mutation that genetically predisposes them to cancer.[41,182-184]

THE ANTICANCER LIVING
GUIDE TO NUTRITION

Food is serious business. It has the power to either nourish and energize us or leave us feeling depleted and exhausted. It is vital that we stop taking our daily decisions about what we eat and drink so lightly. Don't think about what you want for dinner—think about what your body needs. When it comes to what to drink with meals or between meals, default to water. Get beyond your immediate desires (and possibly addictions) and consider what dietary choices will empower your body to stay healthy and resist or overcome disease.

Every bite has the power to contribute positively or negatively to our health. I find focusing on the science the best way to remind me of my priorities and keep me on track. But I'm kind of geeky that way. For you it might be a person you want to live for, or something you hope to do (or see) someday that requires you to maintain or improve your health. As Nella said, she doesn't want to give cancer any advantage, so she eats with that in mind every day.

Dietary Assessment

As in other areas of the Mix of Six, start by evaluating your current diet. When we first started designing the CompLife Study, we teamed up with Zoe Finch Totten, founder and CEO of the Full Yield, Inc., an innovative company uniquely bridging the health-care and food industries.[1] Our focus is to imagine everything you eat and drink in the course of a day as 100 percent, and to ask what percentage of those foods and drinks are health sustaining and what percentage are depleting? The ideal is 90 percent health-sustaining foods and 10 percent health-depleting foods. (One hundred percent healthy is of course even better, but ninety to ten is a good ratio to aim for—more forgiving and more attainable.)

EXAMPLES OF SUSTAINING AND DEPLETING FOODS

Health-Sustaining Foods	Health-Depleting Foods
vegetables	high glycemic index foods (white rice, white bread, white potato, etc.)
fruits	
vegetable proteins (tofu, etc.)	foods with added sugars
legumes and lentils	red and processed meats
fish—wild caught	soda or sugary drinks
organic/free-range chicken and turkey	fried foods
nuts and seeds	potato chips, other highly processed snack foods, and snacks with an excessive ingredient list
whole grains	candy
olive oil	cookies and other high-sugar, highly processed desserts

Directions:

- Keep a log of everything you eat and drink for three to seven days.
- At the end of this self-evaluation, take a close look at the breakdown between healthy and unhealthy foods.

  Highlight everything with added sugar.

  Highlight everything that is white (bread, pasta, etc.) or contains mostly white food.

- How many vegetable servings are you getting a day?

  Recommended five to six servings per day

- How many servings of fruit do you eat a day?

  Recommended two servings per day

- Go back and look at your assumed percentage of healthy versus unhealthy foods.

  Did you overestimate the amount of fruits and vegetables you eat?

Did you underestimate the amount of unhealthy foods in your daily intake?

How close are you to the ninety-to-ten ratio per day?

Your first step is to add anticancer living foods to your diet, not to restrict or take away from what you eat. This single positive action slowly crowds out the depleting food. Retraining your palate takes time, but once you see the good increasing, choosing to cut out addictive foods and drink becomes easier and reinforced by your health-sustaining palate. You will notice then that small quantities of these prior "addictions" become more satisfying. Alternatively, once your palate becomes more sensitive, these previous cravings, when indulged, can taste either much too sweet or much too salty.

Redesigning Your Plate

The hardest thing for Alison and me when we converted to a plant-centered diet was imagining a dinner plate without meat (or pasta) at the center to hold everything else together. The starting point for planning our family meal was identifying the central meat or carb and then thinking about the rest of the plate arranged around that. The difference now is that we think about the two or three vegetables and plant protein we're having, then arrange the plate around them. That's what eating a plant-centered diet means— reimagining your plate with vegetables at the center, as the entrée—the star of the show, not just a supporting role. For details on eating by food groups see Appendix B.

Start with Breakfast: If you're aiming for five to eight servings of fruits and vegetables a day, with more vegetables than fruit (the Japanese daily food pyramid—shaped as a top—suggests five to six servings of vegetables and two fruit, a three-to-one ratio),[2] starting at breakfast is a must:

- If you're having eggs, add parsley and zucchini to the mix. Green onions are also great for your health and go well with eggs, as does a large handful of kale or spinach.
- If you are in the mood for steel-cut oats, add some fruit and have some vegetables on the side. Steel-cut oats are less processed than rolled oats and are classified as whole grains. A Harvard study combining data from fourteen long-term studies that involved more than

786,000 people found that people who ate the most whole grains (like oats, brown rice, barley, and rye) were 20 percent less likely to die of heart disease and 10 percent less likely to die of cancer.[3] For every additional serving of 16 grams of whole grains, the risk of death by heart disease dropped by 9 percent and the risk of death by cancer dropped by 5 percent.

- If you feel like having fruit as a main course, try it with granola containing nuts and yogurt (but make sure your yogurt doesn't have loads of added sugar). Blueberries, raspberries, apples, and pears are loaded with flavonoids, a natural compound, that has been linked with a reduced risk of heart disease, cancer, and diabetes.[4] It is much better to eat whole fruits than drink fruit juice, which is high in sugar and doesn't contain the fiber. It is also important to always pair a fruit with a protein so that the sugars in the fruit are released more slowly.[5]

Preplan for Meals: The key to redesigning your breakfast, lunch, and dinner plates is to plan your vegetables in advance. Focus on the vegetables, as preparing them takes time and is usually what people cut first when planning a meal due to time constraints and energy levels:

- Cook the whole grains (brown rice, quinoa, etc.) and beans at night after dinner is done and the kitchen clean. Put the pot on and spend time with your family relaxing. It can go into the fridge in the pot ready for the next day.
- Prep your vegetables in the morning. Wash and cut them in preparation for cooking in the evening.
- Enlist your family, if available, while they watch TV to clean brussels sprouts or other vegetables.
- Take your lunch to work to avoid eating out too much.
- When leaving for work, bring healthy snacks like a small bag of almonds, so you aren't tempted by the donuts someone is always leaving in the break room.

Ring the Dinner Bell: For many families, dinner is an important social gathering and it is important to have dinner as a family with no devices or televisions on so you can connect with your loved ones. As such, it's a great

OVERCOMING THE VEGETABLE HUMP

A lot of children (and adults) think they don't like vegetables because they've never had them prepared in an appealing way. They've never gotten over the vegetable hump.

In our household, we practice the three-bite rule. Try it three times. If you still don't like it, fine. You will see it on your plate again, but not today and not cooked in the same way. We find that once children take three bites, it's not that hard to get them to finish their vegetables. Also, the mind-set of "just finish your vegetables" doesn't really fit with our way of viewing and interacting with food anymore. Eating nutritious foods is an important part of our health, not just a way to get dessert. The concept that you need to eat "awful food" (vegetables) to get to the good food (dessert) is ultimately self-defeating.

The anticancer guide to eating turns this notion upside down. First, everything on your plate is good for you. Second, vegetables and the vegetable entrée is the centerpiece of the meal. We do a lot to make vegetables appealing, from cooking with enough spice to decorating the dish with a rainbow of colors. It's all about preparation and presentation. Vegetables don't have to (and shouldn't) look like they came out of a can. Even steamed vegetables can be garnished with fresh herbs, drizzled lightly with olive oil and a fresh grind of pepper.

We also have a "fifteen times before you kick it to the curb" rule. That means we will serve a particular vegetable fifteen times in different forms, styles, and recipes, before we decide to move on.

place to introduce a revised anticancer plate that focuses on vegetables. Alison and I often resort to the internet to find new recipes that incorporate a vegetable we're not used to cooking. As you get going with plant-centered cooking, try one new vegetable a week.

VEGETABLES AND DAILY COOKING

The daily grind of preparing a meal can be overwhelming. A strategy that is helpful when cooking vegetables is working in threes when preparing them: one vegetable that requires prep and two that don't. Aim for two to three different vegetables at dinner. Make large amounts and use them the next day on their own, with eggs in the morning, in a salad for lunch, in tacos for dinner.

Look for the "rainbow" of color on your plate. Make sure you include cruciferous vegetables daily:

- Brussels sprouts—need to prep—painless to clean and cut in front of the TV
- Beets—boil or roast—great to cook while getting ready in the morning
- Spinach—quick cooking in sauté pan with olive oil and garlic
- Asparagus—quick cooking—steamed or roasted with olive oil
- Carrots—roasted or sautéed and add spinach and chickpeas to finish
- Red cabbage—sliced very thinly and eaten raw or sliced and sautéed with onion and garlic and fresh herbs
- Broccoli—quick cooking—steam or roast
- Cauliflower—quick cooking—steam or roast
- Kale—wash and remove the ribs in morning—make a salad (massage with pinch of salt) or steam and eat on a multigrain piece of toast rubbed with garlic and drizzled with olive oil

FIND YOUR INNER GREENGROCER

You can't eat healthier until you shop healthier. This might seem obvious, but you would be surprised how many people make a commitment to change their diet and then fall back to their usual purchases at the grocery store—processed food, ready-to-eat meals, frozen pizza, etc. Check recipes before you get in the car. Make a list of all the vegetables you'll need. Check your spice supply. Once you purchase vegetables, you have to eat them or they will go bad. This is encouragement via financial commitment. You paid for those vegetables. You should get your money's worth and eat them, too.

BECOME A LABEL READER

The next time you're in the grocery store and you find yourself tempted by a processed food or drink that used to be part of your regular routine, stop for a minute and read the ingredients. I am continually surprised (although I shouldn't be at this point) by the amount of sugar in every conceivable item in the grocery store. (Four grams is equal to one teaspoon.) In addition to reading the labels of things you used to buy, look through the ingredients and calorie, fat, and sugar content of anything new you are considering. In fact, read the label of every jar/tin/package/bottle you purchase.

EATING OUT

The average American goes out to eat between four and five times a week.[6] We all know it is harder to watch what we eat and know where our food comes from when we buy it prepared in restaurants, diners, and cafés. It is much harder to gauge the amount of sugar, salt, and fat added to our food and drinks and to make healthy choices. According to the CDC's National Center for Health Statistics, on any given day 30 percent of children eat fast food.[7]

Celebrations should not always be accompanied by going out to dinner. We suggest activity-based rewards and celebrations. Even picnics are better than going out to eat, because you know what's in the food you're eating, and you can manage the amount of sugar, salt, and fat.

AVOIDING SUGAR

These days, avoiding sugar isn't as easy as it sounds, and definitely not as easy as it should be. There are more than sixty different names for sugars, including sucrose, cane crystals, cane sugar, corn sweetener, corn syrup, corn syrup solids, crystal dextrose, evaporated cane juice, fructose sweetener, fruit juice concentrates, high-fructose corn syrup, barley malt, dextrose, maltose, rice syrup, and many, many others.

You also want to avoid all artificial ingredients to the extent that is possible. If there is a healthy choice for what you need, choose it. If no healthy option exists, try finding a substitute for that item. The key is to always be actively thinking about your health and the health of your family.

FOR THOSE UNDERGOING CANCER TREATMENT

Maintaining your strength becomes even more important when your system is worn down by chemotherapy, radiation, or surgery. For patients under active cancer treatment, try to maintain protein intake equivalent to 1.2

grams per kilogram per day.[8] When not on treatment, reduce to 0.8 grams per kilogram per day.[9] So, a woman who weighs 130 pounds (59 kilograms) on active cancer treatment needs to eat 70 grams protein a day (1 cup almonds = 30 grams protein; 1 cup cooked soybeans = 30 grams protein; 1 cup chicken breast = 43 grams protein). When not on treatment, the same 130-pound woman needs 47 grams of protein. It is important for people undergoing active treatment to work with a registered dietitian nutritionist certified as a specialist in oncology to make sure they are meeting their dietary needs.

SUGAR SUBSTITUTES

We discussed in detail the dangers of sugar and the unknowns of many sugar substitutes. If your sweet tooth simply cannot be tamed, we recommend using a small amount of natural sweeteners such as honey or maple syrup. Honey has anti-inflammatory and antimicrobial properties and has been shown to improve immune function. Studies in the past five years have indicated that honey has anticancer properties in animal models and cell cultures.[10] Meanwhile, other studies have shown that the phenolic compounds in maple syrup cause a low rise in blood glucose levels and may have an anticancer effect.[11]

Although David Servan-Schreiber touted agave nectar as a healthy alternative sweetener with a low glycemic index, recent research has raised questions about agave. Although it sounds natural, agave is highly processed and contains extremely high amounts of fructose, which enters the bloodstream more slowly than sucrose and remains there longer. High levels of fructose have been related to insulin resistance, high blood pressure, and heart disease.[12]

DAIRY

Dairy causes inflammation.[13] Cancer is a disease of inflammation. Extensive epidemiologic research has linked dairy consumption with increased incidence of prostate cancer.[14] When you do consume dairy, consider paying the extra dollar or two for organic options derived from grass-fed animals. This way, you are reducing the omega-3/omega-6 imbalance that has become pervasive with the mass production of animals fed a primary diet of corn, soy, and grain. Consider nondairy milks such as soy, almond, walnut, cashew, and so on.

SOY AND CANCER

Soy has been proved to have benefits in terms of reducing cancer risk and risk of recurrence. For years, cancer survivors, particularly women with breast cancer, were warned to avoid soy. Much of that reaction was based on animal research, which found that high doses of soy extract caused breast tumors to grow in mice.[15] But a series of large epidemiological studies have found reduced breast cancer risk and improved outcomes when women consume soy, even if they have the genetic mutations that make them at greater risk for breast cancer.[16] A 2012 study that analyzed more than ninety-five hundred breast cancer survivors in the United States and China found that women who ate at least 10 milligrams of soy isoflavones a day (equivalent to one-third cup of soy milk or a quarter cup soybeans) were 25 percent less likely to suffer a recurrence.[16] Another study of Chinese women found that women who ate the most soy were more likely to survive a lung cancer diagnosis.[17]

Because soy is a phytoestrogen, meaning it is a plant-based estrogen, many health-care professionals and cancer survivors think any soy product—or any phytoestrogens for that matter—will stimulate hormone-sensitive cancers to form and grow. But it is important to know that there are two types of estrogen receptors in the body—alpha and beta.[18] Naturally occurring estrogen in the body, released from the ovaries and even excess fat, binds preferentially to estrogen receptor alpha and estrogen receptor alpha stimulation in breast tissue increases cell proliferation and is a risk factor for breast cancer.[19] However, estrogen beta activation has the opposite effect and is thought to counter the proliferative effects of estrogen receptor alpha stimulation.[20] What is important to know is that the phytoestrogenic effect of soy is through binding to estrogen receptor beta.[21] This means the phytoestrogenic effects of soy may actually counter the negative effects of endogenous estrogen on breast tissue and lead to decreases in cell proliferation—one of the cancer hallmarks.

The most recent study on the topic, a multicenter study published in 2017 of 6,235 women with breast cancer enrolled in the Breast Cancer

Family Registry in the United States and Canada, found that women who consumed the highest amount of soy isoflavones (1.5 milligrams daily, equivalent to only a few edamame a day) had a 21 percent reduced all-cause mortality during the ten-year study compared to women who ate the least amount of soy.[22] This result was limited to women who had tumors that were negative for hormone receptors and those who did not receive hormone therapy for their breast cancer. This suggests that soy isoflavones were especially helpful for the women who did not have any hormone treatment for their breast cancer, yet not harmful in the least to those with estrogen positive cancer. The American Cancer Society recommends consuming soy as part of a healthy diet as a whole food, not as a supplement.[23] Soy is a good source of protein and fiber and may decrease cancer risk and improve outcomes for women with breast cancer. Although the jury is out on the merits of non-GMO soybeans versus GMO, many believe it prudent to try and stick with non-GMO by buying organic.

ALCOHOL

Alcohol is listed by the National Toxicology Program as a known human carcinogen.[24] The more someone drinks, the higher their risk of developing certain types of cancers, including head and neck, esophageal, liver, stomach, breast, and colorectal.[25,26]

If you consume alcohol at all, limit yourself to no more than one drink a day for women and not more than two a day for men. However, as alcohol is a known carcinogen, it is perhaps prudent to remove this risk factor and not drink at all. To decrease the sugar spike that comes with alcohol consumption, if you drink, don't drink on an empty stomach. Have a beer, cocktail, or glass of wine with your meal.

COOKING TEMPERATURE

Some oils cooked at high temperature release a chemical called aldehyde, which has been linked to cancer.[27] The oils that are most dangerous in this regard are corn and sunflower oils, especially when heat levels of 350 degrees or higher are maintained for twenty minutes or more. Healthy oils to cook with are canola, olive, coconut, and walnut (although walnut oil is expensive). But do not cook with olive oil at high temperatures, as it has a low smoke point (the point at which the oil will start to emit smoke), and it will oxidize and become unhealthy. Healthy oils to cook with at higher temperatures are canola and avocado.[27]

CANCER AND SUPPLEMENTS

Self-prescribing supplements can be an unsafe and slippery slope. Do you understand your vitamin and mineral deficiencies? If you are deficient in a certain vitamin or mineral, can you get to the correct level with whole foods? In some cases, such as vitamin D, taking a supplement may be necessary. Remember also that some vitamins and minerals are fat-soluble and need to be taken with food, like vitamin D, and others should be taken on an empty stomach. Supplements should be considered like drugs. Take a pill when necessary because a doctor has identified a specific deficiency or a specific reason for taking a pill. But it is always better to achieve your nutritional needs, the necessary vitamins and minerals you need, through whole foods and a well-balanced diet.

CANCER AND BEVERAGES

When you're choosing what to drink at meals or between meals, default to water. Water is the flush button on all the toxins that build up in the digestive tract.[28] Water creates saliva used for digestion; maintains proper membrane moisture levels; promotes the growth, survival, and reproduction of cells; flushes waste (mainly in the form of urine); and lubricates joints.[28] It also aids in the manufacture of hormones and neurotransmitters in the brain, controls body temperature through sweating and respiration, protects the structural integrity of the brain and spinal cord, converts and breaks down food for nutrition, and delivers oxygen throughout the body.[28]

WAYS TO ENCOURAGE WATER DRINKING

- Add a squeeze or two of lemon or orange, a small piece of lemongrass, a sprig of fresh mint, or slice of cucumber.
- Buy a stainless steel or glass water bottle and bring it with you as you go about your day.
- Start each day with a glass of water.

The general rule of thumb is to get at least eight eight-ounce glasses of water a day.[28] Take a moment to think about what that looks like in a given day—how many times do I need to fill my water bottle? Doctors also recommend a better way to gauge your needed water consumption is by the color of your urine.[29] This allows you to keep tabs on what is too much (clear urine with no color) and too little water (dark yellow urine). Keep your urine color light yellow and transparent and you will be appropriately hydrated.

Should you filter your tap water? That depends on where you're getting your water and what contaminants are in it. The Environmental Working Group has put together millions of state water testing records to create a National Drinking Water Database (www.ewg/tapwater). Looking up your municipality is a great place to start. If your water source isn't included in the database, you can ask your local water utility for its latest annual water quality report. (Sometimes these are also available online.)

Once you know what's in your water, you can identify the filter that best matches your needs and your budget. Filters come in six varieties:

- Pitchers
- Faucet mounted
- Faucet integrated
- Countertop
- Under-sink
- Whole house

These different styles are generally broken down into two prominent technologies:

- Carbon filters, which reduce common contaminants such as lead.
- Reverse-osmosis systems, which are costlier but remove contaminants, such as arsenic, that carbon filters don't.

The key is to identify which contaminants you're exposed to via your tap water and then decide on a filter system that best targets those contaminants at a price you can afford.

GREEN TEA

Tea contains polyphenols and flavonoids, both potent antioxidants. Green tea contains three times the catechins of black tea. Catechins are flavonoids being studied for their anticancer potential. In laboratory studies, green tea has been shown to slow or prevent cancer growth in colon, liver, breast, and prostate cells.[30,31] Studies that track people's diets over multiple years have associated regular consumption of green tea with lower risk for colon, bladder, stomach, esophageal, and pancreatic cancers.[30] It is important to note that if you buy bottled green tea, the concentration of catechins varies widely. A study by *Men's Health* magazine in 2010 found that the green tea with the highest amount of EGCG (a type of catechin) ranged from 215 milligrams per bottle to as little as 1 milligram.[32]

COFFEE

The latest research shows that coffee does more good than harm when it comes to cancer risk.[33] In a 2016 report published in *Lancet Oncology*, the World Health Organization's International Agency for Research on Cancer concluded that coffee was unlikely to cause cancer and that regular coffee consumption could protect against uterine and liver cancers.[34] To reach that conclusion, the agency brought together twenty-three international scientists to examine the findings of more than one thousand studies. They found that drinking coffee produced strong antioxidant effects, and in laboratory studies, coffee promoted the death of cancer cells.[34]

THE ANTICANCER LIVING GUIDE NUTRITION SUMMARY (SEE APPENDIX B FOR EATING BY FOOD GROUP)

1. Keep track of everything you eat and drink for a week. Based on your findings, increase your intake of the healthy foods, thereby crowding out the unhealthy foods. Work toward a diet that is 90 percent healthy.
2. Redesign your plate so that every meal includes an assortment of vegetables and a small amount of fruit. Vegetable entrées and vegetables should be the centerpiece of your meal, not just a side.
3. Make eating healthy more convenient. Prep vegetables ahead of time. Double the recipe, so you can have leftovers for a second meal later in the week.
4. Become a healthy shopper. Look up recipes beforehand and shop based on your list. Read labels and beware of added sugars (4 grams equal 1 teaspoon).
5. Celebrate with activities, not with food. Don't think of drinks and dessert as rewards. Instead, reward yourself with a walk or by playing your favorite sport.
6. If you must use sweetener, try honey or maple syrup instead of sugar or sugar substitutes.
7. Limit dairy. Consider nondairy milks like soy or nut.
8. Limit your consumption of alcohol.
9. When it comes to drinks, default to filtered water.
10. Find a type of organic green tea you like and drink it often—at least three cups a day.

CHAPTER TWELVE

The Environment and
the Quest for Health

By now you know I'm a fervent believer that each of us has tremendous influence over our body's ability to heal itself, yet I'm also a realist. There is one aspect of humans and cancer that we are only beginning to discuss, and it's the elephant in the anticancer living room: With our all-consuming embrace of convenience, and our quest to apply science rather than follow its trail to greater wisdom on behalf of humankind, we've built an industrialized infrastructure that has polluted our air, tainted our water, and stripped our land of its resources. While we raced to tame, control, and profit from nature with more potent chemicals and poisons, we have also, it is now clear, poisoned ourselves.

We've been living our lives steeped in chemicals for so long—several generations now—that we simply don't hold on to awareness of it until disaster strikes, like Hurricane Harvey that struck my own home city of Houston in September 2017 and began to affect our health on a daily basis.[1] Then, chemical exposure becomes headline news as toxins are released into the water we drink and air we breathe. Since the 1970s—less than fifty years—more than eighty-seven thousand chemicals have been approved for commercial use.[2] Yet of those thousands upon thousands of chemicals we've developed and unleashed on the world, only just over one thousand have been formally examined and graded for their carcinogenic potential.[3] Of that one thousand, fully five hundred have been found worthy of being graded on a cautiously worded scale: 120 chemicals have been identified as "known" carcinogens; another 81 have been identified as "probable" carcinogens; and another 299 as "possibly" carcinogenic, according to analysis published by the World Health Organization (WHO).[3]

But what about the other 86,600 (give or take) chemicals that are being inhaled, swallowed, or absorbed into the skin in an unfathomable number of combinations that ebb and flow and shift and change as often as the direction of the wind changes? How on earth do we capture data about these unseen substances and figure out if we need to be adding to the master list of known or possible carcinogens? What about the chemicals that may not be directly carcinogenic but may nonetheless modify our internal biology and play a role in the onset of serious diseases, including cancers?

We simply cannot escape our exposure to man-made chemicals. But there is a lot we can do to moderate our exposures. For the most part, it is up to us to become more conscious about the chemicals we are exposed to in the air we breathe, the water we drink, the furniture in our homes, the clothes we wear, and the products we put on our bodies every day. While one-time exposure to chemicals is often considered "safe," many of these products are used every day, and the effects of long-term exposure, especially when combined with other chemicals, is largely unstudied and unknown. It is up to us to proceed through this chemically laden world we live in first and foremost with caution. Some of us may not find this state of affairs optimal and choose to become active at the local or national level. Certainly, prominent disasters affecting thousands of people may contribute to a real change in the way we live with these substances. It's hard to see the silver lining in that, yet we may find ourselves in just that situation.

Our Homes Are Awash in Chemicals

There are so many chemicals packed into every type of household cleaner that to name them all is all but impossible. Every spray bottle filled with heavy-duty cleanser has chemicals in it that are known to be problematic, in terms of relative toxicity.[4,5] It can be irresistible to watch those "cleaning bubbles" hard at work, but it may be worth your while to question the actual convenience they offer.

Toxic chemicals aren't just to be found under our sinks. They're in shampoos, body washes, lotions, hand sanitizers, perfumes, colognes, aftershave, and makeup, even our toothpastes and mouth rinses.[6] We simply cannot get away from them—unless we engage in a conscious, ongoing effort to identify them and find alternatives. Even then, it can be challenging, as chemical manufacturers have caught on to our wish to "go green" and become masterful at masquerading toxic products as being less harmful than they actually are. For instance, have you ever wondered what "fragrance" as an ingredient is? Turns out it is a mix of chemicals that don't have to be disclosed by the manufacturer and often include endocrine-disrupting compounds that can affect our hormone levels over time.[7] Have you ever purchased kitchenware that says on the label "for decorative purposes only"? This means that there is likely lead or another toxic substance in the paint or finish and the bowl or dish should not be used for food storage or presentation.[8,9] Even that cash register receipt you have tucked into your pocket isn't clean; it's laced with bisphenol A or BPA (this is what makes the printed numbers adhere to the paper), a known endocrine disrupter. Research shows that you will have a spike of BPA in your system if you rub your face or eat right after handling a receipt.[10,11]

Clearly, a big part of anticancer living is about becoming a thoughtful consumer and choosing to put your hard-earned dollars toward products, produce, and other purchases that will reduce the number of toxins you and your family are exposed to on a daily basis. As in the other five areas, small steps actually do add up to limit your toxic exposure. In many cases, substitutions are simple and cost effective.

Is Cancer an Industrial Disease?

A team of researchers at the University of Manchester, England, looked at cancer rates spanning millennia, and their findings point to a strong causal link between industrialization and the acceleration of cancer as a leading cause of death. Professors Rosalie David and Michael Zimmerman coauthored a paper published in *Nature Reviews Cancer* in 2010 that studied the time line of cancer prevalence by reviewing the remains of cancer-stricken Egyptian mummies and the data gathered since then.[12] They found "a striking rarity of malignancies in ancient physical remains [that] might indicate that cancer was rare in antiquity, and so poses questions about the role of carcinogenic environmental factors in modern societies." In other words, cancer (or at least the prevalence of cancer) is directly related to our progression into an industrialized society. The implications of this study are what I and others in the field of integrative oncology keep in the forefront of our research and recommendations when thinking about the world we live in: how are environmental toxins affecting our bodies and our ability to stave off disease?

One of the ways that we've been able to track the link between cancer and industrialization is to look at cancer clusters and to learn what they tell us about where our behavior as a society is undermining our best abilities to cure or even prevent the onset of cancer diseases.

The Geography of Cancer

A cancer cluster is defined by the CDC as "a greater-than-expected number of cancer cases that occurs within a group of people in a geographic area over a limited period of time."[13] These are often work related, such as the scrotal cancer that was identified in chimney sweeps in eighteenth-century London or the high incidence of osteosarcoma (a type of bone cancer) among the "radium girls," who painted watch faces with self-luminous paint made with radium in three different factories in the United States in the early twentieth century.[14,15] There are famous legal cases involving suspected man-made causes of cancers such as the Hinkley, California, tainted water case made famous by Erin Brockovich, who discovered that PG&E (Pacific Gas & Electric) had dumped more than three hundred seventy gallons of chromium-tainted waste water into unlined waste ponds.[16] The groundwater became saturated with chromium 6, a chemical used to inhibit rust. Brockovich and the law firm for which she worked as a legal clerk sued PG&E in 1993 and won what was the largest judgment against a corporate polluter at that time. For the next twenty years, the limited scientific data around this type of water contamination was used as a legal football, even as more cases of cancer and other diseases related to the chromium dump were recorded. Finally, in 2014, after the chromium 6 plume had spread hundreds of miles into other water supplies, this chemical was formally recognized as a known carcinogen.[17] Today, Hinkley, California, is a virtual ghost town.

A more recent high-profile cancer cluster is the one that continues to grow in the aftermath of the September 11, 2001, attacks on the United States. As of June 2016, the CDC's World Trade Center Health Program has registered more than fifty-four hundred people diagnosed with cancers thought to have resulted from exposure to carcinogens and pollutants in the aftermath of the attacks.[18] And as time has passed, the rate of reporting has skyrocketed: The latest enrollment *triples* the number of people who had enrolled in 2014, when the registry counted only 1,822 related cancers. Over the last three years, more than fifteen hundred people have been added to the list annually and this number only counts those who have stepped forward to enroll in this federal health program.[19] The hardest hit group is first responders, with 4,692 now receiving health care and medical monitoring through the program. The others are people who lived, worked, or went to school near the World Trade Center. Almost half of the 5,441 enrolled are between the ages of fifty-five and sixty-four.[18] All totaled, those enrolled in the program report 6,378 separate incidences of cancer, which indicates that some people have been diagnosed with more than one type of cancer since their exposure to toxic dust that included an assortment of toxins, including asbestos, lead, PCBs, polyaromatic hydrocarbons (or PAHs), glass fibers, and dioxin to name a few.[20]

One of the few useful things that come with being able to identify these disease clusters is the opportunity it gives scientists to investigate formally the possible correlation between the compromised environment and the on-set of cancer diseases. This has given us the chance to identify known carcin-ogens and to begin to take legislative and social action to limit our exposure to them, despite the well-funded and often aggressive tactics used by many chemical manufacturers to undermine these scientific investigations and to avoid acknowledging their part in poisoning the earth in ways that work against our efforts to prevent cancers and other diseases. More troubling are the low-level exposures to carcinogens that affect the whole planet in the air we breathe. A 2017 paper published in the *New England Journal of Medicine* found that U.S. air pollution levels even at concentrations below the current national standards were associated with increased mortality.[5]

Though cancer deaths in the United States have fallen by more than 20 percent between 1980 and 2015, an examination of the records from the National Center for Health Statistics has allowed researchers to "map" those regional areas where cancer death rates have not followed this trend.[21] For instance:

There is an eighty-five-mile-long corridor along the Mississippi River between New Orleans and Baton Rouge, Louisiana, that's known as "Cancer Alley."[22] This stretch of poorer parishes (counties) is home to more than 150 factories and refineries—and a whole host of pollution-driven diseases, including cancers.

Along the West Texas border with Mexico, there's been a huge uptick in the onset of liver cancers, though researches have not yet been able to pinpoint the cause.[23]

Florida—which is home to seventy-seven Superfund sites (environmental hazardous waste sites), thus ranking it sixth in this category in the country—was projected, in 2016, to rank second in the number of new cancer cases.[24] A recent study published in *Statistics and Public Policy* examined cancer onset rates in Florida from 1986 to 2010 and found a strong association between the presence of these toxic sites and the rising rates of cancer.[24]

The Uphill Battle of Environmental Protection

Organizations like the Environmental Working Group are at the forefront of the movement to advise the public and continue testing chemicals and their impact on humans and to press for involvement from legislators and lawmakers to increase chemical manufacturers' accountability when it comes to public health. The EWG was founded by Ken Cook in 1992, and for the past twenty-six years Cook and his staff have lobbied the U.S. government to align itself with the interests of citizens over chemical-producing corporations.[25] To illustrate how slowly environmental reform happens, one need look only at the Toxic Substances Control Act of 1976 (the TSCA). The law was designed to regulate the introduction of new chemicals or assess existing chemicals as being "safe" before they are released into the marketplace. However, when the law was enacted in 1976, all existing chemicals were deemed safe for use and were "grandfathered" in. It wasn't until 2016 that this law was updated, and the changes made then—even forty years later—were minimal. In an article he published in May 2016, Ken Cook called out the revised law for doing too little "to protect Americans from chemicals that cause cancer and nervous system disorders, impaired fertility, immune system dysfunction, and a host of other health problems."[26] He made special note of what he calls the "Seven Deadly Poisons" that remain in circulation, despite our knowing (for decades, in some cases) how dangerous they are to the public. These poisons are identified as follows:

Asbestos: Despite the direct link between asbestos and lung cancer and other disease being scientifically established, it is still legal and used in the United States even as it is banned in more than fifty other countries.[27] You can still find asbestos in roofing and vinyl materials, brake pads, and other auto parts such as clutches, and it was even recently detected in crayons.

Formaldehyde: This naturally occurring substance becomes carcinogenic in high doses and is found in carpets, wood flooring, hair-straightening products, fingernail polish, paints and varnishes, and household cleaning products. Formaldehyde can damage DNA, and exposure over time—even in low doses—is known to increase cancer risk.[28]

PFCs: Perfluorinated chemicals are nonstick, waterproof, and grease resistant and are used in cookware, weatherproof outerwear, and food packaging. Though a class of these chemicals known as C8s (8 indicates the number of carbon atoms) are no longer made in the United States, C6s still are, and are still in use. These have been linked to cancer and thyroid disease, among other health issues.[29]

Fire Retardants: Chlorinated fire retardants are sprayed onto upholstered furniture and many products made for children, including car seats. They are linked to cancer and hormone disruption.[30]

Vinyl Chloride: This is used to make PVC plastics and many household products, such as shower curtains. Exposure to airborne PVC affects the nervous system and long-term exposure can cause liver damage.[31]

Bisphenol A (BPA): This compound can be found in food and beverage containers—and in people, including babies in the womb. In 2015, California took the step of listing BPA as a female reproductive toxicant.[32]

Phthalates: These compounds make plastics more flexible and are used in PVC plastics, solvents, vinyl flooring, adhesives, and detergents. They are endocrine disrupters and have been linked to diabetes, obesity, and reproductive and thyroid problems.[33,34]

Unfortunately, too little is being done to help reduce the massive chemical load we are exposed to daily. Margaret I. Cuomo, MD, the author of *A*

World Without Cancer: The Making of a New Cure and the Promise of Prevention,[35] spoke with me about the challenges we face in this area. She acknowledged that awareness was the first step, and that an informed public would be better positioned to help demand change: "I think if the public understood the reality that if you buy your face cream or other personal care products in California it will probably be a safer, less-toxic formula than a similar product purchased in Connecticut or New Jersey, they would demand safer products in general." She went on, "They will be outraged, and the pressure applied to the companies will make a difference. I am convinced of it, but the first step is to inform the public." Cuomo believes we are still living in a very 1950s mentality when it comes to environmental regulation of personal care products and food products. "In general, consumers are unaware of the harmfulness of many chemical ingredients in personal care products and their profound effect on our endocrine systems, on fertility, and on everything from obesity to behavior. This is not a small thing. This is a very significant issue."

Environmental Toxins and Endocrine Disruption

Just in the last twenty years or so, a new field has emerged for researching how environmental toxins cause endocrine or hormonal disruption. Rather than being directly linked to the onset of specific cancers like the known fifty-four carcinogens identified by the EPA (such as asbestos, which has been directly linked to the onset of lung cancer and mesothelioma, a type of lung cancer), endocrine disrupters influence our health in different ways by mimicking or enhancing or changing metabolic regulation.[36] Most of us are exposed to a cocktail of environmental toxins on an ongoing daily basis and at a relatively low level of exposure. A class of these toxins known as endocrine-disrupting chemicals (EDCs) can be found in our food, our environment, and in the products we put on our bodies. These compounds interfere with hormone production and metabolism in ways that may—especially over the long term—create biological conditions that make us more susceptible to cancer and other diseases.[35,37,38]

Endocrine disrupters don't work the way classical carcinogens work. Instead, they work like our endocrine system (our natural hormone system), but at extremely low levels that affect the physiology of the body at different times of life and interfere with normal development. Carcinogens cause cellular damage and mutation, whereas endocrine disrupters cause ripples in overall development. We see, for instance, early-onset puberty in both boys and girls when exposed to certain (though often different or uniquely combined) endocrine disrupters in the environment, in food, or in the consumer products these children use. A study by the U.S. Centers for Disease Control and Prevention found that girls exposed to high levels of a solvent used in toilet bowl deodorizers and air fresheners had their first menstrual period seven months earlier than those with lower exposure levels.[39,40] That 2012 research is the culmination of a series of studies that suggest environmental toxins, especially those that mimic hormones, could be responsible for causing changes in humans. The chemical in this particular study, dichlorobenzene, is present in the body of nearly every person tested in the United States.[41]

Meanwhile, a research team headed by Lawrence (Larry) Kushi, ScD, at Kaiser Permanente has been studying whether exposure to environmental chemicals leads to early puberty in more than twelve hundred prepubescent girls in three U.S. cities—New York, Cincinnati, and Oakland. After following the girls for a dozen years, Kushi and his team connected early breast development with two chemicals—triclosan, which is present in toothpaste among many other products, and 2,5-dichorophenol, a chemical used in pesticides and to chlorinate water.[42,43] Those two chemicals were related to girls developing four to nine months sooner. Although Kushi tells me he and his team have "barely scratched the surface" of the data collected so far, in 2016 a request for additional funding for the study was turned down by the National Cancer Institute.

Reports in 2011 and 2012 found that boys in the United States were maturing between six months and two years sooner than they were in the 1970s.[44,45] Researchers aren't clear why this is happening. With girls, they blame estrogen-like chemicals in the environment, such as dichlorobenzene or BPA. But boys exposed to the same chemicals should have an opposite effect—delaying sexual maturation. One possible reason for early puberty in boys could be an increase in rates of obesity, which alter the body's hormone levels. Unfortunately, the risk of both breast and prostate cancer increases with early onset puberty.[46-48]

What makes separating out the effects of different environmental carcinogens and EDCs so challenging is how fluidly and integrally they're threaded throughout virtually every facet of our lifestyle. Janet Gray, PhD, a professor of neuroscience at Vassar College, has been studying endocrine disrupters for the past fifteen years. She explains that our natural hormone system helps maintain "homeostasis," which is systemic hormonal balance. But, over time, endocrine disrupters and chemicals that mimic hormones can cause an imbalance in this delicate system.[37] "When this happens later in life, after our organs are fully developed, we believe it may be influencing brain health issues and certainly the onset of cancers, such as breast cancer," Gray explains. "When endocrine disruption happens to an embryo or a fetus in utero, the long-term consequences can be more dire. Additionally, we pass along this kind of endocrine disruption to future generations, which adds a whole new element to the new field of epigenetics. For example, we have many studies now that show the correlation between women developing breast cancer now and the exposure of their female relatives decades earlier to DDT."

Research on endocrine-disrupting compounds reveals the long-lasting effects of exposure to low levels of endocrine disrupters (whereas when carcinogens are removed, the damage is relatively contained).[49] EDC exposure appears to actually imprint changes on future gene expression (as opposed to gene mutation, which is the effect attributed to classic carcinogens). For example, in 2014 researchers in Chicago found that when male fetuses were exposed to bisphenol A (BPA), the chemical reprogrammed their developing prostate and made them more susceptible to prostate diseases later in life.[50]

This kind of breakthrough in our understanding of the lingering impact of endocrine disrupters should make us all exercise extreme caution when we make choices about what chemicals we expose ourselves to, especially given how "under the radar" the doses of the substances tend to be, and the often-latent appearance of the long-term effects.

A survey by the Environmental Working Group in 2015 found that the average adult uses nine personal care products a day, with 126 unique chemical ingredients.[51] The study, which surveyed more than twenty-three hundred people, found that one in five adults are exposed every day to *all* of the top seven carcinogenic impurities commonly found in personal care products, including formaldehyde, which (as I mentioned) is listed as a known carcinogen by both the International Agency for Research on Cancer and the National Toxicology Program.[3] The study found that women expose themselves to 168 chemicals every day, about twice as many as men. The average man surveyed said he used five to seven personal care products a day.[51] This can include things like deodorant, toothpaste, shampoo, hair gel, shaving cream, aftershave, and lotion. The average woman uses nine to twelve products. The average teenage girl uses seventeen.[52]

For the parents of a fourteen-year-old daughter, this news is especially troubling. Cosmetics such as makeup, moisturizers, and hair care products often contain parabens or phthalates, which are endocrine disrupters. Phthalates have been linked to breast cancer, obesity, infertility, and asthma. In 2014, the U.S. Consumer Product Safety Commission recommended that a number of phthalates be banned from children's toys because studies have connected exposure in rats to abnormalities in the male reproductive tract. The connection is so clear the disorder is called "phthalate syndrome."[53]

Meanwhile, products that promise to protect us from microbes might be doing more harm than good. Many antibacterial soaps, hand sanitizers, and cleaning products contain triclosan. So, while you imagine yourself getting dangerous microbes off your body or out of your house, you might be adding xenoestrogens into your bloodstream and into your environment. A study in 2013 found that triclosan, like several other chemicals we've mentioned, mimics estrogen and could cause the growth of certain types of breast cancer.[54]

While much of the public remains unaware, we are also making rapid strides in our understanding, and our behavior is beginning to change.

The Brighter Side of a Dark Topic

Thanks in part to increased awareness and our improved ability to measure pollutants and draw more direct connections between exposure and disease, change is afoot when it comes to environmental toxins and our ability to recognize and avoid them. For example, it is now possible in most supermarkets (especially in more eco-conscious co-ops and groceries) to find chemical-free versions of virtually every cleaning and beauty product. Nontoxic nail salons are springing up as a natural alternative to what has traditionally been a highly toxic segment of the beauty industry. As public awareness about the dangers of dry-cleaning chemicals grows, more "green" dry cleaners are opening and offering eco-friendly alternatives.

Meanwhile, organic farming is on the rise. Sales of organic produce jumped 23 percent from 2015 to 2016 to $7.6 billion.[55] This is good news for our environment and for our children. Organic farming has been shown to improve water quality in areas of the Midwest at the highest risk for contamination from agricultural runoff. A 2015 study that switched forty children in California to an organic diet for a week found that the levels of pesticides in their urine dropped by almost 50 percent.[56]

Investigative reporting related to environmental hazards has also led to dramatic changes in a number of markets. A *60 Minutes* report in 2015 revealed that laminate flooring from Lumber Liquidators contained high levels of formaldehyde, which led to a multimillion-dollar criminal and civil settlement.[57] In 2014, a food blogger named Vani Hari pointed out that Subway used a chemical found in yoga mats as a bleaching agent and dough conditioner in their breads. The resulting public outcry led Subway to phase out its use of *azodicarbonamide*.[58] Meanwhile, after a number of studies linked the brown coloring in soda to increased cancer risk, many soda manufacturers are starting to phase out the artificial coloring that contains *4-methylimidazole*. In 2011, California required any food or beverage that contains more than 29 milligrams of 4-MEI to include a warning label.[59]

California has been at the forefront of consumer protection when it comes to the public's right to know about chemical ingredients and exposure. In October 2017, Governor Jerry Brown signed the California Cleaning Product Right to Know Act, which requires consumer and industrial cleaning products to list ingredients, including what makes up the innocent-sounding "fragrance," both on the label and online.[60] In New York, Governor Andrew Cuomo is pushing the Household Cleansing Product Information Disclosure Program that would require cleaning product manufacturers to disclose ingredients online.[61]

Meanwhile, some companies aren't waiting for new state rules to increase their transparency. In 2016, SC Johnson launched an air freshener collection that lists every ingredient, including those that make up the "fragrance."[62] Unilever announced plans this year to create a readable Smart-Label that enables buyers to access ingredient information through a smartphone app.[63] And in 2017 Procter & Gamble launched a website that discloses all preservatives in its products.[64] In response to pressure from a coalition of environmental health groups, the Campbell Soup Company announced that it had met a goal to remove all BPA from its soup cans by mid-2017.[65] The lingering question in the Campbell's case is what they used to replace BPA in their cans.

THE HALIFAX PROJECT: Getting to Know Cancer

The Halifax Project is a worldwide collaborative scientific inquiry into the effect of low-dose combinations of chemicals on human health that was inspired by one man, Leroy Lowe, a Canadian educator. Lowe challenged scientists to think differently about the carcinogenic potential of these endocrine disrupters by asking scientists to look at how the "nontoxic chemicals" we are exposed to every day in low doses might cumulatively disrupt multiple systems linked to the carcinogenic process.[66]

The project took place between 2012 and 2015, and it involved more than 350 cancer researchers and scientists from 31 countries.[67] The findings are shedding important light on the link between the environment and cancer. As the group's report concludes: "Our analysis suggests that the cumulative effects of individual (non-carcinogenic) chemicals acting on different pathways, and a variety of related systems, organs, tissues and cells could plausibly conspire to produce carcinogenic synergies."

The information gathered about the general health risks posed by long-term exposure to low levels of endocrine disrupters has set a new course for cancer researchers in terms of looking at environmental toxins as contributing factors to cancer and other diseases, and the papers that have been written, thanks to this project, have helped educate the public in a nonthreatening, action-oriented way.

Dialing Down the Hysteria

It's nearly impossible for any cancer patient to resist wondering if there might have been something in their environment that might have contributed to their disease. David Servan-Schreiber wondered if he might have been affected by the pesticides (specifically atrazine) that were sprayed all over the agricultural fields where he played as a child near Normandy, France. He had two cousins who also played there and ate the foods grown in those fields, both of whom wound up with breast cancer as adults. Atrazine has been found to turn male frogs into female frogs.[68] It is pervasive in the water supply and has been linked to delayed puberty, prostate inflammation, and breast cancer in animal studies.[69,70] Research has found an association between atrazine and prostate cancer, but more study is necessary to make a direct connection.[71]

Contemplating all the pesticides, poisons, EDCs, and toxins that are in our lives is not easy for any of us. In the class on environmental toxins taught through Meg Hirshberg's Anticancer Lifestyle Program, participants jokingly call this the "Holy Crap!" class.[72] While it is important to become informed about chemicals we are routinely exposed to in our environment, it is equally if not more important to not let that knowledge paralyze us from cleaning up our own home environments by buying fewer products that contain hormone-disrupting chemicals and by making proactive changes in our lives to limit our exposure to toxins. While the Holy Crap class is necessary, Hirshberg realizes that being overwhelmed is not an end point. "Very quickly, we move into the practical, empowering information so participants can become more informed consumers," she explains. "We really dial down the hysteria."

It's important that we all understand what we can change and what we cannot when it comes to environmental toxins and anticancer living. We need to collectively become aware of the main known toxins that show up in our air, water, food, and other consumer products (beauty aids, clothing, home-building materials, and household goods).

For example, most of us have no idea what's in our water supply; we simply turn on the tap and take a drink. But because of a few horrible events that get national media attention, we're beginning to take notice. The Flint, Michigan, water crisis gained national attention when the water supply was tainted with dangerous bacteria, factory runoff, and lead.[73] Although many may see this as an isolated event and not relevant to the country as a whole, the EWG in a recent report revealed that an industrial solvent classified as a likely carcinogen, which is also a common impurity in cosmetics and household cleaners, was detected in drinking water supplies for nearly 90 million Americans in forty-five states.[74]

Getting clean water seems like it should be a given for most of us, but it's not as easy as you'd think. Most water bottles made from plastics leech unsafe chemicals like BPA,[75] though many are now BPA-free. While a company may have removed one harmful substance, they may have replaced it with an equally or more harmful substance. For example, BPA has been removed from many products and replaced with bisphenol S (BPS), a chemical that causes the same or worse harm than BPA.[76] A 2013 study by Cheryl Watson at The University of Texas Medical Branch at Galveston found that even small concentrations of BPS can disrupt a cell's normal functioning, which could potentially lead to the same risks associated with the endocrine-disrupting effects of BPA.[77]

When Glenn Sabin decided to forgo conventional treatment after he was diagnosed with CLL (chronic lymphocytic leukemia), one of the first major lifestyle changes he made was to change out the water-filtration system in his home and at the office. "I installed a whole-home softening unit to filter out the bulk of the chlorine and other things, and a reverse-osmosis drinking-water system." Glenn credits his intense focus on clean, toxin-free hydration, along with anticancer eating, sleeping, and living with deep purpose, as vital parts of his own synergistic anticancer living plan.

Proceed with Caution

When you realize the extent to which we live within a chemical-laden environment, it can make you paranoid. We don't want to paralyze you, but we do want you to become more aware of the potential impact of long-term exposure to a variety of chemicals on your health. It is likely that most environmental toxins will never be conclusively tied to cancer, but the list of those that have been is growing and we have no reason to believe it will not continue to grow as we become more adept at tracing chemicals and studying their effects on the human body over time.

Given the lax regulation of chemicals and the reactionary approach of government regulators, it is up to the consumer to be diligent about reading labels and making healthy choices to limit exposure to chemicals and toxins. In our family, we have adopted the Precautionary Principle. Until a chemical is found to be harmless, we try not to use it. When it comes to personal care products, anything that lists on its ingredients "fragrance" includes chemicals, which are likely to be endocrine disrupters, we put them back on the shelf and look for products that have ingredients we recognize, without the parabens or phthalates that can mimic hormones in our bodies. This better-safe-than-sorry approach is the only way in our current deregulated environment to reduce your contact with known and suspected carcinogens that are present in everything from the fire-resistant couch where you relax every evening to endocrine disrupters in the shampoo and other personal care products you use every morning.

Environmental Synergy

The link between environmental exposure and other areas in the Mix of Six is not as clear cut, but emerging data point to connections that may become more definitive with additional research:

- **Obesity:** A study in 2014 found that children exposed to chemicals used to soften plastic were more likely to be obese and at increased risk of diabetes.[78] Researchers at New York University looked at the urine and blood of more than seven hundred fifty adolescents and found increased insulin resistance, a precursor to diabetes, in teenagers with higher levels of di-2-ethylhexyl phthalate or DEHP.[79] Meanwhile, high levels of BPA were connected with being overweight or obese. The rates of obesity were twice as high in teens with the highest BPA levels compared to those with the lowest levels.[80] Researchers speculate that added BPA could throw off hormonal balance and disrupt metabolism, but note that more studies are needed to show a direct link.[81,82]

- **Sleep:** A 2016 study found connections between BPA levels and sleep.[83] Researchers looked at data collected between 2005 and 2010 as part of the National Health and Nutrition Examination Survey. They found that higher BPA levels measured in urine samples corresponded with survey participants who said they got less than six hours of sleep per night. Inadequate sleep has been linked to obesity, diabetes, metabolic syndrome, heart disease, and cancer.

- **Exercise:** A study from the University of Missouri in 2015 found that female mice exposed to BPA or to ethinyl estradiol, the estrogen in birth control pills, were less inclined to engage in physical activity.[84] Researchers exposed mice to the chemicals while they were in the womb and again during weaning through the mother's milk. They found that the exposed mice engaged in less activity at night, when mice are typically more active. The exposed mice moved more slowly, drank less water, and slept more. They also burned more carbs than fats, which many researchers believe is one of the causes of obesity in humans, because the unused fats gradually accumulate in the body.

Moving Toward Cleaner Living

Protecting yourself comes down to a simple philosophy—control what you can control, limit your exposure where you can, and then be active in your community when other environmental dangers come to light. A lot of the environmental contaminants we face are either out of our control or require legislation and activism to change. We think this work is important, but we want you to start with the choices you are making every day. What's in your shampoo or the cleaner you use to clean your bathtub? What about the hair gel you use or the toothpaste you clean your teeth with every night before bed? We suggest starting with the simple things and making a clean sweep of your body and your house. Creating an anticancer environment begins at home and starts with what you are exposing yourself to voluntarily.

THE ANTICANCER LIVING GUIDE
TO DETOXIFY YOUR ENVIRONMENT

In an era when profits often take precedence over precaution, you, the consumer, are responsible for overseeing, monitoring, and controlling (where you can) your exposure to the toxins in your environment. While it is a challenge to avoid *all* exposure to toxins, in the pages that follow we will outline a prescription to reduce your chemical burden utilizing the precautionary principle. When it comes to limiting your chemical exposure, the precautionary principle means that you are maintaining awareness of what you are putting on and in your body and taking steps to avoid exposing yourself unnecessarily to toxins in your household and environment. If you aren't sure whether or not something is harmful, don't risk it. We examine our exposures from the top of our head to the tips of our toes. Then we go from room to room and look at everything we come in contact with—from the products we use to clean the house to the chairs we sit on and the beds we sleep in. Clear your body and your home as much as you can of potentially dangerous chemicals, and protect your children and your community when possible from the ever-expanding realm of toxic exposure. It goes without saying that you should avoid too much sun and never smoke or use e-cigarettes. Sun and smoke are known to contribute to cancer onset, so avoid overexposure to the sun and any exposures to tobacco and the chemicals in e-cigarettes.

Five Pillars for Establishing an Anticancer Environment

1. Reduce your household chemical exposures.
2. Filter your water.
3. Reduce the toxins you put on your body.
4. Reduce the toxins you put in your body.
5. Interact carefully with your larger environment.

Starting the Cleanup

Many find it easiest to move from room to room in their house and eliminate potentially hazardous products as they go. Another way to proceed is to focus on products from the top of your head to the tips of your toes and then products you encounter in your immediate environment, starting with your home.

Keeping Your House Chemical-Free

- Take your shoes off at the door. Streets and lawns are filled with pesticides, herbicides, oil, grease, and other toxic chemicals.
- Open the doors and windows to ventilate your home. New homes especially build up toxins as they are so well sealed.
- Don't use toxic pesticides in your home.
- Swap out your cleaning products for natural, toxin-free cleaners, including products for the laundry, dishwasher soap, and dish soap.
- Go room by room to evaluate your house and what possible chemicals you are using in each room.
- Invest in a vacuum that has a high-efficiency particulate air (HEPA) filter. Vacuum twice a week to remove dust and grime that can carry toxins.
- Houseplants can act as natural air filters. Certain plants are more effective as filters than others. If you have a pet, read about specific plants' possible toxicity to animals. The ASPCA has an informative page on poisonous plants.
- Scented candles can present risks in two ways—the fragrance and the wax. Paraffin, the wax used in most candles, can emit chemicals like benzene and toluene. These substances are known carcinogens.[1,2] Paraffin is a petroleum waste product. Also, many candles have lead core wicks that release lead into the air. The safest candle to use is one made of beeswax. Candles using artificial fragrance will lead to inhalation of a possible endocrine disrupter.[3]
- Use low- or zero-VOC (volatile organic compounds) paint. VOCs are solvents that get released into the air as the paint dries. VOCs can cause acute symptoms, including headaches and dizziness. The long-term effects are less certain, but according to the U.S. Environmental Protection Agency, some VOCs are suspected carcinogens.[4]

- Do not use flame-retardant or stain-resistant chemicals on your furniture, as these chemicals have been classified as carcinogens.[5]
- If carpeting is necessary, air it out for a few days before bringing it into the house. Many carpets and pads contain VOCs and stain repellents that contain perfluorinated chemicals (PFCs). It is ideal to have carpeting free of VOCs and PFCs.
- Avoid air fresheners. As a rule, they are loaded with chemicals of concern, such as EDCs and phthalates.
- For your next mattress and pillow, consider a company that makes these products toxin-free (VOCs and flame retardants). This requires some research and cross-referencing to find companies that are honestly transparent about their practices.

Filter Your Tap Water

- As the majority of chemicals found in U.S. tap water are not regulated, use the precautionary principle and filter your water. There are so many contaminants in water, ranging from chlorine and fluoride and other toxic elements to chemicals (from runoff and manufacturing and household use to diluted prescription drugs and over-the-counter medicines), that filtering is a must in an anticancer living home (check out ewg.org/tap water to see about the water quality in your area).[6]
- A number of filter options are available at different price points. An on-counter water filter or a sink-attachment water filter are cost-effective and easy to use. Don't forget to add filters to showerheads to decrease breathing in aerosolized chemicals from the shower spray that will enter your lungs for transmission into your bloodstream. EWG.org has information on all the options.[7]
- Don't drink water from a plastic bottle. Much of the bottled water on the market is essentially municipal tap water. Also, chemicals such as BPA can leech from the plastic and contaminate the water. Carry a stainless steel or glass bottle with you. Keep it in your bag. Aluminum bottles can have a BPA lining inside, so do your research or stick with glass and stainless steel.

Reduce the Toxins You Put on Your Body

Many companies are seeing the demand for products that contain few if any known toxins. It is now possible to find almost any product in an endocrine-disrupter-free, carcinogen-free version. The next time you visit your hair salon or nail shop, ask about products they carry that are "green." Then go home and look them up online to check what is being said about those products by organizations like EWG (ewg.org/skindeep).

Below is a common list of products men and women use every day. Use the check box to indicate if your current products are toxin-free. It might not be possible to find a completely healthy product, but you can certainly reduce your exposure burden by carefully reading labels and making changes where you can.

Don't discount homemade solutions for many of the items listed below, especially for cleaning and laundering. They are inexpensive, nontoxic, and effective.

Refer to the "chemicals to avoid" list in this section of the book when reviewing ingredients on labels (also see ewg.org/healthy products).

Body Products

❑ Shampoo
❑ Conditioner
❑ Hairstyling product
❑ Soap
❑ Antibacterial hand soap
❑ Toothpaste
❑ Deodorant
❑ Cleanser
❑ Toner
❑ Face cream
❑ Eye cream
❑ Hand cream
❑ Body cream
❑ Perfume

Makeup

- ❑ Makeup remover
- ❑ Eye makeup remover
- ❑ Foundation
- ❑ Primer
- ❑ Powder
- ❑ Concealer
- ❑ Eye shadow
- ❑ Eyeliner
- ❑ Mascara
- ❑ Blush
- ❑ Bronzing powder
- ❑ Lip liner
- ❑ Lipstick or lip gloss

Nail Care

- ❑ Nail polish
- ❑ Nail polish remover
- ❑ Cuticle cream

Hair Salons

- ❑ Hair dye
- ❑ Styling lotion
- ❑ Hair spray
- ❑ Hair gel

Laundry

- ❑ Laundry detergent
- ❑ Fabric softener
- ❑ Fabric-softening sheets
- ❑ Bleaching products
- ❑ Wool dryer balls

Feminine Hygiene Products

- ❑ Sanitary pads
- ❑ Tampons

Sun Protection

- ❑ Sunscreen that is nonaerosol, as aerosolized sprays enter the lungs
- ❑ Lip protection

Bug Spray

- ❑ Nonaerosol bug spray

Household Products

- ❑ Toilet paper
- ❑ Dishwashing liquid
- ❑ Paper towels
- ❑ Air fresheners
- ❑ All-purpose cleaners
- ❑ Toilet bowl cleaners
- ❑ Floor cleaners

Cleaning Products

- ❑ Microfiber cloths that require only water to clean
- ❑ Sponges

Household Cleaning Products

- ❑ Household cleaners
- ❑ Air fresheners
- ❑ Any products with scent

Home Renovations

❑ Low- or zero-VOC paint
❑ Opt for hardwood floors and small washable rugs instead of carpeting
❑ Furniture that contains no stain proofing or flame retardant

Reduce the Toxins You Put in Your Body

Eat Organic

• Eating organic is especially important with the twelve types of produce with the highest amount of pesticide residue: apples, bell peppers, celery, cherries, grapes, lettuce, nectarines, peaches, pears, potatoes, spinach, and strawberries (ewg.org/dirtydozen).[8]

Food Packaging

• Where possible, buy food in glass instead of cans, plastic-lined paper, or plastic.

Food Storage

• Use food containers that are glass, ceramic, or food-grade stainless steel.
• When plastic storage bags are necessary, place the food item in parchment paper and then place the wrapped food inside the plastic bag.

Cookware

• Use food-grade stainless steel, ceramic, and cast-iron cookware.
• Look for cutting boards made of bamboo or wood.
• Avoid microwaving in plastic or Styrofoam.

Interact Carefully with the Larger Environment

As we mentioned, it is important to control what you can and not obsess about what is beyond your control when it comes to environmental toxins.

That said, there are steps we can all take to limit our exposure to potential carcinogens in our larger environment.

Be Careful Using Cell Phones: The connection between exposure to radio-frequency radiation and cancer remains hotly debated. In 2011, the International Agency for Research on Cancer concluded that cell phone use was a possible human carcinogen. But the results from numerous studies have been mixed.[9] When it comes to cell phones, David Servan-Schreiber's warning in *Anticancer* still rings true: "Be careful." As we increase the amount of exposure we have to electromagnetic fields, we are likely to see increases in certain types of cancer, especially in those who have weakened immune systems or genetic predispositions.[10,11] Because our brains are still developing through adolescence, children and teenagers could be more susceptible to the dangers of EMFs.

So, when we say "be careful," this is what we mean:

* Increase the distance between you and your phone, whether that means using a wired earbud when talking, using the speaker function, or keeping your phone away from your body, even when it's on and you're not using it.
* Limit your cell phone use when reception is weak or when you're on the go. EMF emission is strongest when your signal is weak. It is also stronger when your signal is moving from one receiver to the next.

The State of California had considered issuing warnings and guidelines in 2014 for safe cell phone use, but for complex reasons this never reached the public until 2017.[12,13]

Products for the Car: Purchase green products for interior cleaning of your car. Take green products with you to the self-service car wash and use on your car along with your own cleaning rags.

Dry Cleaning: About 85 percent of dry cleaners in the United States use PERC (percholoethylene or tetrachloroethylene), which has been listed as a "likely human carcinogen" by the National Academy of Sciences and shown to cause cancer in animal studies.[14,15]

While the toxicity of PERC to humans remains unclear, we recommend the following precautions when dealing with dry cleaning:

- Remove dry cleaning bags outside of your home or apartment.
- Hang up dry cleaning on a coat rack outside for at least two hours.
- If you live in an apartment, remove the plastic at the dry cleaners and walk your laundry home, airing it out as you go.
- Do not keep the plastic bag over your dry cleaning in your closet.
- Do not leave dry cleaning in your car, as vapors will build up inside the car.

You can also look for "green" dry cleaners. There are a number of processes that have been developed to clean clothes without using PERC, and they include the following:

- **CO_2 Cleaning:** In this cleaning process, perchloroethylene or PERC is replaced by liquid CO_2. The gas form of carbon dioxide is pressurized into a clear liquid in a special machine. After the process is completed, the liquid CO_2 can be pumped into a storage tank and reused. CO_2 cleaning has been endorsed by the EPA.[16,17]
- **Silicone Cleaning:** This method is similar to conventional dry cleaning, but it uses a patented silicone-based solution to remove stains and odors from fabrics. The EPA is still assessing whether the solution, siloxane D5, poses potential risks to human health.
- **Wet Cleaning:** This alternative to dry cleaning is a solvent-free laundering method in which garments are cleaned with water and special detergents in high-tech machines. The EPA has endorsed the method, as it does not use hazardous chemicals or generate chemical waste or air pollution.[18]
- **System K4:** This German technology uses an acetal-based solvent that is reportedly biodegradable and safe for the environment.

THE ANTICANCER LIVING GUIDE
ENVIRONMENTAL SUMMARY

Rid Your House of Toxic Chemicals

* Go room to room and eliminate potentially hazardous products as you go.
* When you enter your house, take your shoes off at the door.
* Use houseplants as natural air filters.
* Opt for hardwood floors or washable rugs instead of carpeting.
* Buy furniture that has no stain proofing or flame retardants.
* Use paint without volatile organic compounds.
* Buy pillows and mattresses that are toxin-free.
* Filter your drinking water.
* Use natural, nontoxic cleaning products (a mixture of vinegar and water is ideal).
* Avoid any products with scent.

Limit Toxins on Your Body

* Check the ingredients of all body products like shampoo, conditioner, toothpaste, and deodorant. Gradually switch to less-toxic options.
* Update your makeup with products that are free of harmful chemicals.
* Reduce your use of chemical-laden hair dyes and artificial products for your hair.
* Buy toxin-free laundry detergent, dishwasher detergent, and dish soap.

Reduce Toxins in Your Body

* Eat organic.
* Store food in glass rather than plastic.
* Use food-grade stainless-steel or cast-iron cookware.
* Use wood cutting boards.

- Put filters on showerheads.
- Don't microwave food in plastic.

Interact Carefully with the Outside World

- Keep your cell phone away from your body.
- Use natural, nontoxic products to clean your car.
- Air out dry cleaning before bringing into your home or closet.
- Look for dry cleaners that use alternative, green technology.

CONCLUDING THOUGHTS

About a year after I first met David Servan-Schreiber, I had the honor and challenge of delivering a speech in his stead. David was scheduled as the keynote speaker at the annual Anderson Network Conference, a patient survivorship conference put on every year at MD Anderson in Houston. That summer, David was suffering through a recurrence of his disease. He called the conference organizers from Paris to say he couldn't make it. He was too sick to travel. Faced with a tight deadline, the organizers asked if I could deliver David's presentation. I had seen it twice, but giving the talk myself was another matter.

That week, David and I were in continual correspondence. He shared his slides, we updated some with the latest research, and we talked through the major points on the phone. We had grown close working to create and fund the Comprehensive Lifestyle Study that was gaining momentum and promised to be one of only a few clinical studies ever to measure the effects of lifestyle change in multiple areas at once. David's support to that point had been key to our progress. On a more personal level, I considered David a like-minded friend who shared my passion about lifestyle as legitimate medicine. I wanted to make sure I honored his message.

The opening day of the conference, the meeting hall was packed. I remember vividly the energizing feeling I had delivering such a powerful, inspiring, and hopeful message to a room full of cancer survivors. They could take an active role in their health. Their lives were not over. They could change their habits and behaviors, starting that very moment, and significantly improve their chances of survival while also improving their quality of life. That day, it felt like David's story of marshaling the body's natural defenses to influence the course of disease became part of me. Since that night, I have given hundreds of talks on the connection between cancer and lifestyle factors, but that first presentation, standing in David's shoes, was a turning point.

Much has changed since then. In the last decade, we've truly stepped onto what I believe is, finally, firm footing when it comes to focusing on prevention as well as treatment of cancer. Almost daily, new research is emerging that shows how much control we actually have over our biological synergy. Our thinking in the oncology world is now finally evolving, too, thanks in no small part to the mapping of the human genome and our new understanding about how human behavior actually has a hand in writing our genomic story.

We now know that we are not at the whim of our ancestry or our genes; we can positively influence the trajectory of our health, at any stage of life, regardless of the presence of disease, and this knowledge (combined with a rapidly growing body of scientific evidence) is changing the conversation about cancer. The approach to treating cancer must include the prevention approaches alongside conventional treatment, and we need to strive to prevent cancer diseases in the first place.

The tough truth is that, at least for the foreseeable future, cancer is going to be part of our lives. But it's also true that more than 50 percent of all cancers are thought to be preventable.[1] In fact, it may be an underestimate. What's more likely is that two-thirds of cancers and most instances of heart disease, stroke, and diabetes could be avoided if we live the way we know we should and follow the anticancer living guidelines to make ourselves and our families healthier, fitter, and more balanced. The research confirms this and gives me hope that we may actually be able to slow the rates of cancer onset. We're also developing tools for measuring the efficacy of lifestyle changes that were once thought "too soft" to measure. Technology and digital imaging are now being deployed to visually diagram population-based epidemiological studies and measure the effect of lifestyle changes on specific biological markers of disease. Genetic heat maps flash when gene behaviors change as a result of lifestyle modifications, and we can measure increasingly sensitive indicators of the presence of cancer or other diseases by using simple blood tests that can detect minute changes in protein loads. These tools of traditional scientific research are now being used in collaboration with written or oral reports to confirm what we've suspected all along: anticancer living matters.

As a colleague recently put it, succinctly, "Cancer is complex, but preventing cancer is not."

What is becoming increasingly clear is that it is not possible to treat our way out of the cancer epidemic. While billions of dollars are going toward more precision-based cancer treatments and early detection as part of the highly touted "Cancer Moonshot" (the important initiative started by former Vice President Joe Biden), cancer prevention through lifestyle change remains the cheapest and most effective method to prevent and improve outcomes. A true partnership of anticancer living and precision medicine is the future of cancer care. It is time to finally move away from a model of disease care to one of true health care.

Living for Health

What motivates people to change is complex, but we often see that cancer is a teachable moment and compels action. Facing the reality of our mortality can certainly be a wake-up call. Most of us know intellectually that we all have a finite time on this earth, but our minds have a sneaky way of keeping us at arm's length from the reality of our own mortality and it's only when we're advanced in age or when we're diagnosed with a disease or illness before then that we become aware that our biological balance, our wholeness and well-being, aren't going to last forever. This awareness brings us back into our bodies, and these moments of clarity are the entry points for change.

But we don't have to wait until we're scared into action to take meaningful steps. Cancer, as complex as it is, is no longer a mystery to us. We now have enough real scientific evidence and information in hand to make the lifestyle changes that will offer us the best chance to keep the diseases of aging, including cancer, at bay. In the last decade, and certainly since the original publication of *Anticancer*, we've begun to crack the code on cancer biology and we're beginning to understand the mechanisms that switch on the deleterious synergy that allows cancers to grow and thrive. The more we know, the more we can do.

Where to Begin

Our lives are complex, busy, and ever changing. Our anticancer living strategies ought to reflect this and be as fluid and as flexible as possible. We believe the most essential place to begin is with social support. It is only when we recognize a different way to live and think "I can do that, too," that we can escape our negative, unhealthy patterns and start to strive for something more. It is only through a supportive community that we can find reinforcement for positive change and reassurance when our own efforts fall short. Once a support network is in place, we can truly start to change our mind-set about our life and our life's purpose. The vast majority of the CompLife Study patients and the long-term cancer survivors we interviewed and feature throughout the book view this mental change as the most critical component of their new way of life, rather than diet or exercise. For many, healing the body became the sole focus and purpose of every daily lifestyle choice, but that emphasis began with an important mental shift that helped them recognize that their daily choices had a real and measurable impact on their health and quality of life.

Our bodies thrive on moderation, calm, and consistency. Unnecessary or repetitive or prolonged stress of any kind can undo our best practices quicker and more dramatically than anything else. This is why once we have our support systems in place we must manage our stress before trying to change our other behaviors around diet, exercise, and sleep. Excess stress will make creating the synergy we hope to achieve by cultivating healthy practices in the other areas of anticancer living impossible. The evidence is also clear that untangling ourselves from stress makes our bodies more resilient and less hospitable to cancer growth.

Putting Yourself First

All the women who have so far signed up for participation in our CompLife Study find this one of the toughest parts of the trial protocol. They're used to taking care of everyone else—kids, spouses, bosses, aging parents—ahead of taking care of themselves. Brucett M. recently attended a retreat with other CompLife women and was able to refocus her efforts on making healthy choices. She said afterward that she had been slipping back into her old ways, putting the needs of others ahead of her own, working too hard, and not getting enough sleep. But this anticancer community helped bring her back to what was important—taking care of herself. "The one thing that struck me the most was the genuine feeling of understanding and encouragement we gave each other," she wrote after the retreat. "It didn't matter if we had just met; you knew it came straight from the heart because that's what we all want for each other—to live long, healthy lives."

Learning to put your own health first does not come easily to most of us, but is especially hard for women, who, universally, are raised to put the needs of others ahead of their own. Once we learn how best to take care of ourselves, we quickly learn that we are even better when it comes to supporting the needs of others.

From Action to Purpose

Living for health means living very deliberately, very pragmatically, and very realistically. Nearly every cancer patient I've met credits the undeniability of the disease with grounding them in reality, sometimes, for the very first time. The things that were once troublesome seem to drop away. The things that are most essential come into sharper focus. Life takes on a new meaning. The body takes on a new meaning. Health and a focused life purpose, rather than fame, success, or other intangibles, become the purpose and the goal.

When we focus on healing ourselves, we often set ourselves on a path that will lead us to fulfilling our true potential in surprising ways. Alison and I hear this over and again from cancer survivors and their advocates. Molly M., who was given six to eighteen months to live, has survived eighteen and a half years and counting with an aggressive brain cancer. At the outset, she described herself as a "physical, emotional, and cognitive wreck." She was half-paralyzed, plagued by full-body seizures, unable to follow or form a sentence, with no memory, and stuck on an extreme emotional roller coaster. Long before neuroplasticity was recognized, Molly told her doctors she was going to "rewire her brain." It took everything she had to persist with her healing regimen. Amazingly, her brain tumor isn't even showing up on MRI scans anymore. When she's not tending to her own health, she's an advocate for healthy living and beating the odds and a support for glioblastoma patients who seek her out for her encouragement and comfort. Her life, she acknowledges, is not what she'd hoped for, but it is rewarding in ways she couldn't have imagined. For Meg Hirshberg, the lack of medical guidance about lifestyle changes that could lower the odds of cancer recurrence inspired her to start a foundation that created in-person and online courses to give patients and those interested in prevention the tools and information they need to live an anticancer lifestyle. Susan Rafte worked to provide emotional support to younger women going through cancer treatment and created a support group for those with metastatic cancer. When Gabe Canales realized the amazing potential of lifestyle change to slow cancer progression or prevent it from forming in the first place, he founded Blue Cure Foundation to educate boys and men about the prevalence of prostate cancer and what they can do to prevent or control it by modifying their lifestyle.

We're not saying that every cancer survivor should devote their life to helping others who face a similar diagnosis or that you need to start a foundation to support cancer prevention. What we do know is that you need to start with yourself to create change and then share that message with others. We see time and again that those with and without cancer are inspired by anticancer living to spread the word, either in a professional way or in a personal way among their family and friends. Alison and I are constantly awed and humbled by the power of this message and its effect on people and their communities.

With that said, it is important to note that these survivors have discovered that cancer is only a small part of who they are; they build lives of rich meaning and purpose around this fact and it keeps them going, quite literally, long after statistical models say they should be gone. When I followed up with Josh M., whom you met in chapter 7 and who has defied the odds and continues to thrive after being diagnosed with an incurable neuroendocrine cancer, he added nuance to the conversation about what constitutes good health care for those with cancer: "I find that too many patients focus on extending a life they're not enjoying. For me, the 'cancer reset' gave me the chance to really define what I mean by a quality life and to begin to pursue that. This is what I think the focus ought to be: on finding the kind of healing that leads to a really profound life upgrade—even if you aren't ever cured."

Another paradox of this shift in perspective is how the process of simplifying one's life (by, for example, leaving a stressful career or radically cleaning up your diet or living environment) brings one a greater sense of meaning, a greater sense of gratitude for the most meaningful things in life, such as family, friends, music, the arts, nature—or even life itself.

Changing the Conversation

Margaret Cuomo, whom you met in the last chapter, recently spoke with me about the challenges of raising awareness about how easy and low-cost lifestyle changes can have a profound preventative impact on one's health. It's difficult to get the message out when it can't be copyrighted or monetized the way drugs are. But she remains hopeful and quite committed to changing the public dialogue. As she puts it, "I am encouraged that people really want to be at their healthiest, at their most vibrant, at their most productive for themselves and for future generations, for their children and their grandchildren. I am confident that the more information we give to the public, the more they'll be able to change, and they'll help us compel companies to develop products that won't harm us consumers."

Her sense of urgency reflects her horror at the notion that our children's generation is the first that may not live as long as we do. "For so many years and in so many cultures—not just American culture—the sign of prosperity and progress is having your children be healthier, taller, smarter, more affluent, and certainly living longer than you did. Now, all of a sudden, we're in a situation where the legacy we're leaving our children is not that, at least in terms of overall health and longevity. We have a social responsibility to address this, and this is why we need to keep getting the anticancer living message out there."

One Step at a Time

Anticancer living is not a static program. In fact, it's no program at all; it's a way of life, and as such, it will evolve and change overtime, just as you do. Yet every incremental change you make that supports your body's innate ability to control disease and promote health will pay dividends in all areas of your life.[2]

Decide that you're going to live as though your life depends on it, because it actually does. You will find that as you step into this kind of self-care, you'll start to feel more vibrantly connected to life and be more available and more present for all that life has to offer you. As one patient said to me, "This isn't work, Lorenzo, this is life!"

But it is pragmatic, and it is grounded in science. There will be nothing miraculous or spontaneous about the health improvements you will experience: They will each be based on cause and effect. Your choices, your action, your good health, the health of the planet. It is all interconnected.

One of the truly amazing impacts of an anticancer lifestyle is the way it can inspire others. Alison and I see the ongoing growth of awareness among our friends and in the friends of our three growing children. Last month, seven years after standing in for David to deliver his keynote speech at the Annual Anderson Network Conference, I gave the opening lecture to launch the conference. On that occasion I chose to share the stage and message of anticancer living with Nella B., one of the CompLife patients whose story we shared in chapter 11. When Nella came into the study, she considered herself well educated about health and nutrition. But what she admitted to the audience was that she only knew 10 percent of what she learned in CompLife and what we are sharing in *Anticancer Living*. She knew she needed to lose weight, but she did not know how to make weight loss, which she had achieved many times, sustainable. She did not know why excess weight was harmful and that fat produces estrogen that feeds her estrogen-positive breast cancer. She knew that eating salad was better than eating a burger, but she did not know that drinking green tea could reduce the growth of new blood vessels her tumor needed to grow and spread. She knew vegetables were good, but she did not know that broccoli could prevent precancerous cells from developing into malignant tumors.

The most stunning change for Nella was the absence of fear that she's experienced; she's no longer afraid of recurrence or cancer proliferation because she feels actively involved in her own cancer care. "I'm first now," she said. "I don't feel like it's [cancer's] got me: I feel like I have it." She described her new relationship with her body in a thrilling way: "I feel more nurturing toward myself, my own body. I have an active relationship with it where I communicate that if it treats me right, I will treat it right. We're working in unison, my body and I, and I fuel it correctly so it can perform correctly."

Watching Nella talk about the importance of adopting a mind-body practice, about how she now reads the labels of all the personal care products she buys and exercises to improve her sleep quality—her complete awakening to anticancer living made me realize that, just like I believe

David passed the torch to me when I gave the speech in his stead seven years ago, it is now my turn to pass the torch to Nella and the many others who are living these healing practices daily. As Nella told the audience that day, it is not fair that so many people go through cancer treatment without knowing how much their lifestyle choices impact their health. Likewise, it is not fair for those of us who don't yet have cancer not to realize that our lifestyle choices influence our quality of life today and our risk of disease in the future.

As Nella concluded her talk, "We're going to have to make integrative medicine part of the treatment plan, so that even the doctors can learn from each other. But it's going to take all of us, right? It's going to take all of us. Can we do it?" And the audience shouted back in unison, "Yes!"

APPENDIX A

The Cancer Hallmarks Explained

While the mapping of the human genome was being completed, two researchers named Douglas Hanahan and Robert Weinberg published an article in 2000, which offered an elegantly simple theory about how cancer cells develop and progress.[1] In their original thesis, Hanahan and Weinberg proposed that there are six basic underlying genetic processes at work that make cancer (a notoriously complex cellular disease) happen. They called this paper the "Hallmarks of Cancer," and they identified the main cellular processes that drive cancer as follows: (1) sustaining proliferative signaling; (2) evading growth suppressors, (3) resisting cell death; (4) enabling replicative immortality; (5) inducing angiogenesis; and (6) activating invasion and metastasis. Several years later, Hanahan and Weinberg added two additional hallmarks—reprogramming energy metabolism and avoiding immune destruction—and two enabling characteristics—genome instability and mutation and tumor-promoting inflammation to their model.[2]

Cancer's Drive to Survive

Proliferative signaling sounds like something you might get a traffic ticket for, but what this essentially refers to is cancer's ability to sustain its own growth so it can continue to spread. This is a fundamental aspect of cancer—uncontrolled cell growth and division. Normal cells are monitored by multiple systems and signals in the body to help keep cell growth and division under control. Cancer cells deregulate the normal signaling from these different systems and allow the cells to grow out of control. Normal cells respond to growth factors that signal the cell to grow and divide or to not grow. Growth factors bind to the surface of cells and the signal to grow is transmitted into the cell and converted to a sequence of biochemical signals, which unleash the genes that promote cell growth and division. Cancer cells highjack these normal signaling pathways to turn them on all the time. In this mode, cells are no longer under control of the normal activation (turning on) and inhibition (turning off) signals and continue growing and dividing unchecked.

Cancer Goes Stealth

At the same time cancer cells are utilizing the body's resources to promote their own growth, they also need to avoid the systems that inhibit cell proliferation (*evading growth suppressors*), including tumor-suppressor genes. The body maintains an intricate balance between growth suppressors, genes that can neutralize powerful *oncogenes* (mutated genes in cancer cells), and factors that maintain healthy cell growth. When the function and signal from tumor-suppressor genes are lost, it means that the cells do not "hear" the message to stop growing. As a result, growth continues out of control. Now that your phone line has been severed, cancer cuts power to your alarm system as well. Your body is left in the dark while cancer progresses.

Cancer as Zombie Vampire

When he was in the advanced stages of brain cancer, David Servan-Schreiber reported growing fears as he was falling asleep that he would be attacked by vampires. He feared that nocturnal monsters immune from death were seeking to cut his own life short. While the vampires in David's dreams were imaginary, the comparison to cancer is apt. Like vampires and zombies roaming city streets at night, cancer cells find ways to circumvent the body's system of cell destruction, so they *resist cell death* and become immortal and mutate indefinitely.

Cell Suicide: One of the most effective ways our system maintains control over inappropriate cell growth and division is through what is called *apoptosis*—spontaneous cell death or cell suicide. Factors within the cell and signals from outside cells can trigger this death-inducing process. Once apoptosis starts to take place, the cell is progressively broken down and then consumed by its neighbors and phagocytic ("cell-eating") cells (think Pac-Man). It is, of course, in the tumor cells' best interest to evade apoptosis, so they can grow unregulated. They do so both through the loss of tumor-suppressor gene function and by increasing the expression of anti-apoptotic genes. By up regulating, or turning on, anti-apoptotic proteins, the cell avoids apoptosis, even though the internal and external processes are sending signals to activate cell death.

Cell Explosion: A second way abnormal cell growth is controlled is through necrosis. Unlike apoptosis, necrotic cells become bloated and explode. A consequence of having the cells explode instead of being "digested" by the system is that the cell death results in the release of certain proteins into the surrounding tissue environment. These include proteins that are pro-inflammatory in nature and recruit inflammatory cells of the immune system to come to the site of the cell explosion and remove necrotic debris. Although this may sound like a good process, first responders rushing to the scene of an accident, recent evidence suggests that *immune inflammatory cells* can sometimes be actively tumor-promoting because they can foster angiogenesis (the formation of new blood vessels) and cell proliferation. In fact, having excessive numbers of cells undergoing necrosis may be a cancer risk factor.

Cancer's Bid for Eternal Life

Normal healthy cells have a limited number of growth-and-division cycles. Cancer cells, on the other hand, have processes activated *enabling replicative immortality*. What typically limits cell growth after successive replications and divisions is either *senescence*, a cell's loss with age of its ability to divide, or cell crisis, which involves cell death (either through apoptosis or other means). If cells evade a state of senescence, then they typically enter a state of crisis and ultimately die. However, cancer cells evade both processes and take on the ability for unlimited replication. This transition is called cell immortalization.

One component within a cell that helps to ensure a cell's integrity is the telomeres, the protective tips on the end of each pair of our twenty-three chromosomes that typically shorten as people age. Elissa Epel, a professor of psychology at the University of California, San Francisco, and coauthor of *The Telomere Effect*, has found that lifestyle choices are related to telomere length, which can be a predictor of disease and longevity. Every time a cell divides, the telomere length shortens. So, at a certain point, the telomere is too short for the cell to continue dividing and it becomes *senescent* (too old to replicate). But, in that state, the environment becomes ripe for cancer. "Once cells get old and get senescent, they become a source for inflammation, which creates a place for cancer to grow," Epel explains. In her research, Epel has found that chronic stress leads to telomere shortening. As telomeres shorten and cells continue to replicate, this can lead to chromosomal instability and damage, a risk factor for mutations. So people who are always stressed can have "older cells" that are more vulnerable to disease at a younger age. Yet, as we will see, healthy lifestyle can slow telomere shortening and reverse the harms of stress on our telomeres.

Telomerase, an enzyme within the nucleus of cells, helps to maintain the integrity of the telomeres. Although largely found at low levels in normal cells, cancer cells and immortalized cells have abnormally high levels of telomerase, allowing the cell to continue to replicate without telomere shortening. Meanwhile, if telomerase levels are low and telomeres get short enough, a successive cell division could lead to a chromosomal aberration. At that point, if the cell does not undergo crisis or apoptosis, a tumor can start to form. Through abnormal telomerase levels and proliferation-associated abnormalities, cells can become immortalized. This allows the cells to avoid a key anticancer defense of senescence and cell death. It is cancer's ticket to eternal life.

Let There Be Blood

Both normal tissues and tumors require a healthy blood supply to help bring in nutrients and oxygen and to remove waste products and carbon dioxide. During the early formation of an embryo and then prenatal development, the vasculature develops when new endothelial cells form together into tubes (*vasculogenesis*), in addition to the sprouting of new vessels (tubes) from existing vessels. This sprouting process is called *angiogenesis*. Once formed, the vascular system remains in place to support the body. Angiogenesis is turned on within the adult body as part of wound healing and female reproductive cycling. But this happens only for a short period of time and then stops. During tumor formation and development, an "angiogenic switch" remains on, allowing new blood vessels to be formed that help maintain the growth of the tumor. This is yet another example of how cancer tricks our normally balanced systems, permanently turning on a switch that was meant to go on and off, creating a constant state of growth, replication, or in this case—blood supply—to keep the cancer cells nourished.

Cancer's Search for a New Home

The spread of cancer from its original site to other parts of the body is usually what makes cancer lethal—*activating invasion and metastasis*. Medical interventions are most successful when cancer is found early and confined to only one site in the body. Although progress has been made at controlling cancer once it has metastasized, this is the area that still poses tremendous challenges and is the primary cause of cancer-related death.

Invasion and metastasis is a multistep process. It begins with the invasion of cancer cells into nearby blood and lymph vessels. This is followed by the cancer cells moving from these transport systems into the other tissues to form microscopic nodules of cancer cells that eventually grow until they become tumors that are large enough to be seen on scans. This last step is called "colonization."

Normally, cells are attached to their scaffolding, the extracellular matrix. If a cell detaches, it is supposed to undergo a process called *anoikis*—a form of programmed cell death. Tumor cells undergo a process that allows them to avoid anoikis, become migratory, and travel throughout the body. They also start to take on stem-cell characteristics, allowing them to land anywhere and adapt to the new surrounding tissues.

Once cancer cells have avoided the body's natural process of cell death and transformed into freely circulating, adaptive cells, they are in search of a new home to "colonize." Cancer cells are not initially adapted to the microenvironment of the tissue where they land. These cells might require hundreds of distinct colonization programs to get activated to allow the cells to grow and thrive. In this state they can also reseed and form additional colonies by further circulating in the body away from the metastatic site.

By adopting an anticancer lifestyle, you are doing everything possible to make the tumor microenvironment inhospitable to tumor growth. This makes it harder for these colonizing cancer cells to settle in and find a new home.

Cancer Siphons Your Tank

Because cancer cells replicate at a higher rate than other cells in the body, it is essential that they have the necessary "fuel" to maintain growth and cellular division—*reprogramming energy metabolism*. Glucose is a key source of fuel to maintain cell growth. Otto Warburg, who won the Nobel Prize in Medicine in 1931, documented a unique feature of cancer cells: even in the presence of oxygen, cancer can reprogram its energy production, by limiting energy generation largely to glycolysis, leading to a process that has been called "aerobic glycolysis."

Energy produced mainly through glycolysis is much less efficient at producing energy for the cell. For the cancer cells to make up for this lack of efficiency in energy production, they require an increase in glucose transporters. Rapidly growing tumor cells have glycolic rates up to two hundred times higher than those of normal cells. This can occur even if oxygen is plentiful. As many tumor types seem to thrive in a microenvironment with low levels of oxygen (hypoxic conditions), efficiently transferring energy through glycolysis allows for increased levels of glucose to enter the cell. A growing tumor can be thought of as a construction site, and as today's researchers explain it, the Warburg effect opens the gates for more trucks to deliver building materials (in the form of glucose molecules) in order to have more energy for cancer to proliferate.

Cancer Goes Undercover

A newly emerged hallmark that has received a lot of attention in the past five years is the ability of cancer cells to *avoid immune destruction*. We know that if components of our immune system are overactive for too long (inflammation), this state can facilitate many hallmark processes. However, the immune system also plays an important role in keeping cancer at bay. T cells are a type of white blood cells that patrol our bodies looking for cells that have been transformed into cancerous cells. The presence of T cells is a good sign for cancer patients. For example, patients with colon and ovarian cancer who have greater infiltration of certain immune cells into the tumor microenvironment have a better prognosis. On the other hand, individuals who have compromised immune systems for extensive periods of time (like people who received an organ transplant or patients with HIV/AIDS) have a higher rate of developing certain cancers. This has led to development of treatments that can boost the immune system.

But as with many of our body's surveillance systems, cancer has found a way to neutralize this immune response. Cancer cells have the capacity to bind receptors on activated T cells and effectively turn them off. The discovery that cancer cells can essentially put the brakes on the immune system has led to a new treatment for cancer, immunotherapy, with what are called checkpoint inhibitors. These drugs help to prevent the cancers cells from turning off the immune system. Checkpoint inhibitors have changed the landscape for cancer treatment and have led to dramatic responses in some patients.

The Green Light for Cancer Growth

The multistep process of *tumorigenesis* (in which cancer cells survive, proliferate, and travel throughout the body), supported by one or more of the hallmark steps listed above, is made possible by two enabling characteristics. The most important is genomic instability, which leads to increased mutations that help trigger the hallmark capabilities. The second enabling characteristic is the inflammatory state of premalignant and malignant cells. This inflammatory state can help promote tumor growth and progression.

Genome Instability and Mutation: How Cancer Is Born

Mutation or another genetic aberration is a necessary first step for engaging and activating the hallmarks. Cancer is a disease of abnormal genes and gene expression. It is the alteration of the genes that sets off tumorigenesis. This can take place due to an inherited genetic phenotype, but as we know, inherited genetic abnormalities are responsible for only 5 to 10 percent of cancers. More often, gene abnormalities come about through gene mutations that you acquire during your lifetime (like from carcinogens in tobacco smoke) or through the modification of expression of nonmutated genes that are influenced by lifestyle factors.

Although spontaneous mutations that lead to cancer are always taking place in the body, genome maintenance systems are active to ensure these mutations remain at as low a rate as possible. It is the shutting down of the genome maintenance process that ultimately allows mutations to form and grow into cancers. Cancer cells themselves can also trigger increased rates of mutation and suppress the genome maintenance systems.

The DNA maintenance machinery, referred to as the "caretakers" of the genome, are a set of genes that help to maintain the integrity of the DNA to decrease persistence of mutations. Defects in these genes will allow mutations to prosper and start the tumorigenic process. If the genes responsible for DNA repair, senescence, or apoptosis are not activated at the time of mutation, then the cells will continue to proliferate unchecked and tumorigenesis begins.

Genome maintenance and repair defects are now recognized as a critical first step *enabling* the start of the tumorigenic process. The vast majority of tumors can be linked back to the instability of the genome as the first step in cancer development. As discussed in part 2, different lifestyle factors are linked with these enabling features. Maintaining the structural integrity of our DNA and decreasing the mutagenic process is the first step in making our body inhospitable to cancer development and growth.

Inflammation: Cancer's Special Sauce

Inflammatory processes have long been recognized as a necessary step in tumorigenesis for most cancers. Nearly all cancer contains immune cells. The presence of some types of immune cells is a good thing, as this indicates the immune system is trying to control the tumor. However, other immune cells can be tumor promoting by causing inflammation. With inflammation, the immune cells release molecules that can promote the hallmark capabilities, including growth factors that sustain proliferative signaling; survival factors that limit cell death; factors that facilitate and increase angiogenesis, invasion, and metastasis; and signals that allow cancer cells to travel through the body. Inflammatory cells also can release chemicals that are mutagenic (cause mutations) that help accelerate the malignant process. Inflammation has been noted at the earliest stages of tumorigenesis and can help in the transition of early malignant cells into full-blown cancer.

The Wound That Never Heals

In the above discussion of the cancer hallmarks and enabling characteristics, each area is presented somewhat in isolation from the other. However, interaction occurs between all the areas and this takes place in what is called the *tumor microenvironment*. The tumor microenvironment is made up of different cell types and proteins that can either foster an environment supportive of cancer growth or an environment that is hostile to cancer growth.

Within the tumor microenvironment are cancer stem cells. These cells, thought to be an originating source of the tumor, are more resistant to treatment than other cancer cells, and help to seed the cancer outside of the primary site in distant organs, leading to metastases. Within the tumor microenvironment are also endothelial cells that can form blood vessels. These cells are critical in the formation of the vascular system to help provide a new vasculature and blood supply to the growing tumor.

It is now clear that inflammation is a double-edged sword. When inflammation becomes chronic, components that were once tumor controlling become tumor promoting. For example, fibroblasts are cells that are critical in the wound-healing process, and they seem to be abundant at tumor sites. What are now termed cancer-associated fibroblasts are known to play a role in cell proliferation, angiogenesis, invasion, and metastasis.

The complex communication that is taking place between these cells in the tumor microenvironment and cells that infiltrate and circulate in the body is what allows a cancer cell to thrive and survive or to be thwarted and die. It is interesting to note that some important processes necessary for cancer to grow—inflammation, recruitment of fibroblasts, increase in angiogenesis—are the same processes that are needed for wound healing. This has led some to suggest that tumors could be viewed as wounds that never heal. What is potentially healthy for a short period of time—inflammation to heal a wound—can become harmful when it becomes a chronic condition.

APPENDIX B

Eating by Food Groups—
A New Pattern

Most of us eat plenty of protein and carbohydrates. We eat fewer or no vegetables, nuts and seeds, beans and legumes, and fruit. The first step to changing your mind-set and making vegetables the star of every meal is to change the way you plan and shop. We look for vegetable recipes that use fresh herbs, allium roots, and a small sprinkling of olive oil.

Vegetable Groups

ALLIUMS

Garlic, onion, leek, green onions, shallots, chives

For those that like the taste—these flavors can be front and center. For those who don't like the taste, they can blend right into dishes and you won't even know they're there. To reduce the strong flavor of garlic and onion without removing the phytochemicals, soak the chopped alliums in water for twenty minutes before cooking:

- Leeks are a perfect base for soups.
- Onions and vegetables roasted are tasty, and roasting brings out the sweetness.
- Garlic can easily be added to every sauté of vegetables, beans and tofu, fish and lean meats.

Alliums have been shown in both epidemiological and laboratory studies to reduce the risk of several types of cancers.[1–3] The naturally occurring organosulfur compounds in alliums could play a role in inhibiting mutations and preventing cancer growth. In one Chinese study, men who had the greatest intake of garlic and scallions (more than 10 grams per day) were 50 percent less likely to get prostate cancer than those who ate the least garlic and scallions (less than 2.2 grams per day).[4] Other studies have shown risk reduction for esophageal, intestinal and stomach cancers, as well as pancreatic, colon, and breast cancers.[3]

CRUCIFEROUS VEGETABLES

Cabbage, brussels sprouts, cauliflower, broccoli, arugula, bok choy, collard greens, kale, mustard greens, radish, turnip, watercress

Research suggests that eating cruciferous vegetable may decrease risk of cancer and progression of disease.[5] Researchers believe that sulforaphane, a compound in cruciferous vegetables, plays a role in cancer prevention as well as slowing cancer growth.[2,6,7]

LOW GLYCEMIC LOAD ROOT VEGETABLES

Sweet potato, turnips, parsnips, carrots, beets

Root vegetables are often overlooked, but they shouldn't be. They are high in vitamin B, which helps protect DNA and lowers cancer risk.[8-10] You'll notice that turnips are considered both root and cruciferous, so they also have sulforaphane. What's more, root vegetables are cheap, they last a lot longer than other vegetables and they can be prepared simply by roasting them for forty minutes to an hour with a bit of olive oil, rosemary or thyme, and of course garlic (added near the end of roasting).

MUSHROOMS

Shiitake, maitake, oyster, button

Mushrooms have been used for millennia as medicine in parts of Asia. They have anti-inflammatory and immune-enhancing qualities. A case-control study in southeast China involving more than one thousand women concluded that mushroom consumption decreased breast cancer risk for both pre- and postmenopausal women.[11] Mushrooms are now being studied and widely recognized for their anticancer compounds, and mushroom extracts are being explored as a possible antitumor medicine.[12] Other mushrooms being investigated for their anticancer properties include *Trametes versicolor* (other names include *Coriolis versicolor*, Yunzhi, turkey tail); *Ganoderma lucidum* (lingzhi or reishi); chaga mushroom (*Inonotus obliquus*); *Cordyceps*; and *Agaricus blazei* Murrill. These mushrooms are not typically available in the supermarket as a whole food and can be found only as supplements. However, I was surprised when one afternoon a few summers ago, I paddled my canoe over to Molly's cottage and found her brewing up a tea with chaga. I had never seen chaga before. It is dense and looks like a piece of petrified wood or clump of dirt. Molly put a few pieces on the stove to boil for twenty minutes. It has a rather earthy flavor, but satisfying. The evidence for the effects of chaga are all preclinical in cell or animal studies, suggesting it boosts the immune system, decreases inflammation, repairs damaged DNA, and increases apoptosis.[13] However, little is known about the appropriate quantities that are safe to consume. Until we know more from ongoing research, it is ideal to consume your mushrooms as a whole food and not in supplement form. Preferentially, eat shiitake and maitake mushrooms (maitake is harder to find in the supermarket), as they likely have a stronger immunological effect over the other conventionally found mushrooms, such as button mushrooms.

BERRIES

Blueberries, blackberries, strawberries, raspberries

According to the American Institute for Cancer Research, berries may be the most beneficial fruit when it comes to cancer prevention.[14] They contain antioxidants that help prevent the cell damage that often precedes cancer, and they block genes associated with inflammation and cancer growth. Dr. Gary Stoner of the Medical College of Wisconsin has researched the role of berries in cancer prevention for more than twenty years.[15] He found that a diet of freeze-dried black raspberries and strawberries cut esophageal cancer rates in rats by 30 to 60 percent and reduced colon cancer by 80 percent.

Researchers also have shown that women who eat plenty of blueberries and strawberries have lower blood pressure and a reduced risk of heart attacks.[16] Although organic berries are expensive, especially when fresh, fresh-frozen maintain many of the nutrients and are more affordable. They pack quite the punch of phytonutrients and are especially potent antioxidants.

FRUIT

Apples, pears, mangos, oranges, grapefruit, cherries, peaches, apricots

Dried fruit can also be much cheaper, but bear in mind that if you wouldn't normally eat five fresh apricots, for example, you wouldn't eat five dried apricots, either. It is easy to overeat fruit when it is dried because the water has been removed. But remember the sugar content is the same as eating the fresh fruit, just concentrated.

NUTS

Walnuts, pecans, peanuts, almonds, Brazil nuts

Although all nuts are part of an anticancer diet,[17,18] walnuts have been the most studied in terms of cancer prevention. Walnuts contain high amounts of phytochemicals called polyphenols, which are powerful antioxidants.[19] Walnuts also contain omega-3 fat, which can help even out your omega-3/omega-6 balance. This is also the reason you won't often find walnuts in nut mixes—the omega-3 makes them more susceptible to going bad.

Nuts and seeds are an easy staple for snacks. The more portable and less refrigeration required, the better. Consider mixing your own nut and seed combinations.

We recommend buying only organic almonds and almond-based products after recent revelations that most almonds sold in the United States are treated with propylene oxide gas, a known carcinogen.[20] This "safety measure" began ten years ago, after a number of salmonella outbreaks were traced to California almonds.[21] Organic almonds are generally treated with a noncarcinogenic process that involves heating the kernel to 200 degrees.

SEEDS—AS TOPPER AND GARNISH OR IN SMOOTHIES

Flaxseed, hemp, sunflower, pumpkin, chia, sesame, cumin, pomegranate

Scientists remain at odds about whether flaxseed can help prevent or help control hormone-related cancers such as breast, prostate, and endometrial.[22,23] Lignans, the phytoestrogens in flaxseed, can change estrogen metabolism. In postmenopausal women, the effect of reducing active estrogen could reduce breast cancer risk. Animal studies have shown that lignans can reduce breast cancer growth, even with estrogen receptor positive breast cancer.[24] Those results suggest that flaxseed could be beneficial, but only when taken in moderation. Flaxseed is also a great plant source for omega-3 fatty acids. Fresh-ground flax-seed consumed as part of a balanced diet (less than three tablespoons per day) adds fiber and healthy micronutrients.

TASTY COMBOS

- Almonds and dried unsweetened apricots
- Dates and pistachios
- Walnuts, goji berries, and a square of chocolate with 70 percent or more cacao (rich in antioxidant and anti-inflammatory polyphenols)
- Unsweetened coconut flakes and walnuts
- Pecans, juice-sweetened cranberries

WHOLE GRAINS

Amaranth (technically a seed, but cooked as a grain), quinoa (technically a seed, but cooked as a grain), farro, Khorasan wheat (kamut), spelt, oats, teff, millet, buckwheat

In a 2015 study, researchers at Harvard School of Public Health found that eating a bowl of quinoa daily reduces the risk of death from cancer by 15 percent. Researchers looked at the diets of more than 367,000 people in eight U.S. states and found that those who ate at least 1.2 ounces of whole grains for every 1,000 calories they consumed reduced their risk of premature death, not only from cancer, but also from heart disease, respiratory disease, and diabetes.[25,26] Researchers believe whole grains have anti-inflammatory properties.[27]

PLANT-BASED PROTEINS

Beans, lentils, pulses (a pulse is the edible seed of plants in the legume family—they grow in pods), tofu

A single serving of legumes provides a significant amount of your daily recommended folate and fiber. Dietary fiber can reduce cancer risk in several ways, including weight control. Gut bacteria also feed on fiber, which may help protect colon cells. Meanwhile, folate helps maintain control of cell growth.[28] Legumes also have phytochemicals that are being studied for their anticancer effects.[29]

PREBIOTICS

Chicory root, Jerusalem artichoke, dandelion greens, raw garlic, raw leeks, raw or cooked onion, raw jicama

Chemotherapy can disrupt the bacterial balance in your gut: your microbiome. Prebiotics can help restore this balance by reestablishing probiotic bacteria like bifidobacteria and lactobacilli.[30] Prebiotics may help inhibit cancer cell formation by improving your microbiome.[31,32] They also reduce the pH of the colon and support the body's production of a fatty acid called butyrate that has been linked to apoptosis.[33] As you recall, one of the cancer hallmarks is disrupting this process so cells that should die stay alive and continue to mutate and grow.

PROBIOTICS

Yogurt, kefir, sauerkraut or other fermented vegetables, dark chocolate, microalgae, miso, pickles, tempeh, kimchi, kombucha

Like prebiotic foods, probiotics help to replenish good bacteria in your gastrointestinal tract and restore balance to your microbiome. In 2013, Chinese researchers found that patients with advanced colorectal adenoma, a precursor to colon cancer, consistently had less healthy gut bacteria.[34] Probiotic foods contain live bacteria, which can reseed your gut with the proper bacterial balance. In exchange, your microbiome will work better to digest your food and convert nutrients and vitamins into forms the body can absorb and use.[35] What's more, maintaining a high diversity of your gut microbiome we know is linked with reduced risk of multiple diseases and will help maintain proper balance and strength of your immune system, decrease inflammation, and will help to keep hormone regulation in balance.[36] Eat fermented or pickled vegetables as condiments in small quantities, as excessive consumption has been linked with stomach cancer. One of my favorite sayings about the microbiome is "Treat your gut like a garden, not like a gutter." Too often we throw anything into our mouths, almost like we're throwing it away, things we know are bad for us and probably should be thrown away. But if you think about how you are maintaining a microbiome garden in your stomach, it can help keep you more conscious about what you eat and how it affects the balance of bacteria in your gut.

(Cancer patients on a neutropenic diet should check with their doctor before consuming fermented foods.)

ANTI-INFLAMMATORY HERBS AND SPICES

Turmeric, ginger, cinnamon, rosemary, sage, oregano, cayenne pepper, basil, thyme, coriander, cardamom, black pepper, clove

Curcumin, the yellow pigment in turmeric, has been the focus of a lot of research for its antioxidant and anti-inflammatory properties.[37] Turmeric extract has been shown to help prevent heart attacks in people who have undergone bypass surgery, and it is being studied as a drug to treat Alzheimer's disease.[38] In terms of cancer, extensive research in animals has shown that curcumin can control cancer growth. A 2011 study by researchers at UCLA's Jonsson Comprehensive Cancer Center found that curcumin suppresses a cell-signaling pathway that helps fuel the growth of head and neck cancer. Researchers also found that, by blocking that signal, curcumin also reduced the amount of pro-inflammatory cytokines in the saliva of participants.[39] Extensive research with all these spices has found that they are potent anti-inflammatory agents.[40,41] Again, it is ideal to consume these spices as a whole food and avoid taking as supplements unless under the direction of a health-care provider.

Environmental Toxin Hit List

Many of these chemicals are commonly used in everyday products. Read labels and learn to recognize harmful ingredients. Keep this list handy as you shop online or in the store.

Endocrine Disrupters

Atrazine—This widely used herbicide has been found to turn male frogs into female frogs.[1] It is pervasive in the water supply and has been linked to delayed puberty, prostate inflammation and breast cancer in animal studies.[2] Research has found an association between atrazine and prostate cancer, but more study is necessary to make a direct connection. [3,4]

BPA—Bisphenol A, or BPA, is a chemical used in the production of plastic. It is found in water bottles, food-storage containers, toys, sippy cups, medical devices, and compact discs. BPA is also used as an epoxy resin to coat bottle tops, food cans, and water-supply pipes. BPA was invented as a medical estrogen, so its exposure is likely to affect hormonal homeostasis in humans. Studies have shown that BPA exposure leads to spikes in blood pressure and could cause obesity.[5] BPA exposure has also been connected to increased cancer risk, brain damage, hormonal problems, and prostate gland issues in developing fetuses and children.[5] Going "BPA-free" may not be a solution. Research shows BPS, the replacement chemical for BPA, has similar effects on the endocrine system.[6]

DDT—Di-chloro-diphenyl-trichloroethane was developed as a synthetic insecticide in the 1940s and was widely used to combat malaria and other insect-borne diseases in both civilian and military populations. Although DDT use in the United States has been limited since the 1970s, it continues to be used in countries where malaria risk is high. DDT is suspected to cause reproductive problems in humans and has been shown to cause liver tumors in animal studies.[7,8]

Dioxin—Dioxins are by-products of industrial processes such as chlorine bleaching of paper pulp, smelting, and the manufacture of certain herbicides. They are classified as persistent organic pollutants. Once they enter the body, mainly through meat, dairy products, fish, and shellfish, they can cause reproductive and developmental problems, damage to the immune system, hormone disruption, and cancer.[9]

Ethinyl Estradiol—The synthetic estrogen used in most oral contraceptive pills. Research arising from the Nurses' Health Study found increased risk of breast cancer in women taking estrogen replacement therapy.[10] Other studies have either found no connection between EE and breast cancer or were inconclusive.[11]

Fragrance/Parfum—Most of the thousands of chemicals listed as fragrances have not been tested for toxicity.[12,13] Fragrances are found in everything from cosmetics and deodorants to laundry detergent, fabric softeners, and cleaning products.[14]

Organophosphates—OPs, created by the reaction between phosphoric acid and alcohol, were originally used as insecticides but were adapted as neurotoxins by the German military in World War II. Since then, they have been used under various brand names as ingredients in lawn and garden sprays. Although more research is required, these chemicals are potentially toxic for young children.[15] Scientists continue to study the long-term effects of low-level exposure to organophosphates on human health.

Parabens—This class of commonly used preservatives help prevent bacterial growth in cosmetics, foods, and pharmaceutical products. They are added to toothpaste, shampoo, deodorant, and other products. A 2014 study found that parabens increased the growth of certain types of breast cancer cells, even at low levels of exposure.[16]

Perchlorate—This compound found in rocket fuel has been discovered as a contaminant in milk and produce. When it gets into the human body it disrupts thyroid function by competing with the nutrient iodine.[17] Ingesting too much perchlorate can alter the hormone balance in your thyroid, which regulates metabolism and is critical for organ and brain development in infants and young children.[17]

Perfluorinated Chemicals—PFCs are used to make nonstick pans, waterproof clothes, and stain-resistant sofas and carpets. During cooking with PFC-coated cookware, the chemicals can escape into food and build up in the body. Research into the impact of PFCs on human health are ongoing, but animal and human studies have shown effects on developing fetuses and young children, decreased fertility, increased cholesterol, immune system effects, and increased cancer risk.[18,19]

Phthalates—Phthalates are a type of chemical that makes plastic both durable and flexible. They are found in products ranging from vinyl flooring and automobiles to rain jackets. Phthalates are also in personal care products such as nail polish, shampoo, soap, and hair spray. Researchers from the University of Michigan School of Public Health found in a 2014 study that exposure to phthalates in personal care products could lower testosterone levels, but more research on human health effects is needed.[20]

PBDEs—Polybrominated diethyl ethers are used as flame-retardants in everything from building materials and electronics to plastics, tiles, and foams. They have been connected to an assortment of health problems, including the disruption of thyroid function, learning impairment, delayed puberty onset, and fetal malformations.[21,22] In animal research, exposure to low levels of PBDE has a greater impact on fetuses and infants compared to adults.[23,24]

Triclosan—An ingredient in many self-described antibacterial products, including hand sanitizers, deodorants, and toothpaste. An animal study in 2014 found that triclosan interferes with a protein that helps flush chemicals out of the body, which over time might lead to liver cancer.[25]

Other Toxins to Avoid

Arsenic—Listed as a known human carcinogen by both the International Agency for Research on Cancer and the U.S. National Toxicology Program, arsenic is one of the world's most toxic elements. While one hopes you won't find it on any list of ingredients, it has historically been used in timber treatment and pesticides and is a by-product of coal-fired power plants, smelting, and mining. High levels of arsenic have also been found in deep-drilled wells.[26]

Coal Tar—Coal tar is a by-product of coke, a solid fuel composed of carbon and coal gas. Coal tar is used to make creosote, which is used as a preservative or antiseptic. According to the Centers for Disease Control and Prevention, coal tar creosote is the most widely used wood preservative in the United States. Coal tar products are used to treat skin diseases such as psoriasis and are used as animal repellents, as well as in insecticides, pesticides, fungicides, and animal dips (a chemical bath meant to protect animals, such as sheep or dogs, from parasites in their fur or on their skin). Occupational exposure to coal tar has been shown to increase the risk of skin, lung, bladder, kidney, and digestive tract cancers.[26]

DEA/TEA/MEA—Ethanolamine compounds are present in an assortment of personal care products, including shampoo, soap, hair dye, lotion, shaving cream, wax, eyeliner, mascara, blush, makeup foundation, and hair conditioner.[27] The European Commission has banned DEA in cosmetics. Ethanolamine compounds have been linked to liver tumors.[28]

Ethoxylated surfactants and 1,4-Dioxane—This by-product results from using ethylene oxide, a known human carcinogen, to make other chemicals less harsh.[29]

Formaldehyde—Listed as a known human carcinogen, formaldehyde is used in the production of solvents, bonding agents, and adhesives. It is found in pressed wood such as plywood and particle board and in foam insulation. Long-term exposure to formaldehyde has been found to increase the risk of leukemia and brain cancer.[26]

Hydroquinone—This is found in skin-whitening and brightening compounds and is a potential carcinogen.[30] Hydroquinone is a benzene derivative.

Lead—Exposure to lead has been linked to tumors of the kidney, brain, and lung.[26] It can be present in old paint, which should be tested before it is sanded or removed. Lead can build up in the body over months and years. People are exposed to lead through paint, gasoline, solder, and consumer products in addition to food, air, water, and soil.

Mercury—A neurotoxin that impairs brain development and has been connected to autism, Alzheimer's, ALS, and multiple sclerosis.[31] Although mercury has not been directly connected to cancer, high doses have been found to harm multiple organs, including the immune system.[31,32] Mercury is found in some types of eye drops and mascara.

Mineral Oil—This by-product of petroleum is found in styling gels, moisturizers, and baby oil. These oils are highly refined. Occupational exposure to less-refined mineral oils have been linked to skin cancer.[33] While more refined liquids used in cosmetics have not been linked to cancer, they do create a film on the skin and prevent the release of toxins.

Oxybenzone—This organic compound, part of the benzophenone family, is included in many types of sunscreen, moisturizers, lip balms, anti-aging creams, conditioners, and lipstick. It has been linked to allergies, cell damage, and hormone disruption.[34]

Paraphenylenediamine (PPD)—This chemical substance is widely used in hair dye. Although PPD has not been directly linked to cancer, multiple studies in the past forty years have shown connections between long-term hair dye use and breast cancer.[35]

PCBs—Polychlorinated biphenyls are a group of chemicals used in everything from electrical equipment and flame-retardants to paints. Although the use of PCBs was restricted and banned in the 1970s and '80s, the chemicals are persistent in the environment and remain present in the air, water, and soil. PCBs have been listed as a probable human carcinogen.[26]

Polyethylene Glycol (PEG)—These chemical compounds used in conditioners, cleansing agents, emulsifiers, and as surfactants often contain impurities, such as ethylene oxide and 1,4-dioxane, which are both recognized as human carcinogens.[36–38]

Silicone-Derived Emollients—These chemicals, which include dimethicone copolyol, cyclomethicone, and dimethicone, coat the skin and prevent it from breathing and releasing toxins. Some emollients have been associated with tumor growth and have been found to build up in the liver and lymph nodes.[39]

Sodium Lauryl Sulfate (or Sodium Lauryl Ether Sulfate)—This chemical is used to create foam in shampoos, toothpastes, conditioners, soaps, cosmetics, and household cleaners. It has not been directly linked to cancer, but it has been found to cause skin and eye irritation.[40]

Talc—Talcum powder is made from talc and is widely used in baby powder, facial powders, and other consumer products. Multiple studies have looked at the connection between talcum powder applied to women's genital area over time and ovarian cancer with mixed results.[41]

Toluene—This clear, colorless solvent occurs naturally in crude oil and is used to make fingernail polish, lacquers, adhesives, rubber, paints, and paint thinners. It is also added to gasoline to increase octane ratings. Toluene affects the nervous system, but it has not been found to cause cancer.[42]

APPENDIX D

Overcoming Barriers
to Behavior Change

Becoming more aware of what exactly you want to change and why you believe you need to make changes are important first steps to successfully pivoting toward a new, healthier path. One of my favorite sayings is, "Energy follows intention." It is only when we develop a clear intention of what we want to change and why we want to change that our energy becomes focused and channeled to help us achieve our objectives.

If this were easy, you would have done it already. That doesn't mean that lifestyle change is impossibly hard; it just means that it takes thought and preparation to climb out of your unhealthy rut and onto your new path forward. You need to deconstruct and analyze what you're doing now and figure out where you are before you can begin taking steps to get where you want to be. To create a successful and sustainable strategy for lifestyle change, first recognize and understand the barriers you face to making the change.

Reframe Your Thoughts

The intent here is to move from the negative to the positive. An abundance of research shows that being positive and optimistic is much more than just a state of mind. In addition to the psychological benefits of reducing depression and anxiety, positive thinking has downstream effects as well, impacting our health and potentially our ability to avoid and overcome disease. In 2016, researchers at the Yale School of Public Health found that people aged fifty and over who had a positive view of aging had lower levels of C-reactive protein, a marker of inflammation that has been related to chronic diseases, including cancer. The study, which looked at more than four thousand people, also found that those with a positive outlook lived significantly longer.

Moving from Can't to Can

Shift focus to what can be accomplished, not to what can't. Remember: Lifestyle changes are not all or nothing. If you can't take big steps, start small. Example: "I can't exercise for thirty minutes today, so I won't exercise at all." Instead say, "I can exercise for twenty minutes today and build up to thirty minutes over the next week." Alternately, try challenging your negative thoughts or conclusions to test their validity. Do you truly not have thirty minutes to exercise? What if you combined your workout with another task you have on your list for the day? Maybe the truth is that you don't want to exercise? What if you went for a walk or spent time being active with your kids or family? What can you do to make exercise more appealing? When you begin to look more closely at negative thoughts, most of the time they don't hold up under questioning. Replace them with more positive ideas that help you move forward and change your lifestyle.

Practice Reframing Your Thoughts

Select a barrier to one of the areas in the Mix of Six: social support, stress-management, quality sleep, physical activity, healthy eating, and avoiding environmental toxins.

Barrier: _____

How could you change how you think about the barrier by reframing it?

_____
_____

FOCUS ON BENEFITS

Make a list of three benefits for each area of the Mix of Six.

Increasing Social Support

_____
_____
_____

Managing Stress

_____
_____
_____

Improving Sleep

_____
_____
_____

Increasing Physical Activity

_____
_____
_____

Eating Healthy Foods

_____

_____

_____

Avoiding Environmental Toxins

_____

_____

_____

Remind yourself regularly why you are making these changes. This will help to sustain the healthy choices now and into the future.

HIGH-RISK EVENTS AND TRIGGERS

Along the way to a healthier life, you will undoubtedly have setbacks, lapses, and relapses. It is important not to feel guilt, shame, or regret about these slipups, as negative emotions end up justifying a return to your old ways. *See, I knew I couldn't do this.* Or *I ate one cup of ice cream, I might as well finish the whole container.* Just because you slip up a bit, doesn't mean you should give up on your goals of that day and your forward movement.

To help you manage and minimize your setbacks, avoid situations in which you are tempted to engage in unhealthy behaviors such as overeating, skipping your mind-body practice, or not getting enough sleep.

Anything that disrupts your standard routine is likely to also disrupt your anticancer lifestyle. Vacations, parties, houseguests, and sickness are all potential pitfalls. Even a change in your work schedule or a new activity, such as having to drive a child to and fro every morning or afternoon can throw off your healthy habits, especially early on.

What are some of the high-risk events in your life?

What steps could you take to minimize the disruption these events bring to your life? If the disruptions can't be avoided, what could you do to minimize their impact?

TRIGGERS

While high-risk events can cause you to revert to your old ways, triggers are situations, people, or encounters that make you want to engage in unhealthy behaviors as a release or reaction. Triggers are everywhere, and we are sometimes unable to avoid them. Sights, sounds, smells, or any stimulus can cause a deeper psychological and emotional reaction that is unexpected and can lead you down a self-destructive path. We have found through experience and our involvement with the CompLife patients that family reunions and gatherings can be triggers (and high-risk events). Recognize these moments and prepare yourself better to handle them or to accept that you're going to have a lapse or setback, and it's not the end of the world. Triggers typically create feelings of frustration, anger, loneliness, anxiety, fear, or regret. But celebrations and achievements can also be a trigger for poor eating, excessive drinking, and ignoring your healthful habits.

What are some of your triggers?

Try and anticipate an upcoming barrier or trigger. What can you do to prepare yourself to manage a trigger that you expect to face in the coming days or weeks?

If you focus on what you can do and come up with a plan, you are more likely to handle triggers and high-risk events without jumping off the proverbial cliff.

When you are facing a barrier, high-risk event, or trigger, do the following:

- Reframe your thought: try not to think negatively.
- Problem solve: what can you do before or during the event or trigger that will stop you from caving to the temptation to eat unhealthfully or skip exercise or your mind-body practice?
- Engage your support system, including your friends and family.
- Focus on benefits: when you are tempted to stray off course of your healthy living plan, focus on the benefits you will receive from your healthier choices to help strengthen your motivation to make better choices.
- Set goals and honor yourself.

VACATION OR HOUSEGUESTS

Traveling and hosting guests are two activities that pose unique challenges when it comes to sustaining an anticancer lifestyle. Traveling, whether for work or vacation, makes it hard to maintain a routine. We tend to not make time for our mind-body practices, making the challenging aspects of travel more stressful. Exercise is often an afterthought, we stay up too late, sleeping in a new bed is not as restful, and eating meal after meal in restaurants is not as healthy as we would like. We are also less in control of our environmental exposures. In order to maintain an anticancer lifestyle some planning ahead is necessary. Houseguests can also make it a challenge to stick to our routines. As much as we love our family and friends, having them at our house or apartment is inevitably disruptive to our daily routine. The quiet moments we savor are suddenly filled with voices and sounds. We spend more meals eating out or catering to the food preferences of our guests and less time exercising. In short, maintaining healthy habits whether on vacation or hosting guests requires careful planning and preparation:

- Find activities that involve walking, like going to parks, monuments, and the like.
- Exercise and do your mind-body practice early in the morning to be sure to fit it into your altered schedule.
- Eat your vegetables first.
- Stay hydrated to avoid mistaking hunger for thirst.
- Have healthy snacks at the ready for houseguests or while vacationing.
- Plan to limit your "cheating" to one day or to a single meal.
- Invite houseguests to go for a walk after dinner or to meditate with you.
- Try to maintain a sleep schedule that you know supports your health.

What is a possible high-risk event or trigger that you'd like to work through before it happens?

Event/trigger: _____

Reframe your thought: _____

Problem solve: _____

Focus on benefits: _____

Enlist support: _____

Set goals: _____

LAPSES AND RELAPSES

A lapse is a single moment or episode during which you revert to a behavior you were trying to change, whether that means staying up late and not getting enough sleep or bingeing on pizza. Lapses happen. Don't beat yourself up about them. Remember why you're making the change. A single setback doesn't mean you are totally off track. It just means that you slipped up. Focus on how the lapse made you feel, physically and emotionally. Remember that negative cost to help keep you on track in the future.

Relapses are when you slip back into old habits, not just once but over time. For example, you fall back into an old habit of eating sugary junk food at nine each night. Just like lapses, relapses can be overcome. As we mentioned, the key is to examine the reasons behind the relapse and figure out what you can do to get back on track. Take time to assess if you have enough and the right kind of support as you address this relapse, and ensure you pay attention to your support as you move forward. Try to stay positive. Feelings of guilt and shame are self-defeating emotions. Encourage yourself with praise and promise. Treat yourself the way you would treat people you love. You wouldn't blame them for relapsing. You would pat them on the back and encourage them to keep trying.

TIPS TO KEEP IN MIND WHEN DEALING
WITH LAPSES AND RELAPSES

* Cognitive distortions, such as all-or-none thinking, frequently make lapses turn into relapses, so it's important to examine your self-talk when a lapse occurs.
* Negativity and self-criticism will only make the situation worse.
* Acknowledge the lapse and plan a positive solution to deal with similar situations in the future so that a lapse does not turn into a relapse.
* Don't make excuses for the lapse (I am on vacation, so it's fine). Acknowledge the lapse and come back to healthy living.
* Practice encouraging yourself.
* Anticancer living is not about being perfect; we all have ups and downs.
* Be conscious of how you are thinking about the lapse or relapse.
* Get back on track by identifying the psychological cause for the setback.
* Start fresh and renew your commitment to choosing a healthier lifestyle. After a relapse, versus a lapse, challenge yourself to commit to healthy living for thirty days straight with no lapses. This may sound challenging, but it can be the ideal way to get back on track and stay on track.
* Identifying the cause for relapse will help you keep an eye out for those situations in the future and plan and prepare ahead.

PRACTICE MAKING A PLAN

Everyone experiences times when it is more difficult to maintain their healthy behaviors. Having a plan for high-risk events and lapses/relapses will help you get back on track.

Consider a situation in which you think you may be at risk for a lapse or relapse in the future. (Example: when on vacation.)

_____

_____

What thoughts might you have during a lapse or relapse?

_____

_____

What is another way you could look at these thoughts?

_____

_____

What are some strategies you can use to avoid the lapse or relapse?

_____

_____

APPENDIX E

Staying Healthy on the Road

Traveling poses unique challenges when it comes to sustaining comprehensive lifestyle change. For one, your regular routine is inevitably disrupted in a variety of ways. You sleep in a bed that's not your own, with different sounds, temperatures, and lighting issues. You wake up in a strange place, on a different schedule, and without your usual options and incentives to stay on track and engage in your mind-body practice. In terms of diet, you spend most meals either eating out or being served food as a guest in someone else's home. You don't have your usual supporters to meet you for physical activity or your dog demanding to be taken for a walk, and you're away from your usual gym or track. Finally, it's more difficult to vet the products you're exposed to in a foreign environment. Whether you're on vacation, visiting relatives, or traveling for work, the risks of being on the road are myriad and deserve special attention.

Plan Ahead

The most important thing you can do when you know you'll be traveling is to anticipate your needs and do your best to prepare in a way that minimizes disruption to your healthy habits. Consider the times when you will be most challenged on the road. This could be during travel days or finding ways to eat right and exercise during a hotel-based conference, a vacation at the beach, or a few days at the house of a close friend or relative.

Social Support

If you're traveling with others or visiting family or friends, engage your fellow travelers or hosts in your plans for healthy living. If someone is game for joining you, it can help to keep you on track and it may forge a deeper bond with that person for years to come. Who knows? Maybe becoming more conscious of their own habits will inspire them to continue a healthier lifestyle after you've returned home. Become an agent for change in your community.

One of the most effective ways to maintain strong social support and continue your own health priorities is to lend a helping hand while visiting friends and family. This simple and deeply appreciated act helps those you care about and keeps you active, also helping to limit eating and drinking in excess. Volunteering your time and engaging in prosocial, eudaimonic behaviors have been shown to have positive impacts on our health. Offering to cook a meal allows you to take on that responsibility from others and to prepare a healthy meal. Cleaning up after a meal, during the day, or asking to be given a special project that a family member has been putting off gives you purpose and supports those you love (as well as keeping you more physically active during your vacation).

Take the time to truly connect with the people around you. That includes strangers on a train or plane or your close friends and family members. Being open to the world around you and empathetic to those who cross your path helps to increase your sense of purpose in life and makes you more likely to feel connected and satisfied.

Mind-Body Practice

You can meditate almost anywhere, but it's nice to find and set up a designated meditation spot if you're staying in the same room or house for more than a day or two. Having a meditation spot encourages you to stick with your daily practice and acts as a visual reminder if you skip a day to get back to sitting, breathing, and fostering calm.

Another meditation practice that works well on the road is mindful walking. This can be done anywhere and is good at airports between flights. This also breaks up the extended sitting time that is somewhat inevitable when you have long flights or flight delays. While everyone is sitting around waiting for the airline worker to announce boarding groups, I am engaged in my mindful walking meditation.

Yoga is also a great tool that requires little or no preparation or accessories, especially if you're in a carpeted room. I like to do a short routine of stretches and poses in airports while waiting for a flight or during layovers or even in the airplane galley on a long-haul flight (although I know we are not supposed to loiter in the walkways).

Sleep

Sleeping on the road is hard, especially if you're moving from place to place, night after night. Researchers at Brown University discovered that, during the first night of sleep at a new location, part of your brain remains active. Even though you might feel safe, your brain is not so sure—likely an adaptive feature we inherited from our Paleolithic ancestors. So, one hemisphere rests while the other hemisphere remains wakeful, just in case. That's why the first night in a new place inevitably leaves you feeling groggy and unrested. But there are steps you can take to make your vacation or travel more restful.

Travel with earplugs, a face mask, and duct tape (instead of bringing a bulky silver roll, wrap some tape around a pen or pencil). You can use the tape to cover LED lights in hotel rooms on televisions, air-conditioning units, or alarm clocks, as these devices emit a considerable amount of light, which can interfere with sleep.

Physical Activity

Staying active on the road requires a little bit of planning and a lot of intention. Once you become aware of how much you sit, you will find that many things can be done just as well while standing. In terms of planning, don't forget to pack workout clothes, or at least tennis shoes so you can walk or hike as part of your traveling routine.

Stay active while you travel. As a general rule, take the stairs rather than the escalators or moving walkways, unless of course you're late for your flight or have a close connection. While waiting, and we certainly wait a lot while traveling, simply walk instead of sitting. On airplanes, I try to choose the aisle seat and stand up and walk the aisles every hour or so to stretch and keep my blood flowing.

Once you've arrived at your destination, find a way to sit less and move more. If you're meeting with just a few people, suggest a walking meeting at a nearby park or green space. People might look at you sideways at first, but I guarantee you'll have a better meeting and people will remember it more if you're on the move. If walking meetings are not possible, stand at the back of the room during a meeting. Take walks with family, friends, and colleagues, especially after meals.

Make a standing desk for your laptop. When I am in hotel rooms, I usually put one of those plastic recycling bins on the desk and place the laptop on top. For me, this is the perfect height. When at someone's house you can use a stack of coffee-table books or stand at a kitchen counter.

Diet

Eating on the road poses obvious challenges. Sometimes you face tables of food you're not supposed to eat or find yourself served a plate of home cooking that is off your diet. While we recommend you stay vigilant, and ideally plan ahead, including telling your host(s) of some of your dietary restrictions, remember it's not the end of the world if you lapse for a night or an afternoon. If it comes down to hurting someone's feeling versus having a lapse, it's sometimes better to take what's given to you. That doesn't mean you have to have seconds or thirds, but sometimes eating on the road, especially in social settings, can be tricky.

When traveling or starting a day on vacation, prepare healthy snacks to bring with you. Try to keep a balance of proteins (nuts and seeds), dried fruit, individual servings of nut butters, dried vegetables (kale, etc.), and minimally processed carbohydrates (things like popcorn, brown rice cakes, and the like).

In restaurants, be creative with the ingredients you see on the menu and don't feel constrained to order the pre-set dishes; become comfortable ordering from the sides. When I'm in a particularly meat-focused restaurant, I'll make my own vegetarian entrée by asking for the kale that comes with the steak, the beans offered with the fried chicken, and the glazed carrots advertised with the fish. Sometimes the waiter or waitress will have to check with the chef, but usually they're able to accommodate me. Also, I'm a good tipper, which I hope makes up for the hassle of my off-the-menu tendencies.

In airports, look at all the ingredients available and create a plant-based meal. This can be easier with some chains than others. For example, Mexican food tends to include beans and vegetables, but go light on the rice, or ask if brown rice is an option. One time when I was in an airport and famished, the closest thing to plant-based food was a pizza chain. I did not want a slice of pizza, but I noticed there were lots of vegetable toppings available. I also saw that they had tinfoil. So I asked if they could simply place lots of veggies with some olive oil on the tinfoil and bake it in the pizza oven for a few minutes. I ended up with a surprisingly delicious and nutritious meal. Although the sales staff was confused about how much to charge me for ingredients that they'd never sold separately, they were amused by my request and had a good laugh about serving pizza vegetables in tinfoil. As I always travel with nuts, I was also able to have my protein needs met. Nuts are almost always available in airports, but read the ingredient list carefully because they often include added sugars and harmful oils, such as soy.

I will often use travel days as a time for a fast. Fasting is part of all cultures and societies dating back thousands of years and has many health benefits. It is important to plan for a twenty-four-hour fast and ensure you remain well hydrated.

Travel with a food-grade stainless-steel beverage container and drink plenty of water when you're on the road, whether you're fasting or not.

Environment

When you're staying in places that you don't know, especially hotels, it's hard to control what chemicals you'll encounter. Sometimes I walk into hotel rooms and the smell of their cleaning products is so strong, it's almost overwhelming. I try to find rooms that have the option of opening the window. I will often turn on fans, open the window, and go out for a few hours. Even if I return to a cold (or hot) room, the ventilation usually helps alleviate some of the chemical buildup. One thing you can control with your environment is what you put on your body, in your hair, and under your arms. Travel with your own toiletries: soap, shampoo, and so forth. When you're on the road, use toxin-free hand sanitizer and wash your hands frequently. If you take fruit to go from a breakfast buffet, be sure to wash it thoroughly as it is likely not organic. Also, keep reading ingredients, even when you're on the road. You might be taking a break from work or at least from home, but your body is still absorbing and processing everything you're putting in and on it. Give it a break, too.

ACKNOWLEDGMENTS

Anticancer living begins with social support, and so too did the writing of this book. We spent two years with what became known as our "ACL Team," forging our way through a process, learning as we went, making missteps and corrections, and always pushing the project forward while staying focused on the ultimate goal and attuned to our central message. The resulting book you now hold in your hands was only possible because of the incredible team of people who lent their expertise to help us shape and deliver *Anticancer Living*.

First and foremost, we are indebted to David Servan-Schreiber for leading the way with his pioneering work in the field of lifestyle and cancer. We thank him for sharing his story and expertise with so many and for making a difference with his passion, dedication, and perseverance during challenging times. He continues to be an inspiration for us all.

Our editor, Carole Desanti, at Viking was a champion of ours from the start. In many ways, it was the closing of one circle and the opening of another. Carole worked with Lorenzo's parents when she was first starting out in publishing; she worked with David on *Anticancer*; and now we, too, have been fortunate to have her serve as our collaborator and guide. With her thoughtful expertise, Carole helped to pull us above the thickets and keep our voice true and our message clear. In addition, we express sincere thanks to all at Viking for believing in our book and working diligently at all stages of the process. Among the many who played a role we thank Christopher Russell and Emily Neuberger, Amy Sun, Louise Braverman, Lindsay Prevette, Juliann (Juli) Barbato, Andrea Schultz, and Brian Tart.

Words seem inadequate to truly express all that our agent, Douglas Abrams of Idea Architects, has done on our behalf. Doug has been our advocate and guide through a process that had few straight lines. He is a master at all he does and really does walk on water. We also extend our sincere thanks to his equally talented team of Lara Love and Kelsey Sheronas and his "brain trust" of creative writers and innovative problem solvers at Idea Architects. We also sincerely thank our foreign rights agents for the tremendous work they have done with *Anticancer Living*—Chandler Crawford and Jo Grossman of the Chandler Crawford Agency, and the team at the Marsh Agency, including Susie Nicklin, Camilla Ferrier, and Jemma McDonagh.

Our message is clearer, brighter, and more compelling thanks to the time and talents of our two collaborative writers. We found a true partner and friend in Stephen Howie, a gifted writer. With his deft skill, Stephen helped us to take this complex and overwhelming topic and make it accessible and engaging. He skillfully brought together all our ideas and kept us true to the message. His humor, patience, and positive attitude supported all our efforts. We also thank Maria McLeod, Stephen's wife, for being our cheerleader and sharing Stephen during this long process. In addition to Stephen, we also collaborated with Emily Heckman, another talented writer. As a member of our writing team, Emily brought a lovely balance and engaging voice to our book. She worked tirelessly to ensure our message was focused and alive. We are forever grateful to Stephen and Emily for their flexibility and total commitment to *Anticancer Living*.

With heartfelt thanks we acknowledge the leading scientists who shared their valuable time and helped us understand the nuances of their respective fields and made sure we got the science right. They were incredibly generous with their time in interviews, emails, follow-up emails, and reading and editing sections of the book. They are listed here in the order they appear: Steve Cole, Elissa Epel, Dean Ornish, Barbara Andersen, David Katz, Susan Lutgendorf, David Spiegel, Michael Lerner, Scott Morris, Martica (Tica) Hall, Michael Irwin, Sonia Ancoli-Israel, Anil Sood, Mike Antoni, Kerry Courneya, Lee Jones, Walter Willett, Cynthia (Cindi) Thomson, Ken Cook, Janet Gray, Lawrence (Larry) Kushi, and Margaret Cuomo. A special thank you to John Pierce, Ali Miller, and Laurie Silver.

We also thank those who believed in our project and helped support the book right from the start by providing advanced praise. In alphabetical order: Neal Barnard, Deepak Chopra, Margaret Cuomo, Patricia Ganz, Gary

Hirshberg, Meg Hirshberg, David Katz, Susan Love, Jun Mao, John Mendel-sohn, Dean Ornish, Kent Osborne, Peter Pisters, David Rosenthal, Franklin Servan-Schreiber, and Andrew Weil. Included in this group are international colleagues who lent their advanced praise: Eran Ben-Arye, Christian Boukaram, Gustav Dobos, Fabio Firenzuoli, R. K. Grover, Xiaomao Guo, Jon Hunter, Michelle Kohn, Shinichi Nitta, H. R. Nagendra, Yogrishi Swami Ramdev, Bashar Saad, Florian Scotte, Paulo de Tarso Ricieri de Lima, and Claudia Witt.

We were fortunate to work with two gifted artists. Lara Crow was flexible and generous with her time, helping us with concepts and ideas while awaiting the birth of her daughter. We were also fortunate to find and work with Laura Beckman, who brought great energy and skill to the illustrations on a very accelerated timeframe.

The CompLife Study at MD Anderson Cancer Center that David Servan-Schreiber and I conceived and that I am in the process of carrying out involves an extensive team of top physicians, scientists, practitioners, and staff. They include Banu Arun, Taylor Austin, Gildy Babiera, Karen Basen-Engquist, Cindy Carmack, Alejandro Chaoul, Lisa Connelly, Robin Haddad, Carol Harrison, Yisheng Li, Smitha Mallaiah, Raghuram Naga-rathna, Patricia Parker, George Perkins, James Reuben, Tina Shih, Amy Spelman, Anil Sood, Peiying Yang, and Sai-ching Yeung.

We are truly inspired by members of the CompLife team who are working directly with study participants and transforming lives before our eyes, including: Robin Haddad, Taylor Austin, Lisa Connelly, Smitha Mallaiah, Sue Thompson (and former dietitians Ali Miller, Deema Simaan, and Joseph Gonzales), and Courtney West.

Who would have envisioned the complexity of finishing all our notes and the Herculean effort it would take. With superstars like Richard Wagner and Laurissa Gann we were able to finish the scientific referencing. Thank you to all those who assisted in this task including: Mary Allen, Aimee Anderson, Taylor Austin, Curtiss Chapman, Michelle Chen, David Farris, Martica Hall, Yoseph Lee, Jewel Ochoa, and Annina Seiler.

We gratefully thank all the cancer patients in CompLife who we interviewed and who so graciously and bravely shared their stories with us: Nella Bea Anderson, Jan Chism, Hashmat Effendi, Michelene Holmes, Jana Lee, Brenda McCalb, Brucett Mojay, Ana Rodriguez, Dawn Howard, and Karan Redus-Cockrell.

To all the cancer survivors we interviewed, some of whom appear in our book, your remarkable knowledge, determination, and example helps shape all of our futures. Thank you for sharing your remarkable stories: Molly Mulloy, Diana Lindsay, Josh Mailman, Glenn Sabin, Meg Hirshberg, Susan Rafte, Dorothy Paterson, Gabe Canales, Deborah Cohan, Elaine Walters, Lourdes Hernandez, Jim Rosborough, Meg Whittmore, Donna Kuethe, Stephen Mosher, Jen Burzycki, Shannon Mann, Sherri Atlas, Carlos Garcia, Catherine Powers-James, and the late Bill Baun. The real-life stories of all these remarkable people are the heart and soul of our book.

We interviewed or spoke to many people for our book who are actively doing the hard work of improving their lifestyle. Each helped to shape and hone our message: Chiara Cohen, Cathy Crath, Deborah Gremillion, Emma Mann, Naomi Rosborough, Anthony Sturm, Alberta Totz, and Ana Trevino-Godfrey.

We would also like to thank the generous support for the CompLife research project. It was financially supported in part by private donations from the Duncan Family Institute with support from Jan and Dan Duncan, the Bosarge Family Foundation, the Thornburg Foundation, Cindy and Rob Citrone, the Lester Family Foundation, the Todd Family Charitable Foundation, Meg and Gary Hirshberg, S3 Partners LLC, Liz and Robert Sloan, Mr. Ricardo Mora, Ms. Maliha Khan, the Andrew & Lillian A. Posey Foundation, Aurora Investment Management LLC, CF Global Trading LLC, Ms. Lynda Arimond and her family through the Not Just Another Cancer Fundraiser, Mr. Ben Latham, and the Rising Tide Foundation. Hundreds of others contributed anywhere from $10 to $5,000 in donations from an open-access philanthropy site that continues to educate the public about the research study. Members of the Houston community also came together to raise funds, including through a concert hosted by Casa Argentina.

We would like to thank Elissa Epel for introducing us to our agent Doug Abrams. It was a pivotal moment. She has been a champion of our project and provided excellent advice throughout the process. We would also like to thank Eliot Schrefer for giving us "Book Publishing 101" at the start of our project and for his and Eric Zahler's support. A special thank you to our friend and colleague Alejandro Chaoul, for helping to educate us about mind-body practices and for his long-standing friendship. As a friend and colleague, Tica Hall inspires us with her true passion and commitment to life and we thank her for her unconditional love, support, and friendship.

Franklin Servan-Schreiber, Pascaline Servan-Schreiber and family have graciously supported our project and been available throughout the writing and publication process.

Thank you to those who took time to give us invaluable feedback on our ideas and manuscript along the way: Ken Cook, Sarah Cortez, Jennifer Mc-Quade, Martica (Tica) Hall, Meg Hirshberg, Sarah Lewis, John Mendelsohn, Karen Mustian, Anil Sood, Steve Cole, Susan Lutgendorf, Richard Wagner, Susan Jefferies, K. Joy Oden, Maura O'Dowd, Cathy Crath, Misty Matin, and Julia Vine.

Thank you to our lifelong friends, Rob Howard and Lisa Howard, for the beautiful jacket and publicity photographs. You were able to make us look better than we could have ever imagined.

The evolution in our thinking and our sustained practice of anticancer living is in large part possible because of our friendships. We thank Shannon, Jamie, Ian, and Emma Mann, along with Cathy, Randy, Jake, Anna, and Cate Crath for inspiring us to make change, remain committed, and to reach out to others with our message. In addition, we thank Maura O'Dowd, Philip Hilder, Ana Trevino-Godfrey, and Jonathan Godfrey. We are especially grateful to all our friends and colleagues who have engaged with us in stimulating conversations, much of which has inspired *Anticancer Living*, including our Houston community and the Canadian contingent in Toronto, Calgary, Montreal, and Georgian Bay.

A special thank you to Gabriel Lopez and his family for allowing us to use their beach house for our writing retreat, and to Cliff Krauss and Paola Cairo for the great conversations, friendship, and letting us crash their beach resort for pool access during that time.

We would like to thank our families for their unconditional love and support of us and this project: Paola and Jon Cohen, Susan and Robert Jefferies, Rachel Jefferies, Mark Jones, Molly Jones, Kate Jones, David Cohen, Haleh Zarkesh, and Rubinaz Cohen. We also thank our extended families for their encouragement and support: Marion and John Hamlin, the Locke, Dempsey, and McFarland families, and all the Italian relatives of the Scaravelli and Passigli families. We thank our children—Alessandro, Luca, and Chiara—for their love and support and for being good-natured about joining us an our anticancer journey and "experimenting" together. Lastly, we thank Vanda Scaravelli (Lorenzo's grandmother), for inspiring us to live the anticancer life.

NOTES

Introduction

1. M. A. Martinez-Gonzalez, A. Sanchez-Tainta, D. Corella, et al., "A provegetarian food pattern and reduction in total mortality in the Prevencion con Dieta Mediterranea (PREDIMED) study," *American Journal of Clinical Nutrition* 100, no. 1 (July 2014): 320S–28S, Erratum, Supplement, *American Journal of Clinical Nutrition* 100, no. 6 (December 2014): 1605.

2. V. Er, J. A. Lane, R. M. Martin, et al., "Adherence to dietary and lifestyle recommendations and prostate cancer risk in the prostate testing for cancer and treatment (ProtecT) trial," *Cancer Epidemiology, Biomarkers and Prevention* 23, no. 10 (October 2014): 206–77.

3. P. F. Innominato, D. Spiegel, A. Ulusakarya, et al., "Subjective sleep and overall survival in chemotherapy-naive patients with metastatic colorectal cancer," *Sleep Medicine* 16, no. 3 (March 2015): 391–98.

4. P. F. Innominato, S. Giacchetti, G. A. Bjarnason, et al., "Prediction of overall survival through circadian rest-activity monitoring during chemotherapy for metastatic colorectal cancer," *International Journal of Cancer* 131, no. 11 (December 2012): 2684–92.

5. P. Cormie, E. M. Zopf, X. Zhang, K. H. Schmitz, "The impact of exercise on cancer mortality, recurrence, and treatment-related adverse effects," *Epidemiologic Reviews* 39, no. 1 (January 2017): 71–92.

6. B. Bortolato, T. N. Hyphantis, S. Valpione, et al., "Depression in cancer: the many biobehavioral pathways driving tumor progression," *Cancer Treatment Reviews* 52 (January 2017): 58–70.

7. B. L. Andersen, H. C. Yang, W. B. Farrar, et al., "Psychologic intervention improves survival for breast cancer patients: a randomized clinical trial," *Cancer* 113, no. 12 (December 2008): 3450–58.

8. J. C. Pairon, P. Andujar, M. Rinaldo, et al., "Asbestos exposure, pleural plaques, and the risk of death from lung cancer," *American Journal of Respiratory and Critical Care Medicine* 190, no. 12 (December 2014): 1413–20.

9. I. A. Ojajarvi, T. J. Partanen, A. Ahlbom, et al., "Occupational exposures and pancreatic cancer: a meta-analysis," *Occupational and Environmental Medicine* 57, no. 5 (May 2000): 316–24.

10. D. Servan-Schreiber, *Anticancer: A New Way of Life* (New York: Viking, 2009).

11. B. Arun, T. Austin, G. V. Babiera, et al., "A comprehensive lifestyle randomized clinical trial: design and initial patient experience," *Integrative Cancer Therapies* 16, no. 1 (March 2017): 3–20.

12. M. L. McCullough, A. V. Patel, L. H. Kushi, et al., "Following cancer prevention guidelines reduces risk of cancer, cardiovascular disease, and all-cause mortality," *Cancer Epidemiology, Biomarkers and Prevention* 20, no. 6 (June 2011): 1089–97.

13. L. J. Rasmussen-Torvik, C. M. Shay, J. G. Abramson, et al., "Ideal cardiovascular health is inversely associated with incident cancer: the atherosclerosis risk in communities study," *Circulation* 127, no. 12 (March 2013): 1270–75.

PART ONE: THE ANTICANCER AGE

Chapter One: The Anticancer Revolution

1. American Institute for Cancer Research, "Nearly 50% of the most common cancers can be prevented," 2017, www.aicr.org/learn-more-about-cancer/infographics/nearly-50-infographic.html.

2. T. Lohse, D. Faeh, M. Bopp, S. Rohrmann, "Adherence to the cancer prevention recommendations of the World Cancer Research Fund/American Institute for Cancer Research and Mortality: a census-linked cohort," *American Journal of Clinical Nutrition* 104, no. 3 (September 2016): 678–85.

3. G. C. Kabat, C. E. Matthews, V. Kamensky, A. R. Hollenbeck, T. E. Rhan, "Adherence to cancer prevention guidelines and cancer incidence, cancer mortality, and total mortality: a prospective cohort study," *American Journal of Clinical Nutrition* 101, no. 3 (March 2015): 558–69.

4. R. L. Siegel, K. D. Miller, A. Jemal, "Cancer statistics, 2017," *CA: A Cancer Journal for Clinicians* 67, no. 1 (January 2017): 7–30.

5. D. Hanahan, R. A. Weinberg, "Hallmarks of cancer: the next generation," *Cell* 144, no. 5 (March 2011): 646–74.

6. G. A. Thomas, B. Cartmel, M. Harrigan, et al., "The effect of exercise on body composition and bone mineral density in breast cancer survivors taking aromatase inhibitors," *Obesity* 25, no. 2 (February 2017): 346–51.

7. M. Inoue-Choi, K. Robien, D. Lazovich, "Adherence to the WCRF/AICR guidelines for cancer prevention is associated with lower mortality among older female cancer survivors," *Cancer Epidemiology Biomarkers & Prevention* 22, no. 5 (May 2013): 792–802.

8. P. Cormie, E. M. Zopf, X. Zhang, K. H. Schmitz, "The impact of exercise on cancer mortality, recurrence, and treatment-related adverse effects," *Epidemiologic Reviews* 39, no. 1 (January 2017): 71–92.

9. S. Wu, S. Powers, W. Zhu, Y. A. Hannun, "Substantial contribution of extrinsic risk factors to cancer development," *Nature* 529, no. 7584 (January 2016): 43–47.

10. World Health Organization, "Cancer," February 2017, www.who.int/mediacentre/factsheets/fs297/en.

11. American Cancer Society, *Cancer Facts & Figures 2017* (Atlanta: American Cancer Society, 2017).

12. M. C. White, D. M. Holman, J. E. Boehm, et al., "Age and cancer risk: a potentially modifiable relationship," *American Journal of Preventive Medicine* 46, no. 3 Supplement 1 (March 2014): S7–15.

13. R. L. Siegel, S. A. Fedewa, W. F. Anderson et al., "Colorectal cancer incidence patterns in the United States, 1974–2013," *Journal of the National Cancer Institute* 109, no. 8 (August 2017).

14. M. R. Cooperberg, J. M. Broering, P. R. Carroll, "Time trends and local variation in primary treatment of localized prostate cancer," *Journal of Clinical Oncology* 28, no. 7 (March 2010): 1117–23.

15. L. J. Esserman, Y. Shieh, E. J. Rutgers, et al., "Impact of mammographic screening on the detection of good and poor prognosis breast cancers," *Breast Cancer Research and Treatment* 130, no. 3 (December 2011): 725–34.

16. D. Katz, "True health initiative, 2017," www.truehealthinitiative.org.

17. J. M. McGinnis, W. H. Foege, "Actual causes of death in the United States," *Journal of the American Medical Association* 270, no. 18 (November 1993): 2207–12.

18. A. H. Mokdad, J. S. Marks, D. F. Stroup, J. L. Gerberding, "Actual causes of death in the United States, 2000," *Journal of the American Medical Association* 291, no. 10 (March 2004): 1238–45.

19. M. Song, E. Giovannucci, "Preventable incidence and mortality of carcinoma associated with lifestyle factors among white adults in the United States," *Journal of the American Medical Association Oncology* 2, no. 9 (September 2016): 1154–61.

20. G. A. Colditz, S. Sutcliffe, "The preventability of cancer: Stacking the deck," *Journal of the American Medical Association Oncology* 2, no. 9 (September 2016): 1131–33.

21. M. Greger, G. Stone, *How Not to Die: Discover the Foods Scientifically Proven to Prevent and Reverse Disease* (New York: Flatiron Books, 2015).

22. Surgeon General's Advisory Committee on Smoking and Health, United States, Public Health Service, Office of the Surgeon General, United States, "Smoking and health: report of the advisory committee of the surgeon general of the public health service," Public Health Service, Office of the Surgeon General, 1964, www.profiles .nlm.nih.gov/NN/B/B/M/Q.

23. F. Islami, L. A. Torre, A. Jemal, "Global trends of lung cancer mortality and smoking prevalence," *Translational Lung Cancer Research* 4, no. 4 (August 2015): 327–38.

24. Australian Bureau of Statistics, "National health survey: First results, 2014–15: Smoking," www.abs.gov.au/ausstats/abs@.nsf/Lookup/bySubject/4364.0.55.001~2014 -15~Main Features~Smoking~24.

25. T. Goldman, "Health policy brief: tobacco taxes," *Health Affairs*, September 19, 2016, www.healthaffairs.org/healthpolicybriefs/brief.php?brief_id=163.

26. K. Lunze, L. Migliorini, "Tobacco control in the Russian Federation—a policy analysis," *BMC Public Health* 13 (January 2013): 64.

27. M. B. Drummond, D. Upson, "Electronic cigarettes: potential harms and benefits," *Annals of the American Thoracic Society* 11, no. 2 (February 2014): 236–42.

28. D. Hammond, J. L. Reid, A. G. Cole, S. T. Leatherdale, "Electronic cigarette use and smoking initiation among youth: longitudinal cohort study," *Canadian Medical Association Journal* 189, no. 43 (October 2017): E1328–36.

29. P. Anand, A. B. Kunnumakara, C. Sundaram, et al., "Cancer is a preventable disease that requires major lifestyle changes," *Pharmaceutical Research* 25, no. 9 (September 2008): 2097–116.

30. D. Chan, "Where do the millions of cancer research dollars go every year?," *Slate*, February 7, 2013, www._/blogs/quora/2013/02/07/where_do_the_millions_of_cancer _research_dollars_go_every_year.html.

31. V. Bouvard, D. Loomis, K. Z. Guyton, et al., "Carcinogenicity of consumption of red and processed meat," *The Lancet Oncology* 16, no. 16 (October 2015): 1599–1600.

32. Y. Jiang, Y. Pan, P. R. Rhea, et al., "A sucrose-enriched diet promotes tumorigenesis in mammary gland in part through the 12-lipoxygenase pathway," *Cancer Research* 76, no. 1 (January 2016): 24–29.

33. Q. Yang, Z. Zhang, E. W. Gregg, et al., "Added sugar intake and cardiovascular diseases mortality among U.S. adults," *Journal of the American Medical Association Internal Medicine* 174, no. 4 (April 2014): 516–24.

34. W. E. Barrington, E. White, "Mortality outcomes associated with intake of fast-food items and sugar-sweetened drinks among older adults in the Vitamins and Lifestyle (VITAL) study," *Public Health Nutrition* 19, no. 18 (December 2016): 3319–26.

35. R. Shavelle, K. Vavra-Musser, J. Lee, J. Brooks, "Life expectancy in pleural and peritoneal mesothelioma," *Lung Cancer International* 2017 (January 2017): 2782590.

36. S. J. Gould, "The median isn't the message," UMass Amherst, www.people.umass.edu/biep540w/pdf/Stephen%20Jay%20Gould.pdf.

37. K. D. Miller, R. L. Siegel, C. C. Lin, et al., "Cancer treatment and survivorship statistics, 2016," *CA: A Cancer Journal for Clinicians* 66, no. 4 (July 2016): 271–89.

38. P. S. Rosenberg, K. A. Barker, W. F. Anderson, "Estrogen receptor status and the future burden of invasive and in situ breast cancers in the United States," *JNCI Journal of the National Cancer Institute* 107, no. 9 (June 2015).

Chapter Two: Our Healing Powers

1. D. Ornish, G. Weidner, W. R. Fair, et al., "Intensive lifestyle changes may affect the progression of prostate cancer," *Journal of Urology* 174, no. 3 (September 2005): 1065–69; discussion 1069–70.

2. D. Romaguera, E. Gracia-Lavedan, A. Molinuevo, et al., "Adherence to nutrition-based cancer prevention guidelines and breast, prostate and colorectal cancer risk in the MCC-Spain case-control study," *International Journal of Cancer* 141, no. 1 (July 2017): 83–93.

3. N. Jankovic, A. Geelen, R. M. Winkels, et al., "Adherence to the WCRF/AICR dietary recommendations for cancer prevention and risk of cancer in elderly from Europe and the United States: a meta-analysis within the CHANCES Project," *Cancer Epidemiology, Biomarkers and Prevention* 26, no. 1 (January 2017): 136–44.

4. P. P. Bao, G. M. Zhao, X. O. Shu et al., "Modifiable lifestyle factors and triple-negative breast cancer survival: a population-based prospective study," *Epidemiology* 26, no. 6 (November 2015): 909–16.

5. C. A. Thomson, M. L. McCullough, B. C. Wertheim, et al., "Nutrition and physical activity cancer prevention guidelines, cancer risk, and mortality in the women's health initiative," *Cancer Prevention Research* 7, no. 1 (January 2014): 42–53.

6. T. Lohse, D. Faeh, M. Bopp, S. Rohrmann, "Adherence to the cancer prevention recommendations of the World Cancer Research Fund/American Institute for Cancer Research and Mortality: a census-linked cohort," *American Journal of Clinical Nutrition* 104, no. 3 (September 2016): 678–85.

7. P. Jallinoja, P. Absetz, R. Kuronen, et al., "The dilemma of patient responsibility for lifestyle change: perceptions among primary care physicians and nurses," *Scandinavian Journal of Primary Health Care* 25, no. 4 (December 2007): 244–49.

8. K. M. Adams, M. Kohlmeier, S. H. Zeisel, "Nutrition education in U.S. medical schools: latest update of a national survey," *Academic Medicine* 85, no. 9 (September 2010): 1537–42.

9. M. Zajenkowski, K. S. Jankowski, D. Kołata, "Let's dance—feel better! Mood changes following dancing in different situations," *European Journal of Sport Science* 15, no. 7 (October 2015): 640–46.

10. V. N. Salimpoor, M. Benovoy, K. Larcher, A. Dagher, R. J. Zatorre, "Anatomically distinct dopamine release during anticipation and experience of peak emotion to music," *Nature Neuroscience* 14, no. 2 (February 2011): 257–62.

11. K. Hojan, E. Kwiatkowska-Borowczyk, E. Leporowska, et al., "Physical exercise for functional capacity, blood immune function, fatigue, and quality of life in high-risk prostate cancer patients during radiotherapy: a prospective, randomized clinical study," *European Journal of Physical & Rehabilitation Medicine* 52, no. 4 (August 2016): 489–501.

12. K. S. Courneya, C. M. Friedenreich, C. Franco-Villalobos, et al., "Effects of supervised exercise on progression-free survival in lymphoma patients: an exploratory follow-up of the help trial," *Cancer Causes and Control* 26, no. 2 (February 2015): 269–76.

13. T. Bouillet, X. Bigard, C. Brami, et al., "Role of physical activity and sport in oncology: scientific commission of the National Federation Sport and Cancer Cami," *Critical Reviews in Oncology-Hematology* 94, no. 1 (April 2015): 74–86.

14. E. M. Zopf, W. Bloch, S. Machtens, et al., "Effects of a 15-month supervised exercise program on physical and psychological outcomes in prostate cancer patients following prostatectomy: the prorehab study," *Integrative Cancer Therapies* 14, no. 5 (September 2015): 409–18.

15. G. Zhu, X. Zhang, Y. Wang, et al., "Effects of exercise intervention in breast cancer survivors: a meta-analysis of 33 randomized controlled trials," *OncoTargets and Therapy* 9 (April 2016): 2153–68.

16. C. Catsburg, A. B. Miller, T. E. Rohan, "Adherence to cancer prevention guidelines and risk of breast cancer," *International Journal of Cancer* 135, no. 10 (November 2014): 2444–52.

17. M. Inoue-Choi, D. Lazovich, A. E. Prizment, K. Robien, "Adherence to the World Cancer Research Fund/American Institute for Cancer Research recommendations for cancer prevention is associated with better health-related quality of life among elderly female cancer survivors," *Journal of Clinical Oncology* 31, no. 14 (May 2013): 1758–66.

18. M. Inoue-Choi, K. Robien, D. Lazovich, "Adherence to the WCRF/AICR guidelines for cancer prevention is associated with lower mortality among older female cancer survivors," *Cancer Epidemiology Biomarkers & Prevention* 22, no. 5 (May 2013): 792–802.

19. American Cancer Society, "ACS guidelines on nutrition and physical activity for cancer prevention," February 5, 2016, www.cancer.org/healthy/eat-healthy-get -active/acs-guidelines-nutrition-physical-activity-cancer-prevention.html.

20. American Institute for Cancer Research, "Recommendations for cancer prevention," 2017, www.aicr.org/reduce-your-cancer-risk/recommendations-for-cancer -prevention.

21. N. Makarem, Y. Lin, E. V. Bandera, P. F. Jacques, N. Parekh, "Concordance with World Cancer Research Fund/American Institute for Cancer Research (WCRF/ AICR) guidelines for cancer prevention and obesity-related cancer risk in the framingham offspring cohort (1991–2008)," *Cancer Causes and Control* 26, no. 2 (February 2015): 277–86.

22. A. C. Vergnaud, D. Romaguera, P. H. Peeters, et al., "Adherence to the World Cancer Research Fund/American Institute for Cancer Research guidelines and risk of death in Europe: results from the European Prospective Investigation into nutrition and cancer cohort study," *American Journal of Clinical Nutrition* 97, no. 5 (May 2013): 1107–20.

23. J. J. Prochaska, J. O. Prochaska, "A review of multiple health behavior change interventions for primary prevention," *American Journal of Lifestyle Medicine* 5, no. 3 (May 2011).

24. S. U. Maier, A. B. Makwana, T. A. Hare, "Acute stress impairs self-control in goal-directed choice by altering multiple functional connections within the brain's decision circuits," *Neuron* 87, no. 3 (August 2015): 621–31.

25. W. E. Barrington, S. A. Beresford, B. A. McGregor, E. White, "Perceived stress and eating behaviors by sex, obesity status, and stress vulnerability: findings from the vitamins and lifestyle (vital) study," *Journal of the Academy of Nutrition and Dietetics* 114, no. 11 (November 2014): 1791–99.

26. A. W. Y. Leung, R. S. M. Chan, M. M. M. Sea, J. Woo, "An overview of factors associated with adherence to lifestyle modification programs for weight management in adults," *International Journal of Environmental Research and Public Health* 14, no. 8 (August 2017): 922.

27. T. Asadollahi, S. Khakpour, F. Ahmadi, et al., "Effectiveness of mindfulness training and dietary regime on weight loss in obese people," *Journal of Medicine and Life* 8, no. 4 (December 2015): 114–24.

28. D. J. Hyman, V. N. Pavlik, W. C. Taylor, G. K. Goodrick, L. Moye, "Simultaneous vs sequential counseling for multiple behavior change," *Archives of Internal Medicine* 167, no. 11 (June 2007): 1152–58.

29. B. Spring, A. King, S. Pagoto, L. Van Horn, J. Fisher, "Fostering multiple healthy lifestyle behaviors for primary prevention of cancer," *American Psychologist* 70, no. 2 (March 2015): 75–90.

30. M. A. Lerner, "Difference Between Healing and Curing," Awaken.org, February 7, 2015, www.awaken.org/read/view.php?tid=1066.

31. D. J. Hauser, N. Schwarz, "The war on prevention: bellicose cancer metaphors hurt (some) prevention intentions," *Personality Health* 14, no. 8 (August 2017): 922.

32. D. Servan-Schreiber, *Anticancer: A New Way of Life* (New York: Viking, 2009).

33. S. K. Lutgendorf, K. De Geest, D. Bender, et al., "Social influences on clinical outcomes of patients with ovarian cancer," *Journal of Clinical Oncology* 30, no. 23 (August 2012): 2885–90.

34. Anticancer Lifestyle Foundation, "Anticancer lifestyle program," 2017, www.anticancerlifestyle.org.

35. P. J. Goodwin, R. T. Chlebowski, "Obesity and cancer: insights for clinicians," *Journal of Clinical Oncology* 34, no. 35 (December 2016): 4197–202.

36. P. Cormie, E. M. Zopf, X. Zhang, K. H. Schmitz, "The impact of exercise on cancer mortality, recurrence, and treatment-related adverse effects," *Epidemiologic Reviews* 39, no. 1 (January 2017): 71–92.

37. M. L. McCullough, A. V. Patel, L. H. Kushi, et al., "Following cancer prevention guidelines reduces risk of cancer, cardiovascular disease, and all-cause mortality," *Cancer Epidemiology, Biomarkers and Prevention* 20, no. 6 (June 2011): 1089–97.

38. P. F. Innominato, D. Spiegel, A. Ulusakarya, et al., "Subjective sleep and overall survival in chemotherapy-naive patients with metastatic colorectal cancer," *Sleep Medicine* 16, no. 3 (March 2015): 391–98.

39. M. Jan, S. E. Bonn, A. Sjolander, et al., "The roles of stress and social support in prostate cancer mortality," *Scandinavian Journal of Urology* 50, no. 1 (August 2016): 47–55.

Chapter Three: What Causes Cancer, Anyway?

1. D. Hanahan, R. A. Weinberg, "Hallmarks of cancer: the next generation," *Cell* 144, no. 5 (March 2011): 646–74.

2. S. Wu, S. Powers, W. Zhu, Y. A. Hannun, "Substantial contribution of extrinsic risk factors to cancer development," *Nature* 529, no. 7584 (January 2016): 43–47.

3. C. Tomasetti, B. Vogelstein, "Variation in cancer risk among tissues can be explained by the number of stem cell divisions," *Science* 347, no. 6217 (January 2015): 78.

4. C. Tomasetti, L. Li, B. Vogelstein, "Stem cell divisions, somatic mutations, cancer etiology, and cancer prevention," *Science* 355, no. 6331 (March 2017): 1330.

5. American Institute for Cancer Research, "The AICR 2015 cancer risk awareness survey report," 2015, www.aicr.org/assets/docs/pdf/education/aicr-awareness-report-2015.pdf.

6. J. E. Garber, K. Offit, "Hereditary cancer predisposition syndromes," *Journal of Clinical Oncology* 23, no. 2 (January 2005): 276–92.

7. P. Lichtenstein, N. V. Holm, P. K. Verkasalo, et al., "Environmental and heritable factors in the causation of cancer—analyses of cohorts of twins from Sweden, Denmark, and Finland," *New England Journal of Medicine* 343, no. 2 (July 2000): 78–85.

8. National Cancer Institute, "BRCA1 and BRCA2: cancer risk and genetic testing," April 1, 2015, www.cancer.gov/about-cancer/causes-prevention/genetics/brca-fact -sheet-q9.

9. American Institute for Cancer Research, "Nearly 50% of the most common cancers can be prevented," 2017, www.aicr.org/learn-more-about-cancer/infographics/nearly -50-infographic.html.

10. International Agency for Research on Cancer, "IARC monographs of the evaluation of carcenogenic risks to humans," World Health Organization, 2017, www.mono graphs.iarc.fr.

11. Centers for Disease Control and Prevention, "Agency for toxic substances and disease registry," November 27, 2017, www.atsdr.cdc.gov.

12. American Association for Cancer Research, "AACR cancer progress report. Preventing cancer: understanding risk factors," www.cancerprogressreport.org/Pages /cpr17-preventing-cancer.aspx.

13. P. Anand, A. B. Kunnumakara, C. Sundaram, et al., "Cancer is a preventable disease that requires major lifestyle changes," *Pharmaceutical Research* 25, no. 9 (September 2008): 2097–116.

14. National Toxicology Program, "Report on carcinogens, fourteenth edition," U.S. Department of Health and Human Services, Public Health Service, 2016b.

15. N. K. LoConte, A. M. Brewster, J. S. Kaur, J. K. Merrill, A. J. Alberg, "Alcohol and cancer: a statement of the American Society of Clinical Oncology," *Journal of Clinical Oncology* (November 2017): JCO2017761155.

16. D. E. Nelson, D. W. Jarman, J. Rehm, et al., "Alcohol-attributable cancer deaths and years of potential life lost in the United States," *American Journal of Public Health* 103, no. 4 (April 2013): 641–48.

17. World Health Organization, "Tobacco Free Initiative (TFI): fact sheet about health benefits of smoking cessation," 2017, www.who.int/tobacco/quitting/benefits/en.

18. A. Parsons, A. Daley, R. Begh, P. Aveyard, "Influence of smoking cessation after diagnosis of early stage lung cancer on prognosis: systematic review of observational studies with meta-analysis," *BMJ* 340 (January 2010).

19. G. Poschl, H. K. Seitz, "Alcohol and cancer," *Alcohol and Alcoholism* 39, no. 3 (June 2004): 155–65.

20. H. Kuper, A. Tzonou, E. Kaklamani, et al., "Tobacco smoking, alcohol consumption and their interaction in the causation of hepatocellular carcinoma," *International Journal of Cancer* 85, no. 4 (February 2000): 498–502.

21. A. Prabhu, K. O. Obi, J. H. Rubenstein, "The synergistic effects of alcohol and tobacco consumption on the risk of esophageal squamous cell carcinoma: a meta-analysis," *American Journal of Gastroenterology* 109, no. 6 (June 2014): 822–27.

22. M. Hashibe, P. Brennan, S. C. Chuang, et al., "Interaction between tobacco and alcohol use and the risk of head and neck cancer: pooled analysis in the inhance consortium," *Cancer Epidemiology, Biomarkers & Prevention* 18, no. 2 (February 2009): 541–50.

23. T. Lohse, D. Faeh, M. Bopp, S. Rohrmann, "Adherence to the cancer prevention recommendations of the World Cancer Research Fund/American Institute for Cancer Research and Mortality: a census-linked cohort," *American Journal of Clinical Nutrition* 104, no. 3 (September 2016): 678–85.

24. A. C. Vergnaud, D. Romaguera, P. H. Peeters, et al., "Adherence to the World Cancer Research Fund/American Institute for Cancer Research guidelines and risk of death in Europe: results from the European Prospective Investigation into nutrition and cancer cohort study," *American Journal of Clinical Nutrition* 97, no. 5 (May 2013): 1107–20.

25. M. Inoue-Choi, K. Robien, D. Lazovich, "Adherence to the WCRF/AICR guidelines for cancer prevention is associated with lower mortality among older female cancer survivors," *Cancer Epidemiology Biomarkers & Prevention* 22, no. 5 (May 2013): 792–802.

26. G. C. Kabat, C. E. Matthews, V. Kamensky, A. R. Hollenbeck, T. E. Rohan, "Adherence to cancer prevention guidelines and cancer incidence, cancer mortality, and total mortality: a prospective cohort study," *American Journal of Clinical Nutrition* 101, no. 3 (March 2015): 558–69.

27. C. A. Thomson, M. L. McCullough, B. C. Wertheim, et al., "Nutrition and physical activity cancer prevention guidelines, cancer risk, and mortality in the Women's Health Initiative," *Cancer Prevention Research* 7, no. 1 (January 2014): 42–53.

28. C. Catsburg, A. B. Miller, T. E. Rohan, "Adherence to cancer prevention guidelines and risk of breast cancer," *International Journal of Cancer* 135, no. 10 (November 2014): 2444–52.

29. A. Nerurkar, "What a Happy Cell Looks Like," February 10, 2015, www.theatlantic.com/health/archive/2015/02/what-a-happy-cell-looks-like/385000.

Chapter Four: A Cell's Quest for Immortality

1. E. Bianconi, A. Piovesan, F. Facchin, et al., "An estimation of the number of cells in the human body," *Annals of Human Biology* 40, no. 6 (December 2013): 463–71.

2. X. Dai, L. Xiang, T. Li, et al., "Cancer hallmarks, biomarkers and breast cancer molecular subtypes," *Journal of Cancer* 10, no. 7 (2016): 1281–94.

3. D. Hanahan, R. A. Weinberg, "Hallmarks of cancer: the next generation," *Cell* 144, no. 5 (March 2011): 646–74.

4. J. R. Aunan, W. C. Cho, K. Soreide, "The biology of aging and cancer: a brief overview of shared and divergent molecular hallmarks," *Aging and Disease* 8, no. 5 (October 2017): 628–42.

5. B. Vogelstein, N. Papadopoulos, V. E. Velculescu, et al., "Cancer genome landscapes," *Science* 339, no. 6127 (March 2013): 1546–58.

6. American Cancer Society, *Cancer Facts & Figures 2017* (Atlanta: American Cancer Society, 2017c).

7. X. Han, J. Wang, Y. Sun, "Circulating tumor DNA as biomarkers for cancer detection," *Genomics, Proteomics & Bioinformatics* 15, no. 2 (April 2017): 59–72.

8. J. Irudayara, "Research could lead to test strips for early cervical cancer detection," March 28, 2017, www.purdue.edu/newsroom/releases/2017/Q1/research-could-lead-to-test-strips-for-early-cervical-cancer-detection.html.

9. For a wonderful history on cancer and cancer treatment, see: S. Mukhergee, *The Emperor of All Maladies: A Biography of Cancer* (New York: Simon and Shuster, 2011).

10. H. S. Ahn, H. J. Kim, H. G. Welch, "Korea's thyroid-cancer 'epidemic'—screening and overdiagnosis," *New England Journal of Medicine* 371, no. 19 (November 2014): 1765–67.

11. J. H. Hayes, M. J. Barry, "Screening for prostate cancer with the prostate-specific antigen test: a review of current evidence," *Journal of the American Medical Association* 311, no. 11 (March 2014): 1143–49.

12. M. R. Cooperberg, J. M. Broering, P. R. Carroll, "Time trends and local variation in primary treatment of localized prostate cancer," *Journal of Clinical Oncology* 28, no. 7 (March 2010): 1117–23.

13. American Cancer Society, "Watchful waiting or active surveillance for prostate cancer," March 11, 2016, www.cancer.org/cancer/prostate-cancer/treating/watchful -waiting.html.

14. T. J. Wilt, M. K. Brawer, K. M. Jones, et al., "Radical prostatectomy versus observation for localized prostate cancer," *New England Journal of Medicine* 367, no. 3 (July 2012): 203–13.

15. J. Hegarty, P. V. Beirne, E. Walsh, et al., "Radical prostatectomy versus watchful waiting for prostate cancer," *Cochrane Database of Systematic Reviews*, no. 11 (November 2010): Cd006590.

16. D. A. Barocas, J. Alvarez, M. J. Resnick, et al., "Association between radiation therapy, surgery, or observation for localized prostate cancer and patient-reported outcomes after 3 years," *Journal of the American Medical Association* 317, no. 11 (March 2017): 1126–40.

17. J. C. Hu, L. Kwan, C. S. Saigal, M. S. Litwin, "Regret in men treated for localized prostate cancer," *Journal of Urology* 169, no. 6 (June 2003): 2279–83.

18. E. J. Groen, L. E. Elshof, L. L. Visser, et al., "Finding the balance between over- and under-treatment of ductal carcinoma in situ (dcis)," *The Breast* 31, Supplement C (February 2017): 274–83.

19. J. R. Benson, I. Jatoi, M. Toi, "Treatment of low-risk ductal carcinoma in situ: is nothing better than something?," *The Lancet Oncology* 17, no. 10 (October 2016): e442–51.

20. L. M. Youngwirth, J. C. Boughey, E. S. Hwang, "Surgery versus monitoring and endocrine therapy for low-risk dcis: the COMET Trial," *Bulletin of the American College of Surgeons* 102, no. 1 (January 2017): 62–63.

21. A. Francis, J. Thomas, L. Fallowfield et al., "Addressing overtreatment of screen detected dcis; the loris trial," *European Journal of Cancer* 51, no. 16 (November 2015): 2296–303.

22. Talk of the Nation, "Science diction: the origin of the word 'cancer,'" National Public Radio, October 22, 2010, www.npr.org/templates/story/story.php?storyId= 130754101.

23. American Cancer Society, "Evolution of cancer treatments: chemotherapy," June 12, 2014, www.cancer.org/cancer/cancer-basics/history-of-cancer/cancer-treatment-chemo .html.

24. National Cancer Institute, "National Cancer Act of 1971," February 16, 2016, www .cancer.gov/about-nci/legislative/history/national-cancer-act-1971.

25. National Human Genome Research Institute, "All about the Human Genome Project (HGP)," October 1, 2015, www.genome.gov/10001772/all-about-the-human -genome-project-hgp.

26. D. Hanahan, R. A. Weinberg, "The hallmarks of cancer," *Cell* 100, no. 1 (January 2000): 57–70.

27. S. K. Lutgendorf, K. DeGeest, L. Dahmoush, et al., "Social isolation is associated with elevated tumor norepinephrine in ovarian carcinoma patients," *Brain, Behavior, and Immunity* 25, no. 2 (February 2011): 250–55.

28. J. M. Zeitzer, B. Nouriani, M. B. Rissling, et al., "Aberrant nocturnal cortisol and disease progression in women with breast cancer," *Breast Cancer Research and Treatment* 158, no. 1 (July 2016): 43–50.

29. Z. Zhang, L. L. Atwell, P. E. Farris, E. Ho, J. Shannon, "Associations between cruciferous vegetable intake and selected biomarkers among women scheduled for breast biopsies," *Public Health Nutrition* 19, no. 7 (May 2016): 1288–95.

30. M. E. Schmidt, A. Meynkohn, N. Habermann, et al., "Resistance exercise and inflammation in breast cancer patients undergoing adjuvant radiation therapy: mediation analysis from a randomized, controlled intervention trial," *International Journal of Radiation Oncology, Biology, Physics* 94, no. 2 (February 2016): 329–37.

31. D. Roy, M. Morgan, C. Yoo, et al., "Integrated bioinformatics, environmental epidemiologic and genomic approaches to identify environmental and molecular links between endometriosis and breast cancer," *International Journal of Molecular Sciences* 16, no. 10 (October 2015): 25285–322.

32. S. W. Cole, A. S. Nagaraja, S. K. Lutgendorf, P. A. Green, A. K. Sood, "Sympathetic nervous system regulation of the tumour microenvironment," *Nature Reviews: Cancer* 15, no. 9 (September 2015): 563–72.

33. S. K. Lutgendorf, E. L. Johnsen, B. Cooper, et al., "Vascular endothelial growth factor and social support in patients with ovarian carcinoma," *Cancer* 95 (August 2002): 808–15.

34. J. M. Saxton, E. J. Scott, A. J. Daley, et al., "Effects of an exercise and hypocaloric healthy eating intervention on indices of psychological health status, hypothalamic-pituitary-adrenal axis regulation and immune function after early-stage breast cancer: a randomised controlled trial," *Breast Cancer Research* 16, no. 2 (April 2014): R39.

35. G. Fisher, T. C. Hyatt, G. R. Hunter, et al., "Effect of diet with and without exercise training on markers of inflammation and fat distribution in overweight women," *Obesity* 19, no. 6 (December 2011): 1131–36.

36. I. Imayama, C. M. Ulrich, C. M. Alfano, et al., "Effects of a caloric restriction weight loss diet and exercise on inflammatory biomarkers in overweight/obese postmenopausal women: a randomized controlled trial," *Cancer Research* 72, no. 9 (May 2012): 2314–26.

37. S. B. Jones, G. A. Thomas, S. D. Hesselsweet, et al., "Effect of exercise on markers of inflammation in breast cancer survivors: the Yale exercise and survivorship study," *Cancer Prevention Research* 6, no. 2 (December 2013).

38. F. K. Tabung, T. T. Fung, J. E. Chavarro, et al., "Associations between adherence to the world cancer research fund/American institute for cancer research cancer prevention recommendations and biomarkers of inflammation, hormonal, and insulin response," *International Journal of Cancer* 140, no. 4 (February 2017): 764–76.

39. A. Boynton, M. L. Neuhouser, M. H. Wener, et al., "Associations between healthy eating patterns and immune function or inflammation in overweight or obese postmenopausal women," *American Journal of Clinical Nutrition* 86, no. 5 (November 2007): 1445–55.

40. K. I. Block, C. Gyllenhaal, L. Lowe, et al., "Designing a broad-spectrum integrative approach for cancer prevention and treatment," *Seminars in Cancer Biology* 35, Supplement (December 2015): S276–304.

41. A. Ruiz-Casado, A. Martin-Ruiz, L. M. Perez, et al., "Exercise and the hallmarks of cancer," *Trends Cancer* 3, no. 6 (June 2017): 423–41.

42. G. J. Koelwyn, D. F. Quail, X. Zhang, R. M. White, L. W. Jones, "Exercise-dependent regulation of the tumour microenvironment," *Nature Reviews: Cancer* 17, no. 10 (September 2017): 620–32.

43. M. Picon-Ruiz, C. Morata-Tarifa, J. J. Valle-Goffin, E. R. Friedman, J. M. Slingerland, "Obesity and adverse breast cancer risk and outcome: mechanistic insights and strategies for intervention," *CA: A Cancer Journal for Clinicians* 67, no. 5 (September 2017): 378–97.

44. W. Demark-Wahnefried, T. J. Polascik, S. L. George, et al., "Flaxseed supplementation (not dietary fat restriction) reduces prostate cancer proliferation rates in men presurgery," *Cancer Epidemiology Biomarkers & Prevention* 17, no. 12 (December 2008): 3577–87.

45. R. Valdes-Ramos, A. D. Benitez-Arciniega, "Nutrition and immunity in cancer," *British Journal of Nutrition* 98, Supplement 1 (October 2007): S127–132.

46. Y. Cao, R. Langer, "A review of Judah Folkman's remarkable achievements in bio-medicine," *Proceedings of the National Academy of Sciences of the United States of America* 105, no. 36 (September 2008): 13203–05.

47. G. H. Lyman, H. L. Moses, "Biomarker tests for molecularly targeted therapies: laying the foundation and fulfilling the dream," *Journal of Clinical Oncology* 34, no. 17 (June 2016): 2061–66.

48. S. C. Sodergren, E. Copson, A. White, et al., "Systematic review of the side effects associated with anti-her2-targeted therapies used in the treatment of breast cancer, on behalf of the eortc quality of life group," *Targeted Oncology* 11, no. 3 (June 2016): 277–92.

49. P. A. Ganz, R. S. Cecchini, T. B. Julian, et al., "Patient-reported outcomes with anastrozole versus tamoxifen for postmenopausal patients with ductal carcinoma in situ treated with lumpectomy plus radiotherapy (nsabp b-35): a randomised, double-blind, phase 3 clinical trial," *The Lancet* 387, no. 10021 (February 2016): 857–65.

50. J. Rotow, T. G. Bivona, "Understanding and targeting resistance mechanisms in NSCLC," *Nature Reviews: Cancer* 17, no. 11 (October 2017): 637–58.

51. N. Shibata, K. Nagai, Y. Morita, et al., "Development of protein degradation inducers of androgen receptor by conjugation of androgen receptor ligands and inhibitor of apoptosis protein ligands," *Journal of Medicinal Chemistry* (June 2017).

52. D. Li, Q. Fu, M. Li, et al., "Primary tumor site and anti-EGFR monoclonal antibody benefit in metastatic colorectal cancer: a meta-analysis," *Future Oncology* 13, no. 12 (May 2017): 1115–27.

53. M. P. Pinto, G. I. Owen, I. Retamal, M. Garrido, "Angiogenesis inhibitors in early development for gastric cancer," *Expert Opinion Investigational Drugs* 26, no. 9 (September 2017): 1007–17.

54. L. E. Fulbright, M. Ellermann, J. C. Arthur, "The microbiome and the hallmarks of cancer," *PLoS Pathogens* 13, no. 9 (September 2017): e1006480.

55. V. Gopalakrishnan, C. N. Spencer, L. Nezi, et al., "Gut microbiome modulates response to anti-PD-1 immunotherapy in melanoma patients," *Science* (November 2017).

56. A. A. Hibberd, A. Lyra, A. C. Ouwehand, et al., "Intestinal microbiota is altered in patients with colon cancer and modified by probiotic intervention," *BMJ Open Gastroenterol* 4, no. 1 (July 2017): e000145.

57. L. E. Wroblewski, R. M. Peek, K. T. Wilson, "Helicobacter pylori and gastric cancer: factors that modulate disease risk," *Clinical Microbiology Reviews* 23, no. 4 (October 2010): 713–39.

58. G. Zeller, J. Tap, A. Y. Voigt, et al., "Potential of fecal microbiota for early-stage detection of colorectal cancer," *Molecular Systems Biology* 10, no. 11 (November 2014): 766.

59. National Cancer Institute, "Targeted cancer therapies," November 6, 2017, www.cancer.gov/about-cancer/treatment/types/targeted-therapies/targeted-therapies-fact-sheet-q6.

60. C. J. Tokheim, N. Papadopoulos, K. W. Kinzler, B. Vogelstein, R. Karchin, "Evaluating the evaluation of cancer driver genes," *Proceedings of the National Academy of Sciences of the United States of America* 113, no. 50 (December 2016): 14330–35.

61. A. L. Wilson, M. Plebanski, A. N. Stephens, "New trends in anti-cancer therapy: combining conventional chemotherapeutics with novel immunomodulators," *Current Medicinal Chemistry* (August 2017).

62. National Cancer Institute, "Human papillomavirus (HPV) vaccines," November 2, 2016, www.cancer.gov/about-cancer/causes-prevention/risk/infectious-agents/hpv-vaccine-fact-sheet.

63. L. E. Markowitz, S. Hariri, C. Lin, et al., "Reduction in human papillomavirus (HPV) prevalence among young women following HPV vaccine introduction in the United States, National Health and Nutrition Examination Surveys, 2003–2010," *Journal of Infectious Diseases* 208, no. 3 (August 2013): 385–93.

64. American Cancer Society, "American Cancer Society recommendations for human papillomavirus (HPV) vaccine use," July 19, 2016, www.cancer.org/cancer/cancer-causes/infectious-agents/hpv/acs-recommendations-for-hpv-vaccine-use.html.

65. American Cancer Society, "American Cancer Society endorses two-dose regimen for HPV vaccination: guideline updated to reflect recent federal recommendation," Science-Daily, February 7, 2017, www.sciencedaily.com/releases/2017/02/170207092811.htm.

66. S. R. Husain, J. Han, P. Au, K. Shannon, R. K. Puri, "Gene therapy for cancer: regulatory considerations for approval," *Cancer Gene Therapy* 22, no. 12 (December 2015): 554–63.

67. A. Trounson, C. McDonald, "Stem cell therapies in clinical trials: progress and challenges," *Cell Stem Cell* 17, no. 1 (July 2015): 11–22.

Chapter Five: The Epigenetics of Prevention

1. S. Wu, S. Powers, W. Zhu, Y. A. Hannun, "Substantial contribution of extrinsic risk factors to cancer development," *Nature* 529, no. 7584 (January 2016): 43–47.

2. M. Gerlinger, A. J. Rowan, S. Horswell, et al., "Intratumor heterogeneity and branched evolution revealed by multiregion sequencing," *New England Journal of Medicine* 366, no. 10 (March 2012): 883–92.

3. D. Ornish, J. Lin, J. M. Chan, et al., "Effect of comprehensive lifestyle changes on telomerase activity and telomere length in men with biopsy-proven low-risk prostate cancer: 5-year follow-up of a descriptive pilot study," *The Lancet Oncology* 14, no. 11 (October 2013): 1112–20.

4. D. Ornish, M. J. Magbanua, G. Weidner, et al., "Changes in prostate gene expression in men undergoing an intensive nutrition and lifestyle intervention," *Proceedings of the National Academy of Sciences of the United States of America* 105, no. 24 (June 2008): 8369–74.

5. W. Demark-Wahnefried, E. A. Platz, J. A. Ligibel, et al., "The role of obesity in cancer survival and recurrence," *Cancer Epidemiology, Biomarkers & Prevention* 21, no. 8 (June 2012): 1244–59.

6. L. Delgado-Cruzata, W. Zhang, J. A. McDonald, et al., "Dietary modifications, weight loss, and changes in metabolic markers affect global DNA methylation in Hispanic, African American, and Afro-Caribbean breast cancer survivors," *Journal of Nutrition* 145, no. 4 (April 2015): 783–90.

7. Z. Li, W. J. Aronson, J. R. Arteaga, et al., "Feasibility of a low-fat/high-fiber diet intervention with soy supplementation in prostate cancer patients after prostatectomy," *European Journal of Clinical Nutrition* 62, no. 4 (April 2008): 526–36.

8. S. K. Lutgendorf, K. DeGeest, L. Dahmoush, et al., "Social isolation is associated with elevated tumor norepinephrine in ovarian carcinoma patients," *Brain, Behavior, and Immunity* 25, no. 2 (February 2011): 250–55.

9. Y. C. Yang, M. K. McClintock, M. Kozloski, T. Li, "Social isolation and adult mortality: the role of chronic inflammation and sex differences," *Journal of Health and Social Behavior* 54, no. 2 (June 2013): 183–203.

10. E. Motevaseli, A. Dianatpour, S. Ghafouri-Fard, "The role of probiotics in cancer treatment: emphasis on their in vivo and in vitro anti-metastatic effects," *International Journal of Molecular Cellular Medicine* 6, no. 2 (Spring 2017): 66–76.

11. K. L. Chen, P. Jung, E. Kulkoyluoglu-Cotul, et al., "Impact of diet and nutrition on cancer hallmarks," *Journal of Cancer Prevention & Current Research* 7, no. 4 (February 2017): 00240.

12. A. Ruiz-Casado, A. Martin-Ruiz, L. M. Perez, et al., "Exercise and the hallmarks of cancer," *Trends in Cancer* 3, no. 6 (June 2017): 423–41.

13. L. Cohen, S. W. Cole, A. K. Sood, et al., "Depressive symptoms and cortisol rhythmicity predict survival in patients with renal cell carcinoma: role of inflammatory signaling," *PloS One* 7, no. 8 (August 2012): e42324.

14. J. Lin, J. A. Blalock, M. Chen, et al., "Depressive symptoms and short telomere length are associated with increased mortality in bladder cancer patients," *Cancer Epidemiology, Biomarkers & Prevention* 24, no. 2 (February 2015): 336–43.

15. L. E. Carlson, T. L. Beattie, J. Giese-Davis, et al., "Mindfulness-based cancer recovery and supportive-expressive therapy maintain telomere length relative to controls in distressed breast cancer survivors," *Cancer* 121, no. 3 (February 2015): 476–84.

16. M. R. Irwin, R. Olmstead, E. C. Breen, et al., "Tai chi, cellular inflammation, and transcriptome dynamics in breast cancer survivors with insomnia: a randomized controlled trial," *Journal of the National Cancer Institute Monographs* 2014, no. 50 (November 2014): 295–301.

17. M. K. Bhasin, J. A. Dusek, B. H. Chang, et al., "Relaxation response induces temporal transcriptome changes in energy metabolism, insulin secretion and inflammatory pathways," *PloS One* 8, no. 5 (May 2013): e62817.

18. S. W. Cole, "Human social genomics," *Plos Genetics* 10, no. 8 (August 2014): e1004601.

19. S. W. Cole, L. C. Hawkley, J. M. Arevalo, et al., "Social regulation of gene expression in human leukocytes," *Genome Biology* 8, no. 9 (September 2007): R189.

20. S. W. Cole, M. E. Levine, J. M. Arevalo, et al., "Loneliness, eudaimonia, and the human conserved transcriptional response to adversity," *Psychoneuroendocrinology* 6 (December 2015): 11–17.

21. S. W. Cole, G. Conti, J. M. Arevalo, et al., "Transcriptional modulation of the developing immune system early life social adversity," *Proceedings of the National Academy of Sciences of the United States of America* 109, no. 50 (December 2012): 20578–83.

22. V. J. Felitti, R. F. Anda, D. Nordenberg, et al., "Relationship of childhood abuse and household dysfunction to many of the leading causes of death in adults. The adverse childhood experiences (ACE) study," *American Journal of Preventive Medicine* 14, no. 4 (May 1998): 245–58.

23. M. Kelly-Irving, B. Lepage, D. Dedieu, et al., "Childhood adversity as a risk for cancer: findings from the 1958 British birth cohort study," *BMC Public Health* 13 (August 2013): 767.

24. K. Hughes, M. A. Bellis, K. A. Hardcastle, et al., "The effect of multiple adverse childhood experiences on health: a systematic review and meta-analysis," *The Lancet Public Health* 2, no. 8 (August 2017): e356–66.

25. M. H. Antoni, S. K. Lutgendorf, B. Blomberg, et al., "Cognitive-behavioral stress management reverses anxiety-related leukocyte transcriptional dynamics," *Biological Psychiatry* 71, no. 4 (February 2012a): 366–72.

26. BLUEPRINT Epigenome, "A blueprint of haemtopoietic epigenomes," 2017, www.blueprint-epigenome.eu.

27. Johns Hopkins University School of Medicine, "Center for the Epigenetics of Common Human Disease," 2017, www.hopkinsmedicine.org/epigenetics/index.html.

28. Cancer Quest, "Interview with Dr. Jean-Pierre Issa," 2016, www.cancerquest.org/media-center/cancer-research-interviews/dr-jean-pierre-issa.

29. R. Yehuda, L. M. Bierer, "Transgenerational transmission of cortisol and PTSD risk," *Progress in Brain Research* 167 (November 2008): 121–35.

30. R. Yehuda, N. P. Daskalakis, L. M. Bierer, et al., "Holocaust exposure induced intergenerational effects on fkbp5 methylation," *Biological Psychiatry* 80, no. 5 (September 2016): 372–80.

31. M. P. Groot, R. Kooke, N. Knoben, et al., "Effects of multi-generational stress exposure and offspring environment on the expression and persistence of transgenerational effects in arabidopsis thaliana," *PloS One* 11, no. 3 (March 2016): e0151566.

32. A. Klosin, E. Casas, C. Hidalgo-Carcedo, T. Vavouri, B. Lehner, "Transgenerational transmission of environmental information in C. elegans," *Science* 356, no. 6335 (April 2017): 320–23.

33. B. M. Herrera, S. Keildson, C. M. Lindgren, "Genetics and epigenetics of obesity," *Maturitas* 69, no. 1 (May 2011): 41–49.

34. M. V. Veenendaal, R. C. Painter, S. R. de Rooij, et al., "Transgenerational effects of prenatal exposure to the 1944–45 Dutch famine," *BJOG: An International Journal of Obstetrics and Gynaecology* 120, no. 5 (April 2013): 548–53.

35. E. H. Blackburn, E. S. Epel, "Telomeres and adversity: too toxic to ignore," *Nature* 490, no. 7419 (October 2012): 169–71.

36. K. Rogers, "Epigenetics: a turning point in our understanding of heredity," *Scientific American*, January 16, 2012, www.blogs.scientificamerican.com/guest-blog/epigenetics-a-turning-point-in-our-understanding-of-heredity/#.

37. American Cancer Society, "DES exposure: questions and answers," June 10, 2015, www.cancer.org/cancer/cancer-causes/medical-treatments/des-exposure.html.

38. L. Titus-Ernstoff, R. Troisi, E. E. Hatch, et al., "Offspring of women exposed in utero to diethylstilbestrol (DES): a preliminary report of benign and malignant pathology in the third generation," *Epidemiology* 19, no. 2 (March 2008): 251–57.

39. M. K. Skinner, M. Manikkam, C. Guerrero-Bosagna, "Epigenetic transgenerational actions of environmental factors in disease etiology," *Trends in Endocrinology and Metabolism* 21, no. 4 (April 2010): 214–22.

40. F. Perera, J. Herbstman, "Prenatal environmental exposures, epigenetics, and disease," *Reproductive Toxicology* 31, no. 3 (January 2011): 363–73.

41. J. M. Gray, S. Rasanayagam, C. Engel, J. Rizzo, "State of the evidence 2017: an update on the connection between breast cancer and the environment," *Environmental Health* 16, no. 1 (September 2017): 94.

42. Z. M. Zhao, B. Zhao, Y. Bai, et al., "Early and multiple origins of metastatic lineages within primary tumors," *Proceedings of the National Academy of Sciences of the United States of America* 113, no. 8 (February 2016): 2140–45.

43. Z. Kashef, "Yale study examines evolution of cancer," YaleNews, February 8, 2016, www.news.yale.edu/2016/02/08/yale-study-examines-evolution-cancer.

Chapter Six: Synergy and the Mix of Six

1. S. W. Cole, A. S. Nagaraja, S. K. Lutgendorf, P. A. Green, A. K. Sood, "Sympathetic nervous system regulation of the tumour microenvironment," *Nature Reviews: Cancer* 15, no. 9 (September 2015): 563–72.

2. S. K. Lutgendorf, B. L. Andersen, "Biobehavioral approaches to cancer progression and survival: mechanisms and interventions," *American Psychologist* 70, no. 2 (March 2015): 186–97.

3. C. P. Fagundes, K. W. Murdock, D. A. Chirinos, P. A. Green, "Biobehavioral pathways to cancer incidence, progression, and quality of life," *Current Directions in Psychological Science* (November 2017).

4. R. J. Davidson, B. S. McEwen, "Social influences on neuroplasticity: stress and interventions to promote well-being," *Nature Neuroscience* 15, no. 5 (April 2012): 689–95.

5. S. Sephton, D. Spiegel, "Circadian disruption in cancer: a neuroendocrine-immune pathway from stress to disease?," *Brain, Behavior, and Immunity* 17, no. 5 (October 2003): 321–28.

6. M. R. Irwin, "Why sleep is important for health: a psychoneuroimmunology perspective," *Annual Review of Psychology* 66, no. 1 (January 2015): 143–72.

7. M. R. Irwin, R. Olmstead, J. E. Carroll, "Sleep disturbance, sleep duration, and inflammation: a systematic review and meta-analysis of cohort studies and experimental sleep deprivation," *Biological Psychiatry* 80, no. 1 (July 2016): 40–52.

8. I. M. Lee, E. J. Shiroma, F. Lobelo, et al., "Effect of physical inactivity on major non-communicable diseases worldwide: an analysis of burden of disease and life expectancy," *The Lancet* 380, no. 9838 (July 2012): 219–29.

9. L. Cohen, A. Jefferies, "Comprehensive lifestyle change: harnessing synergy to improve cancer outcomes," *Journal of the National Cancer Institute Monographs*, no. 52 (November 2017).

10. D. Romaguera, E. Gracia-Lavedan, A. Molinuevo, et al., "Adherence to nutrition-based cancer prevention guidelines and breast, prostate and colorectal cancer risk in the MCC-Spain case-control study," *International Journal of Cancer* 141, no. 1 (July 2017): 83–93.

11. F. Bravi, J. Polesel, W. Garavello, et al., "Adherence to the World Cancer Research Fund/American Institute for Cancer research recommendations and head and neck cancers risk," *Oral Oncology* 6 (January 2017): 59–64.

12. A. C. Vergnaud, D. Romaguera, P. H. Peeters, et al., "Adherence to the World Cancer Research Fund/American Institute for Cancer Research guidelines and risk of death in Europe: results from the European Prospective Investigation into nutrition and cancer cohort study," *American Journal of Clinical Nutrition* 97, no. 5 (May 2013): 1107–20.

13. B. L. Andersen, W. B. Farrar, D. M. Golden-Kreutz, et al., "Psychological, behavioral, and immune changes after a psychological intervention: a clinical trial," *Journal of Clinical Oncology* 22, no. 17 (September 2004): 3570–80.

14. B. L. Andersen, H. C. Yang, W. B. Farrar, et al., "Psychologic intervention improves survival for breast cancer patients: a randomized clinical trial," *Cancer* 113, no. 12 (December 2008): 3450–58.

15. B. L. Andersen, L. M. Thornton, C. L. Shapiro, et al., "Biobehavioral, immune, and health benefits following recurrence for psychological intervention participants," *Clinical Cancer Research* 16, no. 12 (June 2010): 3270–78.

16. B. L. Andersen, W. B. Farrar, D. Golden-Kreutz, et al., "Distress reduction from a psychological intervention contributes to improved health for cancer patients," *Brain, Behavior, and Immunity* 21, no. 7 (October 2007): 953–61.

17. B. L. Andersen, R. A. Shelby, D. M. Golden-Kreutz, "RCT of a psychological intervention for patients with cancer: I. Mechanisms of change," *Journal of Consulting and Clinical Psychology* 75, no. 6 (December 2007): 927–38.

18. D. Ornish, G. Weidner, W. R. Fair, et al., "Intensive lifestyle changes may affect the progression of prostate cancer," *Journal of Urology* 174, no. 3 (September 2005): 1065–69; discussion 1069–70.

19. D. Ornish, J. Lin, J. M. Chan, et al., "Effect of comprehensive lifestyle changes on telomerase activity and telomere length in men with biopsy-proven low-risk prostate cancer: 5-year follow-up of a descriptive pilot study," *The Lancet Oncology* 14, no. 11 (October 2013): 1112–20.

20. D. Ornish, M. J. Magbanua, G. Weidner, et al., "Changes in prostate gene expression in men undergoing an intensive nutrition and lifestyle intervention," *Proceedings of the National Academy of Sciences of the United States of America* 105, no. 24 (June 2008): 8369–74.

21. D. Lemanne, K. I. Block, B. R. Kressel, V. P. Sukhatme, J. D. White, "A case of complete and durable molecular remission of chronic lymphocytic leukemia following treatment with epigallocatechin-3-gallate, an extract of green tea," *Cureus* 7, no. 12 (December 2015): e441.

22. G. Sabin, D. Lemanne. *n of 1: One Man's Harvard-Documented Remission of Incurable Cancer Using Only Natural methods* (Silver Spring, MD: FON Press, 2016).

PART TWO: THE MIX OF SIX

Chapter Seven: The Foundation Is Love and Social Support

1. N. D. Anderson, T. Damianakis, E. Kroger, et al., "The benefits associated with volunteering among seniors: a critical review and recommendations for future research," *Psychological Bulletin* 140, no. 6 (November 2014): 1505–33.

2. M. A. Okun, E. W. Yeung, S. Brown, "Volunteering by older adults and risk of mortality: a meta-analysis," *Psychology and Aging* 28, no. 2 (June 2013): 564–77.

3. C. E. Jenkinson, A. P. Dickens, K. Jones, et al., "Is volunteering a public health intervention? A systematic review and meta-analysis of the health and survival of volunteers," *BMC Public Health* 13, no. 1 (August 2013): 773.

4. L. Ayalon, "Volunteering as a predictor of all-cause mortality: what aspects of volunteering really matter?," *International Psychogeriatrics* 20, no. 5 (October 2008): 1000–1013.

5. B. E. Kok, K. A. Coffey, M. A. Cohn, et al., "How positive emotions build physical health: perceived positive social connections account for the upward spiral between positive emotions and vagal tone," *Psychological Science* 24, no. 7 (July 2013): 1123–32.

6. J. Dyavanapalli, O. Dergacheva, X. Wang, D. Mendelowitz, "Parasympathetic vagal control of cardiac function," *Current Hypertension Reports* 18, no. 3 (March 2016): 22.

7. S. W. Porges, J. A. Doussard-Roosevelt, A. K. Maiti, "Vagal tone and the physiological regulation of emotion," *Monographs of the Society for Research in Child Development* 59, no. 2–3 (February 1994): 167–86.

8. L. S. Smith, P. A. Dmochowski, D. W. Muir, B. S. Kisilevsky, "Estimated cardiac vagal tone predicts fetal responses to mother's and stranger's voices," *Developmental Psychobiology* 49, no. 5 (July 2007): 543–47.

9. J. F. Thayer, S. S. Yamamoto, J. F. Brosschot, "The relationship of autonomic imbalance, heart rate variability and cardiovascular disease risk factors," *International Journal of Cardiology* 141, no. 2 (May 2010): 122–31.

10. J. M. Dekker, E. G. Schouten, P. Klootwijk, et al., "Heart rate variability from short electrocardiographic recordings predicts mortality from all causes in middle-aged and elderly men: the Zutphen study," *American Journal of Epidemiology* 145, no. 10 (May 1997): 899–908.

11. X. Zhou, Z. Ma, L. Zhang, et al., "Heart rate variability in the prediction of survival in patients with cancer: a systematic review and meta-analysis," *Journal of Psychosomatic Research* 89 (October 2016): 20–25.

12. A. Kogan, C. Oveis, E. W. Carr, et al., "Vagal activity is quadratically related to prosocial traits, prosocial emotions, and observer perceptions of prosociality," *Journal of Personality and Social Psychology* 107, no. 6 (December 2014): 1051–63.

13. B. H. Gottlieb, E. D. Wachala, "Cancer support groups: a critical review of empirical studies," *Psycho-Oncology* 16, no. 5 (May 2007): 379–400.

14. L. M. Hoey, S. C. Ieropoli, V. M. White, M. Jefford, "Systematic review of peer-support programs for people with cancer," *Patient Education and Counseling* 70, no. 3 (March 2008): 315–37.

15. B. Nausheen, Y. Gidron, R. Peveler, R. Moss-Morris, "Social support and cancer progression: a systematic review," *Journal of Psychosomatic Research* 67, no. 5 (November 2009): 403–15.

16. B. N. Uchino, "Social support and health: a review of physiological processes potentially underlying links to disease outcomes," *Journal of Behavioral Medicine* 29, no. 4 (August 2006): 377–87.

17. C. L. Decker, "Social support and adolescent cancer survivors: a review of the literature," *Psycho-Oncology* 16, no. 1 (January 2007): 1–11.

18. S. Hughes, L. M. Jaremka, C. M. Alfano, et al., "Social support predicts inflammation, pain, and depressive symptoms: longitudinal relationships among breast cancer survivors," *Psychoneuroendocrinology* 42 (April 2014): 38–44.

19. M. Karin, F. R. Greten, "NF-kappaB: linking inflammation and immunity to cancer development and progression," *Nature Reviews: Immunology* 5, no. 10 (October 2005): 749–59.

20. D. Ribatti, "Inflammation and Cancer," in *Inflammation and Angiogenesis* (Cham, Switzerland: Springer International Publishing, 2017), 17–24.

21. C. H. Kroenke, Y. L. Michael, E. M. Poole, et al., "Postdiagnosis social networks and breast cancer mortality in the after breast cancer pooling project," *Cancer* 123, no. 7 (April 2017): 1228–37.

22. E. L. Garcia, J. R. Banegas, A. G. Perez-Regadera, R. H. Cabrera, F. Rodriguez-Artalejo, "Social network and health-related quality of life in older adults: a population-based study in spain," *Quality of Life Research* 14, no. 2 (March 2005): 511–20.

23. M. Gonzalez-Saenz de Tejada, A. Bilbao, M. Bare, et al., "Association between social support, functional status, and change in health-related quality of life and changes in anxiety and depression in colorectal cancer patients," *Psycho-Oncology* 26, no. 9 (September 2017): 1263–69

24. C. Stout, J. Marrow, E. N. Brandt Jr., S. Wolf, "Unusually low incidence of death from myocardial infarction. Study of an Italian American community in Pennsylvania," *Journal of the American Medical Association* 188 (June 1964): 845–49.

25. B. Egolf, J. Lasker, S. Wolf, L. Potvin, "The Roseto effect: a 50-year comparison of mortality rates," *American Journal of Public Health* 82, no. 8 (August 1992): 1089–92.

26. D. Buettner, *The Blue Zones: 9 Lessons for Living Longer from the People Who've Lived the Longest* (Washington, D.C.: National Geographic, 2012).

27. M. Suzuki, D. C. Willcox, B. Willcox, "Okinawa centenarian study: investigating healthy aging among the world's longest-lived people," in *Encyclopedia of Geropsychology*, ed. Nancy A. Pachana (Singapore: Springer Singapore, 2017), 1–5.

28. K. L. Weihs, S. J. Simmens, J. Mizrahi, et al., "Dependable social relationships predict overall survival in stages II and III breast carcinoma patients," *Journal of Psychosomatic Research* 59, no. 5 (November 2005): 299–306.

29. J. G. Trudel, N. Leduc, S. Dumont, "Perceived communication between physicians and breast cancer patients as a predicting factor of patients' health-related quality of life: a longitudinal analysis," *Psycho-Oncology* 23, no. 5 (May 2014): 531–38.

30. S. Swartzman, J. N. Booth, A. Munro, F. Sani, "Posttraumatic stress disorder after cancer diagnosis in adults: a meta-analysis," *Depression and Anxiety* 34, no. 4 (April 2017): 327–39.

31. D. J. Goldsmith, G. A. Miller, "Conceptualizing how couples talk about cancer," *Health Communication* 29, no. 1 (February 2014): 51–63.

32. Y. C. Yang, M. K. McClintock, M. Kozloski, T. Li, "Social isolation and adult mortality: the role of chronic inflammation and sex differences," *Journal of Health and Social Behavior* 54, no. 2 (June 2013): 183–203.

33. S. L. Gomez, S. Shariff-Marco, M. DeRouen, et al., "The impact of neighborhood social and built environment factors across the cancer continuum: current research, methodological considerations, and future directions," *Cancer* 121, no. 14 (July 2015): 2314–30.

34. A. A. Aizer, M. H. Chen, E. P. McCarthy, et al., "Marital status and survival in patients with cancer," *Journal of Clinical Oncology* 31, no. 31 (November 2013): 3869–76.

35. J. Holt-Lunstad, T. B. Smith, M. Baker, T. Harris, D. Stephenson, "Loneliness and social isolation as risk factors for mortality: a meta-analytic review," *Perspectives on Psychological Science* 10, no. 2 (March 2015): 227–37.

36. A. Strachman, S. L. Gable, "What you want (and do not want) affects what you see (and do not see): avoidance social goals and social events," *Personality & Social Psychology Bulletin* 32, no. 11 (November 2006): 1446–58.

37. J. D. Creswell, M. R. Irwin, L. J. Burklund, et al., "Mindfulness-based stress reduction training reduces loneliness and pro-inflammatory gene expression in older adults: a small randomized controlled trial," *Brain, Behavior, and Immunity* 26, no. 7 (October 2012): 1095–1101.

38. L. F. You, J. R. Yeh, M. C. Su, "Expression profiles of loneliness-associated genes for survival prediction in cancer patients," *Asian Pacific Journal of Cancer Prevention* 15, no. 1 (February 2014): 185–190.

39. S. W. Cole, "Social regulation of human gene expression: Mechanisms and implications for public health," *American Journal of Public Health* 103 Supplement 1 (October 2013): S84–92.

40. S. W. Cole, L. C. Hawkley, J. M. Arevalo, et al., "Social regulation of gene expression in human leukocytes," *Genome Biology* 8, no. 9 (September 2007): R189.

41. D. R. Jutagir, B. B. Blomberg, C. S. Carver, et al., "Social well-being is associated with less pro-inflammatory and pro-metastatic leukocyte gene expression in women after surgery for breast cancer," *Breast Cancer Research and Treatment* 165, no. 1 (August 2017): 169–80.

42. J. M. Knight, J. D. Rizzo, B. R. Logan, et al., "Low socioeconomic status, adverse gene expression profiles, and clinical outcomes in hematopoietic stem cell transplant recipients," *Clinical Cancer Research* 22, no. 1 (January 2016): 69–78.

43. M. G. Cuneo, A. Schrepf, G. M. Slavich, et al., "Diurnal cortisol rhythms, fatigue and psychosocial factors in five-year survivors of ovarian cancer," *Psychoneuroendocrinology* 84 (October 2017): 139–42.

44. S. K. Lutgendorf, K. DeGeest, L. Dahmoush, et al., "Social isolation is associated with elevated tumor norepinephrine in ovarian carcinoma patients," *Brain, Behavior, and Immunity* 25, no. 2 (February 2011): 250–55.

45. S. K. Lutgendorf, A. K. Sood, B. Anderson, et al., "Social support, psychological distress, and natural killer cell activity in ovarian cancer," *Journal of Clinical Oncology* 23, no. 28 (October 2005): 7105–13.

46. E. S. Costanzo, S. K. Lutgendorf, A. K. Sood, et al., "Psychosocial factors and interleukin-6 among women with advanced ovarian cancer," *Cancer* 104, no. 2 (July 2005): 305–13.

47. S. K. Lutgendorf, K. De Geest, D. Bender, et al., "Social influences on clinical outcomes of patients with ovarian cancer," *Journal of Clinical Oncology* 30, no. 23 (August 2012): 2885–90.

48. K. A. Muscatell, N. I. Eisenberger, J. M. Dutcher, S. W. Cole, J. E. Bower, "Links between inflammation, amygdala reactivity, and social support in breast cancer survivors," *Brain, Behavior, and Immunity* 53 (March 2016): 34–38.

49. K. S. Madden, M. J. Szpunar, E. B. Brown, "Early impact of social isolation and breast tumor progression in mice," *Brain, Behavior, and Immunity* 30 Supplement (March 2013): S135–41.

50. B. Nausheen, N. J. Carr, R. C. Peveler, et al., "Relationship between loneliness and proangiogenic cytokines in newly diagnosed tumors of colon and rectum," *Psychosomatic Medicine* 72, no. 9 (November 2010): 912–16.

51. S. K. Lutgendorf, E. L. Johnsen, B. Cooper, et al., "Vascular endothelial growth factor and social support in patients with ovarian carcinoma," *Cancer* 95 (August 2002): 808–15.

52. C. P. Fagundes, L. M. Jaremka, R. Glaser, et al., "Attachment anxiety is related to Epstein-Barr virus latency," *Brain, Behavior, and Immunity* 41 (October 2014): 232–38.

53. M. Lekander, C. J. Furst, S. Rotstein, H. Blomgren, M. Fredrikson, "Social support and immune status during and after chemotherapy for breast cancer," *Acta Oncologica* 35, no. 1 (July 1996): 31–37.

54. L. M. Tomfohr, K. M. Edwards, J. W. Madsen, P. J. Mills, "Social support moderates the relationship between sleep and inflammation in a population at high risk for developing cardiovascular disease," *Psychophysiology* 52, no. 12 (December 2015): 1689–97.

55. Y. C. Yang, T. Li, S. M. Frenk, "Social network ties and inflammation in U.S. adults with cancer," *Biodemography and Social Biology* 60, no. 1 (May 2014): 21–37.

56. P. T. Marucha, T. R. Crespin, R. A. Shelby, B. L. Andersen, "TNF-alpha levels in cancer patients relate to social variables," *Brain, Behavior, and Immunity* 19, no. 6 (November 2005): 521–25.

57. A. Hinzey, M. M. Gaudier-Diaz, M. B. Lustberg, A. C. DeVries, "Breast cancer and social environment: getting by with a little help from our friends," *Breast Cancer Research* 18, no. 1 (May 2016): 54.

58. S. K. Lutgendorf, K. DeGeest, L. Dahmoush, et al., "Social isolation is associated with elevated tumor norepinephrine in ovarian carcinoma patients," *Brain, Behavior, and Immunity* 25, no. 2 (February 2011): 250–55.

59. S. W. Cole, M. E. Levine, J. M. Arevalo, et al., "Loneliness, eudaimonia, and the human conserved transcriptional response to adversity," *Psychoneuroendocrinology* 62 (December 2015): 11–17.

60. G. M. Slavich, S. W. Cole, "The emerging field of human social genomics," *Clinical Psychological Science* 1, no. 3 (July 2013): 331–48.

61. J. T. Cacioppo, S. Cacioppo, J. P. Capitanio, S. W. Cole, "The neuroendocrinology of social isolation," *Annual Review of Psychology* 66 (January 2015): 733–67.

62. S. W. Cole, "Social regulation of human gene expression: mechanisms and implications for public health," *American Journal of Public Health* 103, Supplement 1 (October 2013): S84–92.

63. S. K. Lutgendorf, K. DeGeest, C. Y. Sung, et al., "Depression, social support, and beta-adrenergic transcription control in human ovarian cancer," *Brain, Behavior, and Immunity* 23, no. 2 (February 2009): 176–83.

64. S. K. Lutgendorf, P. H. Thaker, J. M. Arevalo, et al., "Biobehavioral modulation of the exosome transcriptome in ovarian carcinoma," *Cancer* (November 2017).

65. D. R. Jutagir, B. B. Blomberg, C. S. Carver, et al., "Social well-being is associated with less pro-inflammatory and pro-metastatic leukocyte gene expression in women after surgery for breast cancer," *Breast Cancer Research and Treatment* 165, no. 1 (August 2017): 169–80.

66. J. M. Knight, J. D. Rizzo, B. R. Logan, et al., "Low socioeconomic status, adverse gene expression profiles, and clinical outcomes in hematopoietic stem cell transplant recipients," *Clinical Cancer Research* 22, no. 1 (January 2016): 69–78.

67. S. W. Cole, L. C. Hawkley, J. M. Arevalo, et al., "Social regulation of gene expression in human leukocytes," *Genome Biology* 8, no. 9 (September 2007): R189.

68. I. Barrera, D. Spiegel, "Review of psychotherapeutic interventions on depression in cancer patients and their impact on disease progression," *International Review of Psychiatry* 26, no. 1 (February 2014): 31–43.

69. D. Spiegel, "Minding the body: psychotherapy and cancer survival," *British Journal of Health Psychology* 19, no. 3 (September 2014): 465–85.

70. J. Giese-Davis, Y. Brandelli, C. Kronenwetter, et al., "Illustrating the multi-faceted dimensions of group therapy and support for cancer patients," *Healthcare (Basel)* 4, no. 3 (August 2016).

71. A. J. Cunningham, C. V. Edmonds, G. P. Jenkins, et al., "A randomized controlled trial of the effects of group psychological therapy on survival in women with metastatic breast cancer," *Psycho-Oncology* 7, no. 6 (December 1998): 508–17.

72. J. Giese-Davis, K. Collie, K. M. Rancourt, et al., "Decrease in depression symptoms is associated with longer survival in patients with metastatic breast cancer: a secondary analysis," *Journal of Clinical Oncology* 29, no. 4 (February 2011): 413–20.

73. D. Spiegel, G. R. Morrow, C. Classen, et al., "Group psychotherapy for recently diagnosed breast cancer patients: a multicenter feasibility study," *Psycho-Oncology* 8, no. 6 (December 1999): 482–93.

74. D. Spiegel, J. R. Bloom, H. C. Kraemer, E. Gottheil, "Effect of psychosocial treatment on survival of patients with metastatic breast cancer," *The Lancet* (October 1989): 888–91.

75. F. I. Fawzy, A. L. Canada, N. W. Fawzy, "Malignant melanoma: effects of a brief, structured psychiatric intervention on survival and recurrence at 10-year follow-up," *Archives of General Psychiatry* 60, no. 1 (January 2003): 100–103.

76. A. J. Cunningham, "Group psychological therapy: an integral part of care for cancer patients," *Integrative Cancer Therapies* 1, no. 1 (March 2002): 67–75; discussion 75.

77. D. Spiegel, "The Connection: Mind Your Body," 2014, www.theconnection.tv/dr-david-spiegel-ph-d.

78. *Commonweal*, "Commonweal," 2017, www.commonweal.org.

79. Caringbridge, "About us," www.caringbridge.org/about-us.

80. R. J. Leider, *Power of Purpose: Find Meaning, Live Longer, Better* (Oakland, CA: Berrett-Koehler Publishers, 2015).

81. B. L. Fredrickson, K. M. Grewen, K. A. Coffey, et al., "A functional genomic perspective on human well-being," *Proceedings of the National Academy of Sciences of the United States of America* 110, no. 33 (August 2013): 13684–89.

82. S. Cohen, "Social relationships and health," *American Psychologist* 59, no. 8 (November 2004): 676–84.

83. Harvard Medical School, "Harvard study of adult development," 2015, www.adultdevelopmentstudy.org.

84. R. J. Waldinger, M. S. Schulz, "What's love got to do with it?: social functioning, perceived health, and daily happiness in married octogenarians," *Psychology and Aging* 25, no. 2 (June 2010): 422–31.

85. L. Mineo, "Good genes are nice, but joy is better: Harvard study, almost 80 years old, has proved that embracing community helps us live longer, and be happier," *Harvard Gazette*, April 11, 2017, www.news.harvard.edu/gazette/story/2017/04/over-nearly-80-years-harvard-study-has-been-showing-how-to-live-a-healthy-and-happy-life.

86. R. J. Waldinger, S. Cohen, M. S. Schulz, J. A. Crowell, "Security of attachment to spouses in late life: concurrent and prospective links with cognitive and emotional wellbeing," *Clinical Psychological Science* 3, no. 4 (June 2015): 516–29.

87. D. G. Cruess, M. H. Antoni, B. A. McGregor, et al., "Cognitive-behavioral stress management reduces serum cortisol by enhancing benefit finding among women being treated for early stage breast cancer," *Psychosomatic Medicine* 62, no. 3 (June 2000): 304–08.

88. P. Cabral, H. B. Meyer, D. Ames, "Effectiveness of yoga therapy as a complementary treatment for major psychiatric disorders: a meta-analysis," *Primary Care Companion for CNS Disorders* 13, no. 4 (July 2011).

89. K. D. Chandwani, G. Perkins, H. R. Nagendra, et al., "Randomized, controlled trial of yoga in women with breast cancer undergoing radiotherapy," *Journal of Clinical Oncology* 32, no. 10 (April 2014): 1058–65.

90. C. G. Ratcliff, K. Milbury, K. D. Chandwani, et al., "Examining mediators and moderators of yoga for women with breast cancer undergoing radiotherapy," *Integrative Cancer Therapies* 15, no. 3 (September 2016): 250–62.

91. B. A. McGregor, M. H. Antoni, A. Boyers, et al., "Cognitive-behavioral stress management increases benefit finding and immune function among women with early-stage breast cancer," *Journal of Psychosomatic Research* 56, no. 1 (January 2004): 1–8.
92. V. Frankl, *Man's Search for Meaning: An Introduction to Logotherapy* (Boston: Beacon Press, 2006).
93. R. M. Ryan, E. L. Deci, "On happiness and human potentials: A review of research on hedonic and eudaimonic well-being," *Annual Review of Psychology* 52 (February 2001): 141–66.
94. L. Z. Davis, G. M. Slavich, P. H. Thaker, et al., "Eudaimonic well-being and tumor norepinephrine in patients with epithelial ovarian cancer," *Cancer* 121, no. 19 (October 2015): 3543–50.
95. S. K. Nelson-Coffey, M. M. Fritz, S. Lyubomirsky, S. W. Cole, "Kindness in the blood: a randomized controlled trial of the gene regulatory impact of prosocial behavior," *Psychoneuroendocrinology* 81 (July 2017): 8–13.
96. S. B. Fleishman, P. Homel, M. R. Chen, et al., "Beneficial effects of animal-assisted visits on quality of life during multimodal radiation-chemotherapy regimens," *Journal of Community and Supportive Oncology* 13, no. 1 (January 2015): 22–26.
97. M. Wheeler, "Be happy: your genes may thank you for it," July 29, 2013, www.newsroom.ucla.edu/releases/don-t-worry-be-happy-247644.
98. Church Health, "About Church Health," 2017, www.churchhealth.org/about-church-health.
99. Anticancer Lifestyle Foundation, "Anticancer Lifestyle Program," 2017, www.anticancerlifestyle.org.

The Anticancer Living Guide to Love and Social Support

1. Stagen Leadership Academy: www.stagen.com/academy/overview.
2. C. E. Jenkinson, A. P. Dickens, K. Jones, et al., "Is volunteering a public health intervention? A systematic review and meta-analysis of the health and survival of volunteers," *BMC Public Health* 13, no. 1 (August 2013): 773.

Chapter Eight: Stress and Resilience

1. S. K. Lutgendorf, B. L. Andersen, "Biobehavioral approaches to cancer progression and survival: mechanisms and interventions," *American Psychologist* 70, no. 2 (March 2015): 186–97.
2. R. Glaser, J. K. Kiecolt-Glaser, "Stress-induced immune dysfunction: implications for health," *Nature Reviews Immunology* 5, no. 3 (March 2005): 243–51.
3. S. W. Cole, A. S. Nagaraja, S. K. Lutgendorf, P. A. Green, A. K. Sood, "Sympathetic nervous system regulation of the tumour microenvironment," *Nature Reviews: Cancer* 15, no. 9 (September 2015): 563–72.
4. J. W. Eng, K. M. Kokolus, C. B. Reed, et al., "A nervous tumor microenvironment: the impact of adrenergic stress on cancer cells, immunosuppression, and immunotherapeutic response," *Cancer, Immunology, and Immunotherapy* 63, no. 11 (November 2014): 1115–28.
5. M. R. Hara, J. J. Kovacs, E. J. Whalen, et al., "A stress response pathway regulates DNA damage through beta2-adrenoreceptors and beta-arrestin-1," *Nature* 477, no. 7364 (August 2011): 349–53.
6. H. Lavretsky, P. Siddarth, N. Nazarian, et al., "A pilot study of yogic meditation for family dementia caregivers with depressive symptoms: effects on mental health, cognition, and telomerase activity," *International Journal of Geriatric Psychiatry* 28, no. 1 (March 2013): 57–65.

7. K. D. Chandwani, G. Perkins, H. R. Nagendra, et al., "Randomized, controlled trial of yoga in women with breast cancer undergoing radiotherapy," *Journal of Clinical Oncology* 32, no. 10 (April 2014): 1058–65.

8. M. J. Cordova, M. B. Riba, D. Spiegel, "Post-traumatic stress disorder and cancer," *The Lancet Psychiatry* 4, no. 4 (April 2017): 330–38.

9. American Psychiatric Association, *Diagnostic and Statistical Manual of Mental Disorders (DSM-5°)* (Washington, D.C.: American Psychiatric Publishing, 2013).

10. K. D. Stein, K. L. Syrjala, M. A. Andrykowski, "Physical and psychological long-term and late effects of cancer," *Cancer* 112, no. 11 Supplement (June 2008): 2577–92.

11. PDQ Supportive and Palliative Care Editorial Board, "Cancer-Related Post-traumatic Stress (PDQ°): Health Professional Version, in PDQ Cancer Information Summaries," National Cancer Institute (US), January 7, 2015, www.ncbi.nlm.nih.gov/books/NBK65728.

12. A. M. H. Krebber, L. M. Buffart, G. Kleijn, et al., "Prevalence of depression in cancer patients: a meta-analysis of diagnostic interviews and self-report instruments," *Psycho-Oncology* 23, no. 2 (February 2014): 121–30.

13. J. Walker, C. Holm Hansen, P. Martin, et al., "Prevalence of depression in adults with cancer: a systematic review," *Annals of Oncology* 24, no. 4 (April 2013): 895–900.

14. R. Caruso, M. G. Nanni, M. Riba, et al., "Depressive spectrum disorders in cancer: prevalence, risk factors and screening for depression: a critical review," *Acta Oncologica* 56, no. 2 (February 2017): 146–55.

15. A. J. Mitchell, M. Chan, H. Bhatti, et al., "Prevalence of depression, anxiety, and adjustment disorder in oncological, haematological, and palliative-care settings: a meta-analysis of 94 interview-based studies," *The Lancet Oncology* 12, no. 2 (February 2011): 160–74.

16. M. McCartney, "The fight is on: military metaphors for cancer may harm patients," *British Medical Journal* 349 (August 2014).

17. N. M. Wiggins, "Stop using military metaphors for disease," *British Medical Journal* 345 (July 2012).

18. M. A. Lerner, *Choices in Healing: Integrating the Best of Conventional and Complementary Approaches* (Cambridge, MA: MIT Press, 1994).

19. E. Blackburn, E. Epel, *The Telomere Effect: A Revolutionary Approach to Living Younger, Healthier, Longer* (London: Grand Central Publishing, 2017).

20. D. Servan-Schreiber, *Not the Last Goodbye: Reflections on Life, Death, Healing and Cancer* (London: Pan Macmillan, 2012).

21. H. Benson, J. W. Lehmann, M. S. Malhotra, et al., "Body temperature changes during the practice of g-Tum-mo yoga," *Nature* 295, no. 5846 (January 1982): 234–36.

22. A. Lutz, H. A. Slagter, J. D. Dunne, R. J. Davidson, "Attention regulation and monitoring in meditation," *Trends in Cognitive Sciences* 12, no. 4 (March 2008): 163–69.

23. A. Lutz, L. L. Greischar, N. B. Rawlings, M. Ricard, R. J. Davidson, "Long-term meditators self-induce high-amplitude gamma synchrony during mental practice," *Proceedings of the National Academy of Sciences of the United States of America* 101, no. 46 (November 2004): 16369–73.

24. A. Lutz, J. Brefczynski-Lewis, T. Johnstone, R. J. Davidson, "Regulation of the neural circuitry of emotion by compassion meditation: effects of meditative expertise," *PloS One* 3, no. 3 (March 2008): e1897.

25. J. Kabat-Zinn, *Full Catastrophe Living: Using the Wisdom of Your Body and Mind to Face Stress, Pain, and Illness* (New York: Delta, 2005).

26. R. J. Davidson, J. Kabat-Zinn, J. Schumacher, et al., "Alterations in brain and immune function produced by mindfulness meditation," *Psychosomatic Medicine* 65, no. 4 (August 2003): 564–70.

27. B. K. Hölzel, E. A. Hoge, D. N. Greve, et al., "Neural mechanisms of symptom improvements in generalized anxiety disorder following mindfulness training," *NeuroImage: Clinical* 2 (March 2013): 448–58.

28. M. A. Rosenkranz, R. J. Davidson, D. G. Maccoon, et al., "A comparison of mindfulness-based stress reduction and an active control in modulation of neurogenic inflammation," *Brain, Behavior, and Immunity* 27, no. 1 (January 2013): 174–84.

29. K. Luu, P. A. Hall, "Hatha yoga and executive function: a systematic review," *Journal of Alternative and Complementary Medicine* 22, no. 2 (February 2015): 125–33.

30. M. K. Leung, W. K. W. Lau, C. C. H. Chan, et al., "Meditation-induced neuroplastic changes in amygdala activity during negative affective processing," *Social Neuroscience* (April 2017): 1–12.

31. I. Buric, M. Farias, J. Jong, C. Mee, I. A. Brazil, "What is the molecular signature of mind-body interventions? A systematic review of gene expression changes induced by meditation and related practices," *Frontiers in Immunology* 8 (June 2017): 670.

32. J. D. Creswell, M. R. Irwin, L. J. Burklund, et al., "Mindfulness-based stress reduction training reduces loneliness and pro-inflammatory gene expression in older adults: a small randomized controlled trial," *Brain, Behavior, and Immunity* 26, no. 7 (October 2012): 1095–1101.

33. J. F. Carlson, T. L. Beattie, J. Giese-Davis, et al., "Mindfulness-based cancer recovery and supportive-expressive therapy maintain telomere length relative to controls in distressed breast cancer survivors," *Cancer* 121, no. 3 (February 2015): 476–84.

34. F. Zeidan, A. L. Adler-Neal, R. E. Wells, et al., "Mindfulness-meditation-based pain relief is not mediated by endogenous opioids," *Journal of Neuroscience* 36, no. 11 (March 2016): 3391–97.

35. D. C. Johnson, N. J. Thom, E. A. Stanley, et al., "Modifying resilience mechanisms in at-risk individuals: a controlled study of mindfulness training in marines preparing for deployment," *American Journal of Psychiatry* 171, no. 8 (August 2014): 844–53.

36. B. Rees, F. Travis, D. Shapiro, R. Chant, "Reduction in posttraumatic stress symptoms in Congolese refugees practicing transcendental meditation," *Journal of Traumatic Stress* 26, no. 2 (April 2013): 295–98.

37. J. S. Brooks, T. Scarano, "Transcendental meditation in the treatment of post-Vietnam adjustment," *Journal of Counseling & Development* 64, no. 3 (November 1985): 212–15.

38. B. Arun, T. Austin, G. V. Babiera, et al., "A comprehensive lifestyle randomized clinical trial: design and initial patient experience," *Integrative Cancer Therapies* 16, no. 1 (March 2017): 3–20.

39. M. Moreno-Smith, S. K. Lutgendorf, A. K. Sood, "Impact of stress on cancer metastasis," *Future Oncology* 6, no. 12 (December 2010): 1863–81.

40. A. K. Sood, S. K. Lutgendorf, "Stress influences on anoikis," *Cancer Prevention Research* 4, no. 4 (April 2011): 481–85.

41. G. N. Armaiz-Pena, S. W. Cole, S. K. Lutgendorf, A. K. Sood, "Neuroendocrine influences on cancer progression," *Brain, Behavior, and Immunity* 30 Supplement (March 2013): S19–25.

42. P. H. Thaker, L. Y. Han, A. A. Kamat, et al., "Chronic stress promotes tumor growth and angiogenesis in a mouse model of ovarian carcinoma," *Nature Medicine* 12, no. 8 (August 2006): 939–44.

43. S. J. Creed, C. P. Le, M. Hassan, et al., "Beta2-adrenoceptor signaling regulates invadopodia formation to enhance tumor cell invasion," *Breast Cancer Research* 17, no. 1 (November 2015): 145.

44. S. W. Cole, A. K. Sood, "Molecular pathways: beta-adrenergic signaling in cancer," *Clinical Cancer Research* 18, no. 5 (March 2012): 1201–6.

45. A. K. Sood, G. N. Armaiz-Pena, J. Halder, et al., "Adrenergic modulation of focal adhesion kinase protects human ovarian cancer cells from anoikis," *Journal of Clinical Investigation* 120, no. 5 (May 2010): 1515–23.

46. K. Sanada, M. Alda Diez, M. Salas Valero, et al., "Effects of mindfulness-based interventions on biomarkers in healthy and cancer populations: a systematic review," *BMC Complementary and Alternative Medicine* 17, no. 1 (February 2017): 125.

47. K. A. Biegler, A. K. Anderson, L. B. Wenzel, K. Osann, E. L. Nelson, "Longitudinal change in telomere length and the chronic stress response in a randomized pilot biobehavioral clinical study: implications for cancer prevention," *Cancer Prevention Research* 5, no. 10 (October 2012): 1173–82.

48. S. K. Lutgendorf, P. H. Thaker, J. M. Arevalo, et al., "Biobehavioral modulation of the exosome transcriptome in ovarian carcinoma," *Cancer* (November 2017).

49. E. S. Epel, E. H. Blackburn, J. Lin, et al., "Accelerated telomere shortening in response to life stress," *Proceedings of the National Academy of Sciences of the United States of America* 101, no. 49 (December 2004): 17312–15.

50. L. M. Pyter, "The influence of cancer on endocrine, immune, and behavioral stress responses," *Physiology and Behavior* 166 (November 2016): 4–13.

51. M. F. Bevans, E. M. Sternberg, "Caregiving burden, stress, and health effects among family caregivers of adult cancer patients," *Journal of the American Medical Association* 307, no. 4 (January 2012): 398–403.

52. J.-P. Gouin, R. Glaser, W. B. Malarkey, D. Beversdorf, J. Kiecolt-Glaser, "Chronic stress, daily stressors, and circulating inflammatory markers," *Health Psychology* 31, no. 2 (September 2012): 264–68.

53. J. K. Kiecolt-Glaser, J. R. Dura, C. E. Speicher, O. J. Trask, R. Glaser, "Spousal caregivers of dementia victims: longitudinal changes in immunity and health," *Psychosomatic Medicine* 53, no. 4 (August 1991): 345–62.

54. R. Glaser, J. Sheridan, W. B. Malarkey, R. C. MacCallum, J. K. Kiecolt-Glaser, "Chronic stress modulates the immune response to a pneumococcal pneumonia vaccine," *Psychosomatic Medicine* 62, no. 6 (December 2000): 804–7.

55. R. Schulz, S. R. Beach, "Caregiving as a risk factor for mortality: the caregiver health effects study," *Journal of the American Medical Association* 282, no. 23 (December 1999): 2215–19.

56. R. Glaser, J. K. Kiecolt-Glaser, R. H. Bonneau, et al., "Stress-induced modulation of the immune response to recombinant hepatitis B vaccine," *Psychosomatic Medicine* 54, no. 1 (February 1992): 22–29.

57. H. M. Derry, C. P. Fagundes, R. Andridge, et al., "Lower subjective social status exaggerates interleukin-6 responses to a laboratory stressor," *Psychoneuroendocrinology* 38, no. 11 (November 2013): 2676–85.

58. Y. J. Ko, Y. M. Kwon, K. H. Kim, et al., "High-sensitivity C-reactive protein levels and cancer mortality," *Cancer Epidemiology, Biomarkers & Prevention* 21, no. 11 (November 2012): 2076–86.

59. L. Guo, S. Liu, S. Zhang, et al., "C-reactive protein and risk of breast cancer: a systematic review and meta-analysis," *Scientific Reports* 5 (May 2015): 10508.

60. J. Zacho, A. Tybjaerg-Hansen, B. G. Nordestgaard, "C-reactive protein and all-cause mortality—the Copenhagen City Heart Study," *European Heart Journal* 31, no. 13 (July 2010): 1624–32.

61. L. Cohen, S. W. Cole, A. K. Sood, et al., "Depressive symptoms and cortisol rhythmicity predict survival in patients with renal cell carcinoma: role of inflammatory signaling," *PloS One* 7, no. 8 (August 2012): e42324.

62. S. W. Cole, M. E. Levine, J. M. Arevalo, et al., "Loneliness, eudaimonia, and the human conserved transcriptional response to adversity," *Psychoneuroendocrinology* 62 (December 2015): 11–17.

63. S. W. Cole, "Human social genomics," *Plos Genetics* 10, no. 8 (August 2014): e1004601.

64. L. M. Jaremka, C. P. Fagundes, J. Peng, et al., "Loneliness promotes inflammation during acute stress," *Psychological Science* 24, no. 7 (April 2013): 10.1177 /0956797612464059.

65. M. Moieni, M. R. Irwin, I. Jevtic, et al., "Trait sensitivity to social disconnection enhances pro-inflammatory responses to a randomized controlled trial of endotoxin," *Psychoneuroendocrinology* 62 (December 2015): 336–42.

66. J. E. Bower, G. Greendale, A. D. Crosswell, et al., "Yoga reduces inflammatory signaling in fatigued breast cancer survivors: a randomized controlled trial," *Psychoneuroendocrinology* 43 (January 2014): 20–29.

67. M. R. Irwin, R. Olmstead, E. C. Breen, et al., "Tai chi, cellular inflammation, and transcriptome dynamics in breast cancer survivors with insomnia: a randomized controlled trial," *Journal of the National Cancer Institute Monographs* 2014, no. 50 (November 2014): 295–301.

68. M. H. Antoni, S. K. Lutgendorf, B. Blomberg, et al., "Cognitive-behavioral stress management reverses anxiety-related leukocyte transcriptional dynamics," *Biological Psychiatry* 71, no. 4 (February 2012a): 366–72.

69. K. M. Ziol-Guest, G. J. Duncan, A. Kalil, W. T. Boyce, "Early childhood poverty, immune-mediated disease processes, and adult productivity," *Proceedings of the National Academy of Sciences of the United States of America* 109, Supplement 2 (October 2012): 17289–93.

70. K. B. Ehrlich, G. E. Miller, E. Chen, "Childhood adversity and adult physical health," in *Developmental Psychopathology* (New York: John Wiley, 2010).

71. K. Hughes, M. A. Bellis, K. A. Hardcastle, et al., "The effect of multiple adverse childhood experiences on health: a systematic review and meta-analysis," *The Lancet Public Health* 2, no. 8 (August 2017): e356–66.

72. Centers for Disease Control and Prevention, "Adverse childhood experiences (ACES)," April 1, 2016, www.cdc.gov/violenceprevention/acestudy/index.html.

73. V. J. Felitti, R. F. Anda, D. Nordenberg, et al., "Relationship of childhood abuse and household dysfunction to many of the leading causes of death in adults. The adverse childhood experiences (ACE) study," *American Journal of Preventive Medicine* 14, no. 4 (May 1998): 245–58.

74. Centers for Disease Control and Prevention, "About the CDC-Kaiser ACE Study," April 1, 2016, www.cdc.gov/violenceprevention/acestudy/about.html.

75. Centers for Disease Control and Prevention, "About behavioral risk factor surveillance system ACE data," April 1, 2016, www.cdc.gov/violenceprevention/acestudy /ace_brfss.html.

76. E. B. Raposa, J. E. Bower, C. L. Hammen, J. M. Najman, P. A. Brennan, "A developmental pathway from early life stress to inflammation: the role of negative health behaviors," *Psychological Science* 25, no. 6 (June 2014): 1268–74.

77. J. Bick, O. Naumova, S. Hunter, et al., "Childhood adversity and DNA methylation of genes involved in the hypothalamus–pituitary–adrenal axis and immune system: whole-genome and candidate-gene associations," *Development and Psychopathology* 24, no. 4 (November 2012): 1417–25.

78. C. Pretty, D. D. O'Leary, J. Cairney, T. J. Wade, "Adverse childhood experiences and the cardiovascular health of children: a cross-sectional study," *BMC Pediatrics* 13 (December 2013): 208.

79. N. J. Burke, J. L. Hellman, B. G. Scott, C. F. Weems, V. G. Carrion, "The impact of adverse childhood experiences on an urban pediatric population," *Child Abuse and Neglect* 35, no. 6 (June 2011): 408–13.

80. C. P. Fagundes, M. E. Lindgren, C. L. Shapiro, J. K. Kiecolt-Glaser, "Child maltreatment and breast cancer survivors: social support makes a difference for quality of

life, fatigue, and cancer stress," *European Journal of Cancer* 48, no. 5 (March 2012): 728–36.

81. J. E. Bower, A. D. Crosswell, G. M. Slavich, "Childhood adversity and cumulative life stress: risk factors for cancer-related fatigue," *Clinical Psychological Science* 2, no. 1 (January 2014).

82. L. Witek Janusek, D. Tell, K. Albuquerque, H. L. Mathews, "Childhood adversity increases vulnerability for behavioral symptoms and immune dysregulation in women with breast cancer," *Brain, Behavior, and Immunity* 30, Supplement (June 2013): S149–62.

83. T. J. Han, J. C. Felger, A. Lee, et al., "Association of childhood trauma with fatigue, depression, stress, and inflammation in breast cancer patients undergoing radiotherapy," *Psycho-Oncology* 25, no. 2 (February 2016): 187–93.

84. C. C. Conley, B. T. Bishop, B. L. Andersen, "Emotions and emotion regulation in breast cancer survivorship," *Healthcare* 4, no. 3 (August 2016): 56.

85. A. L. Stanton, S. Danoff-Burg, C. L. Cameron, et al., "Emotionally expressive coping predicts psychological and physical adjustment to breast cancer," *Journal of Consulting and Clinical Psychology* 68, no. 5 (October 2000): 875–82.

86. M. A. Killingsworth, D. T. Gilbert, "A wandering mind is an unhappy mind," *Science* 330, no. 6006 (November 2010): 932.

87. G. M. Slavich, M. R. Irwin, "From stress to inflammation and major depressive disorder: a social signal transduction theory of depression," *Psychological Bulletin* 140, no. 3 (January 2014): 774–815.

88. R. A. Sansone, L. A. Sansone, "Gratitude and well being: the benefits of appreciation," *Psychiatry* 7, no. 11 (November 2010): 18–22.

89. R. A. Emmons, M. E. McCullough, "Counting blessings versus burdens: an experimental investigation of gratitude and subjective well-being in daily life," *Journal of Personality and Social Psychology* 84, no. 2 (February 2003): 377–89.

90. M. Jackowska, J. Brown, A. Ronaldson, A. Steptoe, "The impact of a brief gratitude intervention on subjective well-being, biology and sleep," *Journal of Health Psychology* 21, no. 10 (October 2015): 2207–17.

91. L. S. Redwine, B. L. Henry, M. A. Pung, et al., "Pilot randomized study of a gratitude journaling intervention on heart rate variability and inflammatory biomarkers in patients with stage B heart failure," *Psychosomatic Medicine* 78, no. 6 (July–August 2016): 667–76.

92. M. E. McCullough, J. A. Tsang, R. A. Emmons, "Gratitude in intermediate affective terrain: links of grateful moods to individual differences and daily emotional experience," *Journal of Personality and Social Psychology* 86, no. 2 (February 2004): 295–309.

93. M. E. McCullough, R. A. Emmons, J. A. Tsang, "The grateful disposition: a conceptual and empirical topography," *Journal of Personality and Social Psychology* 82, no. 1 (January 2002): 112–27.

94. M. H. Antoni, J. M. Lehman, K. M. Kilbourn, et al., "Cognitive-behavioral stress management intervention decreases the prevalence of depression and enhances benefit finding among women under treatment for early-stage breast cancer," *Health Psychology* 20, no. 1 (January 2001): 20–32.

95. J. M. Stagl, S. C. Lechner, C. S. Carver, et al., "A randomized controlled trial of cognitive-behavioral stress management in breast cancer: survival and recurrence at 11-year follow-up," *Breast Cancer Research and Treatment* 154, no. 2 (November 2015): 319–28.

96. M. H. Antoni, S. K. Lutgendorf, B. Blomberg, et al., "Cognitive-behavioral stress management reverses anxiety-related leukocyte transcriptional dynamics," *Biological Psychiatry* 71, no. 4 (February 2012a): 366–72.

97. J. M. Stagl, L. C. Bouchard, S. C. Lechner, et al., "Long-term psychological benefits of cognitive-behavioral stress management for women with breast cancer: 11-year follow-up of a randomized controlled trial," *Cancer* 121, no. 11 (June 2015): 1873–81.

98. E. J. Rodriquez, S. E. Gregorich, J. Livaudais-Toman, E. J. Perez-Stable, "Coping with chronic stress by unhealthy behaviors," *Journal of Aging and Health* (May 2016): 898264316645548.

99. American Psychological Association, "Americans engage in unhealthy behaviors to manage stress," February 23, 2006, www.apa.org/news/press/releases/2006/01/stress-management.aspx.

100. J. K. Kiecolt-Glaser, D. L. Habash, C. P. Fagundes, et al., "Daily stressors, past depression, and metabolic responses to high-fat meals: a novel path to obesity," *Biological Psychiatry* 77, no. 7 (April 2015): 653–60.

101. E. Puterman, J. Lin, J. Krauss, E. H. Blackburn, E. S. Epel, "Determinants of telomere attrition over one year in healthy older women: stress and health behaviors matter," *Molecular Psychiatry* 20, no. 4 (July 2015): 529–35.

102. A. A. Prather, E. Puterman, J. Lin, et al., "Shorter leukocyte telomere length in midlife women with poor sleep quality," *Journal of Aging Research* 2011 (November 2011): 721390.

103. E. Puterman, J. Lin, E. Blackburn, et al., "The power of exercise: buffering the effect of chronic stress on telomere length," *PloS One* 5, no. 5 (May 2010): e10837.

104. Q. Sun, L. Shi, J. Prescott, et al., "Healthy lifestyle and leukocyte telomere length in U.S. Women," *PloS One* 7, no. 5 (July 2012): e38374.

The Anticancer Living Guide to Stress Reduction

1. M. R. Irwin, R. Olmstead, E. C. Breen, et al., "Cognitive behavioral therapy and tai chi reverse cellular and genomic markers of inflammation in late-life insomnia: a randomized controlled trial," *Biological Psychiatry* 78, no. 10 (November 2015a): 721–29.

2. M. H. Antoni, L. C. Bouchard, J. M. Jacobs, et al., "Stress management, leukocyte transcriptional changes and breast cancer recurrence in a randomized trial: an exploratory analysis," *Psychoneuroendocrinology* 74 (December 2016): 269–77.

3. More about Molly's Meditation: Molly M. gained tremendous knowledge from the program Alistair Cunningham developed in Toronto, Canada, called the Healing Journey Program. Program material is available online at www.healingjourney.ca. She practices a combination of relaxation, imagery, and meditation that includes calling up her ancestors and enlisting their help to prevent cancer cells from growing and spreading within her body. Molly is quick to point out that her visual imagery—for example, imagining leprechauns (from the lore of her Irish grandmother) cutting the blood supply to every tumor cell, cauterizing the cells, and then corking them so they cannot spread messages to the rest of her body that they need more blood—doesn't work for everyone.

4. M. Shahriari, M. Dehghan, S. Pahlavanzadeh, A. Hazini, "Effects of progressive muscle relaxation, guided imagery and deep diaphragmatic breathing on quality of life in elderly with breast or prostate cancer," *Journal of Education and Health Promotion* 6 (May 2017): 1.

5. Z. Chen, Z. Meng, K. Milbury, et al., "Qigong improves quality of life in women undergoing radiotherapy for breast cancer: results of a randomized controlled trial," *Cancer* 119, no. 9 (January 2013): 10.1002/cncr.27904.

6. R. Jahnke, L. Larkey, C. Rogers, J. Etnier, F. Lin, "A comprehensive review of health benefits of qigong and tai chi," *American Journal of Health Promotion* 24, no. 6 (July–August 2010): e1–25.

7. K. D. Chandwani, G. Perkins, H. R. Nagendra, et al., "Randomized, controlled trial of yoga in women with breast cancer undergoing radiotherapy," *Journal of Clinical Oncology* 32, no. 10 (April 2014): 1058–65.

8. J. K. Kiecolt-Glaser, J. M. Bennett, R. Andridge, et al., "Yoga's impact on inflammation, mood, and fatigue in breast cancer survivors: a randomized controlled trial," *Journal of Clinical Oncology* 32, no. 10 (April 2014): 1040–49.

9. K. M. Mustian, M. Janelsins, L. J. Peppone, C. Kamen, "Yoga for the treatment of insomnia among cancer patients: Evidence, mechanisms of action, and clinical recommendations," *Oncology & Hematology Review* 10, no. 2 (October 2014): 164–68.

10. S. C. Danhauer, E. L. Addington, S. J. Sohl, A. Chaoul, L. Cohen, "Review of yoga therapy during cancer treatment," *Supportive Care in Cancer* 25, no. 4 (April 2017): 1357–72.

11. C. G. Ratcliff, K. Milbury, K. D. Chandwani, et al., "Examining mediators and moderators of yoga for women with breast cancer undergoing radiotherapy," *Integrative Cancer Therapies* 15, no. 3 (September 2016): 250–62.

12. M. J. Mackenzie, A. J. Wurz, Y. Yamauchi, L. A. Pires, S. N. Culos-Reed, "Yoga helps put the pieces back together: a qualitative exploration of a community-based yoga program for cancer survivors," *Evidence-Based Complementary and Alternative Medicine* 2016 (December 2016): 1832515.

13. V. Scaravelli, *Awakening the Spine: Yoga for Health, Vitality, and Energy*, 2nd ed. (London: Pinter & Martin, 2012).

14. S. Blaschke, "The role of nature in cancer patients' lives: A systematic review and qualitative meta-synthesis," *BMC Cancer* 17 (May 2017): 370.

15. Section on Integrative Medicine, "Mind-body therapies in children and youth," *Pediatrics* 138, no. 3 (September 2016).

16. Y. G. Yoo, D. J. Lee, I. S. Lee, et al., "The effects of mind subtraction meditation on depression, social anxiety, aggression, and salivary cortisol levels of elementary school children in South Korea," *Journal of Pediatric Nursing* 31, no. 3 (May–June 2016): e185–97.

17. X. Zeng, C. P. K. Chiu, R. Wang, T. P. S. Oei, F. Y. K. Leung, "The effect of loving-kindness meditation on positive emotions: a meta-analytic review," *Frontiers in Psychology* 6 (November 2015): 1693.

18. S. G. Hofmann, P. Grossman, D. E. Hinton, "Loving-kindness and compassion meditation: potential for psychological interventions," *Clinical Psychology Review* 31, no. 7 (July 2011): 1126–32.

19. B. L. Fredrickson, M. A. Cohn, K. A. Coffey, J. Pek, S. M. Finkel, "Open hearts build lives: positive emotions, induced through loving-kindness meditation, build consequential personal resources," *Journal of Personality and Social Psychology* 95, no. 5 (November 2008): 1045–62.

20. D. J. Kearney, C. A. Malte, C. McManus, et al., "Loving-kindness meditation for posttraumatic stress disorder: a pilot study," *Journal of Traumatic Stress* 26, no. 4 (August 2013): 42–34.

21. T. Triplett, R. Santos, S. Rosenbloom, "American driving survey 2014–2015 AAA Foundation for Traffic Safety," September 2016, www.aaafoundation.org /sites/default/files/AmericanDrivingSurvey2015.pdf.

Chapter Nine: The Need for Rest and Recovery

1. M. H. Kryger, T. Roth, W. C. Dement, *Principles and Practice of Sleep Medicine* (Philadelphia: Elsevier, 2016).

2. C. Dibner, U. Schibler, U. Albrecht, "The mammalian circadian timing system: organization and coordination of central and peripheral clocks," *Annual Review of Physiology* 72 (February 2010): 517–49.

3. M. R. Irwin, R. Olmstead, J. E. Carroll, "Sleep disturbance, sleep duration, and inflammation: a systematic review and meta-analysis of cohort studies and experimental sleep deprivation," *Biological Psychiatry* 80, no. 1 (July 2016): 40–52.

4. Y. Komada, S. Asaoka, T. Abe, Y. Inoue, "Short sleep duration, sleep disorders, and traffic accidents," *IATSS Research* 37, no. 1 (July 2013): 1–7.

5. F. P. Cappuccio, D. Cooper, L. D'Elia, P. Strazzullo, M. A. Miller, "Sleep duration predicts cardiovascular outcomes: a systematic review and meta-analysis of prospective studies," *European Heart Journal* 32, no. 12 (June 2011): 1484–92.

6. F. P. Cappuccio, L. D'Elia, P. Strazzullo, M. A. Miller, "Sleep duration and all-cause mortality: a systematic review and meta-analysis of prospective studies," *Sleep* 33, no. 5 (May 2010): 585-92.

7. S. R. Patel, F. B. Hu, "Short sleep duration and weight gain: a systematic review," *Obesity* 16, no. 3 (March 2008): 643–53.

8. L. A. Zuurbier, A. I. Luik, A. Hofman, et al., "Fragmentation and stability of circadian activity rhythms predict mortality: the Rotterdam Study," *American Journal of Epidemiology* 181, no. 1 (January 2015): 54–63.

9. T. Dekker, "The Guls Horne-Booke, 1609," in: *Renascence Editions*, University of Oregon (2003). Text transcribed by Risa S. Bear, July 2003, from the 1904 Temple Classics edition, http://www.luminarium.org/renascence-editions/dekker2.html.

10. S. Chung, G. H. Son, K. Kim, "Circadian rhythm of adrenal glucocorticoid: its regulation and clinical implications," *Biochimica et Biophysica Acta (BBA)—Molecular Basis of Disease* 1812, no. 5 (May 2011): 581–91.

11. B. Wood, M. S. Rea, B. Plitnick, M. G. Figueiro, "Light level and duration of exposure determine the impact of self-luminous tablets on melatonin suppression," *Applied Ergonomics* 44, no. 2 (March 2013): 237–40.

12. Y. Yang, J. C. Shin, D. Li, R. An, "Sedentary behavior and sleep problems: a systematic review and meta-analysis," *International Journal of Behavioral Medicine* 24, no. 4 (August 2017): 481–92.

13. M. A. de Assis, E. Kupek, M. V. Nahas, F. Bellisle, "Food intake and circadian rhythms in shift workers with a high workload," *Appetite* 40, no. 2 (April 2003): 175–83.

14. D. M. Arble, J. Bass, A. D. Laposky, M. H. Vitaterna, F. W. Turek, "Circadian timing of food intake contributes to weight gain," *Obesity* 17, no. 11 (September 2009): 2100–2102.

15. B. J. Taylor, K. A. Matthews, B. P. Hasler, et al., "Bedtime variability and metabolic health in midlife women: the SWAN Sleep Study," *Sleep* 39, no. 2 (February 2016): 457–65.

16. K. G. Baron, K. J. Reid, "Circadian misalignment and health," *International Review of Psychiatry* 26, no. 2 (April 2014): 139–54.

17. H. S. Dashti, F. A. J. L. Scheer, P. F. Jacques, S. Lamon-Fava, J. M. Ordovás, "Short sleep duration and dietary intake: epidemiologic evidence, mechanisms, and health implications," *Advances in Nutrition* 6, no. 6 (November 2015): 648–59.

18. M. Hastings, J. S. O'Neill, E. S. Maywood, "Circadian clocks: regulators of endocrine and metabolic rhythms," *Journal of Endocrinology* 195, no. 2 (November 2007): 187–98.

19. C. E. Kline, "The bidirectional relationship between exercise and sleep: implications for exercise adherence and sleep improvement," *American Journal of Lifestyle Medicine* 8, no 6 (November–December 2014): 375–79.

20. M. Wilking, M. Ndiaye, H. Mukhtar, N. Ahmad, "Circadian rhythm connections to oxidative stress: implications for human health," *Antioxid Redox Signal* 19, no. 2 (July 2013): 192–208.

21. D. J. Buysse, "Sleep health: can we define it? does it matter?," *Sleep* 37, no. 1 (January 2014): 9–17.

22. Centers for Disease Control and Prevention, "Perceived insufficient rest or sleep among adults—United States, 2008," *Morbidity and Mortality Weekly Report*, October 29, 2009, www.cdc.gov/mmwr/preview/mmwrhtml/mm5842a2.htm.

23. M. Z. Hossin, "From habitual sleep hours to morbidity and mortality: existing evidence, potential mechanisms, and future agenda," *Sleep Health* 2, no. 2 (June 2016): 146–53.

24. National Sleep Foundation, "Lack of sleep is affecting Americans, finds the national sleep foundation," December 2014, www.sleepfoundation.org/media-center/press -release/lack-sleep-affecting-americans-finds-the-national-sleep-foundation.

25. D. Leger, B. Poursain, D. Neubauer, M. Uchiyama, "An international survey of sleeping problems in the general population," *Current Medical Research and Opinion* 24, no. 1 (January 2008): 307–17.

26. R. C. Anafi, R. Pellegrino, K. R. Shockley, et al., "Sleep is not just for the brain: transcriptional responses to sleep in peripheral tissues," *BMC Genomics* 14 (May 2013): 362.

27. H. M. Ollila, S. Utge, E. Kronholm, et al., "Trib1 constitutes a molecular link between regulation of sleep and lipid metabolism in humans," *Translational Psychiatry* 2 (March 2012): e97.

28. Y. Takahashi, D. M. Kipnis, W. H. Daughaday, "Growth hormone secretion during sleep," *Journal of Clinical Investigation* 47, no. 9 (September 1968): 2079–90.

29. M. B. Davidson, "Effect of growth hormone on carbohydrate and lipid metabolism," *Endocrine Reviews* 8, no. 2 (May 1987): 115–31.

30. D. H. Bovbjerg, "Circadian disruption and cancer: sleep and immune regulation," *Brain, Behavior, and Immunity* 17 Supplement 1 (February 2003): S48–50.

31. R. V. Puram, M. S. Kowalczyk, C. G. de Boer, et al., "Core circadian clock genes regulate leukemia stem cells in AML," *Cell* 165, no. 2 (April 2016): 303–16.

32. L. Fu, N. M. Kettner, "The circadian clock in cancer development and therapy," *Progress in Molecular Biology and Translational Science* 119 (August 2013): 221–82.

33. F. Hakim, Y. Wang, S. X. L. Zhang, et al., "Fragmented sleep accelerates tumor growth and progression through recruitment of tumor-associated macrophages and tlr4 signaling," *Cancer Research* 74, no. 5 (January 2014): 1329–37.

34. J. H. Lee, A. Sancar, "Circadian clock disruption improves the efficacy of chemotherapy through p73-mediated apoptosis," *Proceedings of the National Academy of Sciences of the United States of America* 108, no. 26 (June 2011): 10668–72.

35. A. Grundy, J. M. Schuetz, A. S. Lai, et al., "Shift work, circadian gene variants and risk of breast cancer," *Cancer Epidemiology* 37, no. 5 (October 2013): 606–12.

36. S. Dimitrov, L. Besedovsky, J. Born, T. Lange, "Differential acute effects of sleep on spontaneous and stimulated production of tumor necrosis factor in men," *Brain, Behavior, and Immunity* 47 (July 2015): 201–10.

37. J. M. Krueger, J. A. Majde, F. Obal, "Sleep in host defense," *Brain, Behavior, and Immunity* 17, Supplement 1 (February 2003): S41–47.

38. C. S. Moller-Levet, S. N. Archer, G. Bucca, et al., "Effects of insufficient sleep on circadian rhythmicity and expression amplitude of the human blood transcriptome," *Proceedings of the National Academy of Sciences of the United States of America* 110, no. 12 (March 2013): E1132–41.

39. L. Cohen, S. W. Cole, A. K. Sood, et al., "Depressive symptoms and cortisol rhythmicity predict survival in patients with renal cell carcinoma: role of inflammatory signaling," *PloS One* 7, no. 8 (August 2012): e42324.

40. S. E. Sephton, E. Lush, E. A. Dedert, et al., "Diurnal cortisol rhythm as a predictor of lung cancer survival," *Brain, Behavior, and Immunity* 30, Supplement (March 2013): S163–70.

41. S. E. Sephton, R. M. Sapolsky, H. C. Kraemer, D. Spiegel, "Diurnal cortisol rhythm as a predictor of breast cancer survival," *Journal of the National Cancer Institute* 92, no. 12 (June 2000): 994–1000.

42. P. Philip, C. Chaufton, L. Orriols, et al., "Complaints of poor sleep and risk of traffic accidents: a population-based case-control study," *PloS One* 9, no. 12 (December 2014): e114102.

43. R. C. Cox, B. O. Olatunji, "A systematic review of sleep disturbance in anxiety and related disorders," *Journal of Anxiety Disorders* 37, Supplement C (January 2016): 104–29.

44. J. Fernandez-Mendoza, S. Shea, A. N. Vgontzas, et al., "Insomnia and incident depression: role of objective sleep duration and natural history," *Journal of Sleep Research* 24, no. 4 (August 2015): 390–98.

45. L. Zhai, H. Zhang, D. Zhang, "Sleep duration and depression among adults: a meta-analysis of prospective studies," *Depression and Anxiety* 32, no. 9 (September 2015): 664–70.

46. P. L. Franzen, P. J. Gianaros, A. L. Marsland, et al., "Cardiovascular reactivity to acute psychological stress following sleep deprivation," *Psychosomatic Medicine* 73, no. 8 (November 2011): 679–82.

47. B. J. Taylor, L. A. Irish, L. M. Martire, et al., "Avoidant coping and poor sleep efficiency in dementia caregivers," *Psychosomatic Medicine* 77, no. 9 (November–December 2015): 1050–57.

48. F. Bianchini, R. Kaaks, H. Vainio, "Overweight, obesity, and cancer risk," *The Lancet Oncology* 3, no. 9 (September 2002): 565–74.

49. J. M. Siegel, "Rapid eye movement sleep," in *Principles and Practice of Sleep Medicine*, eds. M. H. Kryger, T. Roth, and W. C. Demen (Philadelphia: Elsevier, 2016), 78–85.

50. C. A. Everson, C. D. Laatsch, N. Hogg, "Antioxidant defense responses to sleep loss and sleep recovery," *American Journal of Physiology—Regulatory, Integrative and Comparative Physiology* 288, no. 2 (February 2005): R374.

51. M. Adamczyk-Sowa, K. Pierzchala, P. Sowa, et al., "Melatonin acts as antioxidant and improves sleep in MS patients," *Neurochemical Research* 39, no. 8 (August 2014): 1585–93.

52. T. C. Erren, R. J. Reiter, "A generalized theory of carcinogenesis due to chronodisruption," *Neuroendocrinology Letters* 29, no. 6 (December 2008): 815–21.

53. J. Noguti, M. L. Andersen, C. Cirelli, D. A. Ribeiro, "Oxidative stress, cancer, and sleep deprivation: is there a logical link in this association?," *Sleep and Breathing* 17, no. 3 (September 2013): 905–10.

54. K. Straif, R. Baan, Y. Grosse, et al., "Carcinogenicity of shift-work, painting, and fire-fighting," *The Lancet Oncology* 8, no. 12 (December 2007): 1065–66.

55. H. Zhao, J. Y. Yin, W. S. Yang, et al., "Sleep duration and cancer risk: a systematic review and meta-analysis of prospective studies," *Asian Pacific Journal of Cancer Prevention* 14, no. 12 (January 2013): 7509–15.

56. L. Besedovsky, T. Lange, J. Born, "Sleep and immune function," *Pflügers Archiv: European Journal of Physiology* 463, no. 1 (November 2012): 121–37.

57. M. Jackowska, M. Hamer, L. A. Carvalho, et al., "Short sleep duration is associated with shorter telomere length in healthy men: findings from the Whitehall II cohort study," *PloS One* 7, no. 10 (November 2012): e47292.

58. D. P. Venancio, D. Suchecki, "Prolonged REM sleep restriction induces metabolic syndrome-related changes: mediation by pro-inflammatory cytokines," *Brain, Behavior, and Immunity* 47 (July 2015): 109–17.

59. G. Hurtado-Alvarado, E. Dominguez-Salazar, L. Pavon, J. Velazquez-Moctezuma, B. Gomez-Gonzalez, "Blood-brain barrier disruption induced by chronic sleep loss:

low-grade inflammation may be the link," *Journal of Immunology Research* 2016 (October 2016): 4576012.

60. C. Clifford, "Olympic hero Michael Phelps says the secret to his success is one most people overlook," February 17, 2017, www.cnbc.com/2017/02/14/olympic-hero -michael-phelps-says-this-is-the-secret-to-his-success.html.

61. N. Hinde, "Revealed: the diets of Olympic athletes, including Michael Phelps, Usain, Bolt and Adam Peaty," October 8, 2016, www.huffingtonpost.co.uk/entry /diets-of-olympians-michael-phelps-adam-peaty-louis-smith-nicola-adams_uk _57ab0b99e4b0b3afa75cba85.

62. Z. McCann, "Sleep tracking brings new info to athletes," June 1, 2012, www.espn.com /blog/playbook/tech/post/_/id/797/sleep-tracking-brings-new-info-to-athletes.

63. E. A. Copenhaver, A. B. Diamond, "The value of sleep on athletic performance, injury, and recovery in the young athlete," *Pediatric Annals* 46, no. 3 (March 2017): e106–11.

64. S. Kolling, T. Wiewelhove, C. Raeder, et al., "Sleep monitoring of a six-day microcycle in strength and high-intensity training," *European Journal of Sports Science* 16, no. 5 (August 2016): 507–15.

65. Fatigue Science, "Five areas sleep has the greatest impact on athletic performance," September 23, 2015, www.fatiguescience.com/blog/5-ways-sleep-impacts-peak -athletic-performance/.

66. J. M. Jones, "In U.S., 40% get less than recommended amount of sleep," December 19, 2013, www.news.gallup.com/poll/166553/less-recommended-amount-sleep.aspx.

67. M. Hirshkowitz, K. Whiton, S. M. Albert, et al., "National Sleep Foundation's sleep time duration recommendations: methodology and results summary," *Sleep Health* 1, no. 1 (March 2015): 40–43.

68. N. F. Watson, M. S. Badr, G. Belenky, et al., "Recommended amount of sleep for a healthy adult: a joint consensus statement of the American Academy of Sleep Medicine and Sleep Research Society," *Journal of Clinical Sleep Medicine* 11, no. 6 (June 2015): 591–92.

69. M. A. Carskadon, "Sleep in adolescents: the perfect storm," *Pediatric Clinics of North America* 58, no. 3 (June 2011): 637–47.

70. S. J. Crowley, C. Acebo, M. A. Carskadon, "Sleep, circadian rhythms, and delayed phase in adolescence," *Sleep Medicine* 8, no. 6 (September 2007): 602–12.

71. National Sleep Foundation, "Sleep in America poll: teens and sleep summary of findings," 2006, www.sleepfoundation.org/sleep-polls-data/sleep-in-america-poll /2006-teens-and-sleep.

72. C. E. Basch, C. H. Basch, K. V. Ruggles, S. Rajan, "Prevalence of sleep duration on an average school night among 4 nationally representative successive samples of American high school students, 2007–2013," *Preventing Chronic Disease* 11 (December 2014): E216.

73. A. Winsler, A. Deutsch, R. D. Vorona, P. A. Payne, M. Szklo-Coxe, "Sleepless in Fairfax: the difference one more hour of sleep can make for teen hopelessness, suicidal ideation, and substance use," *Journal of Youth and Adolescence* 44, no. 2 (February 2015): 362–78.

74. M. M. Mitler, M. A. Carskadon, C. A. Czeisler, et al., "Catastrophes, sleep, and public policy: consensus report," *Sleep* 11, no. 1 (February 1988): 100–9.

75. National Transportation Safety Board, "Organizational factors in Metro-North railroad accidents," 2014, www.ntsb.gov/safety/safety-studies/documents/SIR1404.pdf.

76. Institute of Medicine Committee on Sleep Medicine Research, "The National Academies collection: reports funded by National Institutes of Health," in *Sleep Disorders and Sleep Deprivation: An Unmet Public Health Problem*, eds. H. R. Colten and B. M. Altevogt (Washington, D.C.: National Academies Press, 2006).

77. Y. Chong, C. D. Fryer, Q. Gu, "Prescription sleep aid use among adults: United States, 2005–2010," *NCHS Data Brief* no. 127 (August 2013): 1–8.
78. M. Hafner, M. Stepanek, J. Taylor, W. M. Troxel, C. Van Stolk, "Why sleep matters—the economic costs of insufficient sleep: a cross-country comparative analysis," RAND Corporation, 2016, www.rand.org/pubs/research_reports/RR1791.html.
79. E. Van Cauter, K. Spiegel, E. Tasali, R. Leproult, "Metabolic consequences of sleep and sleep loss," *Sleep Medicine* 9 Supplement 1, no. 1 (September 2008): S23–28.
80. F. P. Cappuccio, F. M. Taggart, N. B. Kandala, et al., "Meta-analysis of short sleep duration and obesity in children and adults," *Sleep* 31, no. 5 (May 2008): 619–26.
81. K. Spiegel, E. Tasali, P. Penev, E. Van Cauter, "Brief communication: sleep curtailment in healthy young men is associated with decreased leptin levels, elevated ghrelin levels, and increased hunger and appetite," *Annals of Internal Medicine* 141, no. 11 (December 2004): 846–50.
82. J. A. Mitchell, D. Rodriguez, K. H. Schmitz, J. Audrain-McGovern, "Sleep duration and adolescent obesity," *Pediatrics* 131, no. 5 (May 2013): e1428–34.
83. C. Sabanayagam, A. Shankar, "Sleep duration and cardiovascular disease: results from the national health interview survey," *Sleep* 33, no. 8 (August 2010): 1037–42.
84. Z. Shan, H. Ma, M. Xie, et al., "Sleep duration and risk of type 2 diabetes: a meta-analysis of prospective studies," *Diabetes Care* 38, no. 3 (March 2015): 529–37.
85. P. H. Finan, P. J. Quartana, M. T. Smith, "The effects of sleep continuity disruption on positive mood and sleep architecture in healthy adults," *Sleep* 38, no. 11 (November 2015): 1735–42.
86. R. G. Kent, B. N. Uchino, M. R. Cribbet, K. Bowen, T. W. Smith, "Social relationships and sleep quality," *Annals of Behavioral Medicine* 49, no. 6 (December 2015): 912–17.
87. J. Minkel, M. Moreta, J. Muto, et al., "Sleep deprivation potentiates HPA axis stress reactivity in healthy adults," *Health Psychology* 33, no. 11 (November 2014): 1430–34.
88. J. F. Dewald-Kaufmann, F. J. Oort, A. M. Meijer, "The effects of sleep extension on sleep and cognitive performance in adolescents with chronic sleep reduction: an experimental study," *Sleep Medicine* 14, no. 6 (June 2013): 510–17.
89. H. P. Van Dongen, G. Maislin, J. M. Mullington, D. F. Dinges, "The cumulative cost of additional wakefulness: dose-response effects on neurobehavioral functions and sleep physiology from chronic sleep restriction and total sleep deprivation," *Sleep* 26, no. 2 (March 2003): 117–26.
90. J. W. Noh, K. B. Kim, J. H. Lee, et al., "Association between sleep duration and injury from falling among older adults: a cross-sectional analysis of Korean community health survey data," *Yonsei Medical Journal* 58, no. 6 (November 2017): 1222–28.
91. M. Wittmann, J. Dinich, M. Merrow, T. Roenneberg, "Social jetlag: misalignment of biological and social time," *Chronobiology International* 23, no. 1–2 (May 2006): 497–509.
92. Y. Liu, A. G. Wheaton, D. P. Chapman, et al., "Prevalence of healthy sleep duration among adults—United States, 2014," *MMWR: Morbidity and Mortality Weekly Report* 65, no. 6 (February 2016): 137–41.
93. M. A. Grandner, S. P. Drummond, "Who are the long sleepers? Towards an understanding of the mortality relationship," *Sleep Medicine Reviews* 11, no. 5 (October 2007): 341–60.
94. L. B. Strand, M. K. Tsai, D. Gunnell, et al., "Self-reported sleep duration and coronary heart disease mortality: a large cohort study of 400,000 Taiwanese adults," *International Journal of Cardiology* 207 (March 2016): 246–51.
95. P. J. Magistretti, I. Allaman, "A cellular perspective on brain energy metabolism and functional imaging," *Neuron* 86, no. 4 (May 2015): 883–901.

96. M. E. Raichle, D. A. Gusnard, "Appraising the brain's energy budget," *Proceedings of the National Academy of Sciences of the United States of America* 99, no. 16 (August 2002): 10237–39.

97. L. Xie, H. Kang, Q. Xu, et al., "Sleep drives metabolite clearance from the adult brain," *Science* 342, no. 6156 (October 2013): 373–77.

98. B. A. Mander, S. M. Marks, J. W. Vogel, et al., "Beta-amyloid disrupts human nREM slow waves and related hippocampus-dependent memory consolidation," *Nature Neuroscience* 18, no. 7 (July 2015): 1051–57.

99. K. E. Sprecher, R. L. Koscik, C. M. Carlsson, et al., "Poor sleep is associated with CSF biomarkers of amyloid pathology in cognitively normal adults," *Neurology* 89, no. 5 (August 2017): 445–53.

100. J. M. Tarasoff-Conway, R. O. Carare, R. S. Osorio, et al., "Clearance systems in the brain—implications for Alzheimer disease," *Nature Reviews: Neurology* 11, no. 8 (July 2015): 457–70.

101. J. Backhaus, J. Born, R. Hoeckesfeld, et al., "Midlife decline in declarative memory consolidation is correlated with a decline in slow wave sleep," *Learning and Memory* 14, no. 5 (May 2007): 336–41.

102. T. Blackwell, K. Yaffe, S. Ancoli-Israel, et al., "Poor sleep is associated with impaired cognitive function in older women: the study of osteoporotic fractures," *Journals of Gerontology: Series A* 61, no. 4 (April 2006): 405–10.

103. E. Hita-Yanez, M. Atienza, J. L. Cantero, "Polysomnographic and subjective sleep markers of mild cognitive impairment," *Sleep* 36, no. 9 (September 2013): 1327–34.

104. Y. S. Ju, S. J. Ooms, C. Sutphen, et al., "Slow wave sleep disruption increases cerebrospinal fluid amyloid-beta levels," *Brain* 140, no. 8 (August 2017): 2104–11.

105. N. F. Watson, D. Buchwald, J. J. Delrow, et al., "Transcriptional signatures of sleep duration discordance in monozygotic twins," *Sleep* 40, no. 1 (January 2017): zsw01.

106. K. L. Knutson, E. Van Cauter, "Associations between sleep loss and increased risk of obesity and diabetes," *Annals of the New York Academy of Sciences* 1129 (July 2008): 287–304.

107. M. Nagai, S. Hoshide, K. Kario, "Sleep duration as a risk factor for cardiovascular disease—a review of the recent literature," *Current Cardiology Reviews* 6, no. 1 (February 2010): 54–61.

108. C. L. Thompson, L. Li, "Association of sleep duration and breast cancer oncotype DX recurrence score," *Breast Cancer Research and Treatment* 134, no. 3 (August 2012): 1291–95.

109. C. L. Thompson, E. K. Larkin, S. Patel, et al., "Short duration of sleep increases risk of colorectal adenoma," *Cancer* 117, no. 4 (February 2011): 841–47.

110. P. F. Innominato, S. Giacchetti, G. A. Bjarnason, et al., "Prediction of overall survival through circadian rest-activity monitoring during chemotherapy for metastatic colorectal cancer," *International Journal of Cancer* 131, no. 11 (December 2012): 2684–92.

111. M. Hall, D. J. Buysse, M. A. Dew, et al., "Intrusive thoughts and avoidance behaviors are associated with sleep disturbances in bereavement-related depression," *Depression and Anxiety* 6, no. 3 (December 1998): 106–12.

112. M. H. Hall, M. D. Casement, W. M. Troxel, et al., "Chronic stress is prospectively associated with sleep in midlife women: the Swan sleep study," *Sleep* 38, no. 10 (October 2015): 1645–54.

113. M. Hall, A. Baum, D. J. Buysse, et al., "Sleep as a mediator of the stress-immune relationship," *Psychosomatic Medicine* 60, no. 1 (January–February 1998): 48–51.

114. M. Hall, R. Vasko, D. Buysse, et al., "Acute stress affects heart rate variability during sleep," *Psychosomatic Medicine* 66, no. 1 (January–February 2004): 56–62.

115. A. A. Prather, D. Janicki-Deverts, N. E. Adler, M. Hall, S. Cohen, "Sleep habits and susceptibility to upper respiratory illness: the moderating role of subjective socioeconomic status," *Annals of Behavioral Medicine* 51, no. 1 (February 2017): 137–46.

116. E. Fonad, T.-B. R. Wahlin, B. Winblad, A. Emami, H. Sandmark, "Falls and fall risk among nursing home residents," *Journal of Clinical Nursing* 17, no. 1 (January 2008): 126–34.

117. C. M. Morin, R. R. Bootzin, D. J. Buysse, et al., "Psychological and behavioral treatment of insomnia: update of the recent evidence (1998–2004)," *Sleep* 29, no. 11 (November 2006): 1398–1414.

118. C. M. Morin, C. Colecchi, J. Stone, R. Sood, D. Brink, "Behavioral and pharmacological therapies for late-life insomnia: a randomized controlled trial," *Journal of the American Medical Association* 281, no. 11 (March 1999): 991–99.

119. C. M. Morin, A. Vallières, B. Guay, et al., "Cognitive behavioral therapy, singly and combined with medication, for persistent insomnia: a randomized controlled trial," *Journal of the American Medical Association* 301, no. 19 (May 2009): 2005–15.

120. C. H. Bastien, C. M. Morin, M. C. Ouellet, F. C. Blais, S. Bouchard, "Cognitive-behavioral therapy for insomnia: comparison of individual therapy, group therapy, and telephone consultations," *Journal of Consulting and Clinical Psychology* 72, no. 4 (August 2004): 653–59.

121. L. M. Ritterband, F. P. Thorndike, L. A. Gonder-Frederick, et al., "Efficacy of an internet-based behavioral intervention for adults with insomnia," *Archives of General Psychiatry* 66, no. 7 (July 2009): 692–98.

122. J. A. Johnson, J. A. Rash, T. S. Campbell, et al., "A systematic review and meta-analysis of randomized controlled trials of cognitive behavior therapy for insomnia (CBT-I) in cancer survivors," *Sleep Medicine Reviews* 27, no. Supplement C (June 2016): 20–28.

123. L. M. Ritterband, E. T. Bailey, F. P. Thorndike, et al., "Initial evaluation of an internet intervention to improve the sleep of cancer survivors with insomnia," *Psycho-Oncology* 21, no. 7 (April 2012): 695–705.

124. J. Savard, H. Ivers, M. H. Savard, C. M. Morin, "Long-term effects of two formats of cognitive behavioral therapy for insomnia comorbid with breast cancer," *Sleep* 39, no. 4 (April 2016): 813–23.

125. M. R. Irwin, R. Olmstead, C. Carrillo, et al., "Tai chi chih compared with cognitive behavioral therapy for the treatment of insomnia in survivors of breast cancer: a randomized, partially blinded, noninferiority trial," *Journal of Clinical Oncology* 35, no. 23 (August 2017): 2656–65.

126. M. R. Irwin, R. Olmstead, E. C. Breen, et al., "Cognitive behavioral therapy and tai chi reverse cellular and genomic markers of inflammation in late life insomnia: a randomized controlled trial," *Biological Psychiatry* 78, no. 10 (February 2015b): 721–29.

127. D. S. Black, G. A. O'Reilly, R. Olmstead, E. C. Breen, M. R. Irwin, "Mindfulness meditation and improvement in sleep quality and daytime impairment among older adults with sleep disturbances: a randomized clinical trial," *Journal of the American Medical Association Internal Medicine* 175, no. 4 (April 2015): 494–501.

128. K. M. Mustian, L. K. Sprod, M. Janelsins, et al., "Multicenter, randomized controlled trial of yoga for sleep quality among cancer survivors," *Journal of Clinical Oncology* 31, no. 26 (September 2013): 3233–41.

129. K. D. Chandwani, G. Perkins, H. R. Nagendra, et al., "Randomized, controlled trial of yoga in women with breast cancer undergoing radiotherapy," *Journal of Clinical Oncology* 32, no. 10 (April 2014): 1058–65.

130. A. Chaoul, K. Milbury, A. Spelman, et al., "Randomized trial of Tibetan yoga in patients with breast cancer undergoing chemotherapy," *Cancer* (September 2017).

131. National Comprehensive Cancer Network, "Cancer-related fatigue (version 1.2014)," January 6, 2014, www.williams.medicine.wisc.edu/fatigue.pdf.

132. American Cancer Society, "Chemotherapy side effects," February 15, 2016, www.cancer.org/treatment/treatments-and-side-effects/treatment-types/chemotherapy/chemotherapy-side-effects.html.

133. American Cancer Society, "Side effects of targeted cancer therapy drugs," June 6, 2016, www.cancer.org/treatment/treatments-and-side-effects/treatment-types/targeted-therapy/side-effects.html.

134. American Cancer Society, "Risks of cancer surgery," April 19, 2016, www.cancer.org/treatment/treatments-and-side-effects/treatment-types/surgery/risks-of-cancer-surgery.html.

135. J. E. Bower, "Cancer-related fatigue: mechanisms, risk factors, and treatments," *Nature Reviews: Clinical Oncology* 11, no. 10 (August 2014): 597–609.

136. S. Ancoli-Israel, M. Rissling, A. Neikrug, et al., "Light treatment prevents fatigue in women undergoing chemotherapy for breast cancer," *Supportive Care in Cancer* 20, no. 6 (June 2012): 1211–19.

137. J. A. Johnson, S. N. Garland, L. E. Carlson, et al., "Bright light therapy improves cancer-related fatigue in cancer survivors: a randomized controlled trial," *Journal of Cancer Survivorship* (November 2017).

138. J. F. Meneses-Echávez, E. González-Jiménez, R. Ramírez-Vélez, "Supervised exercise reduces cancer-related fatigue: a systematic review," *Journal of Physiotherapy* 61, no. 1 (January 2015): 3–9.

139. S. A. Johns, L. F. Brown, K. Beck-Coon, et al., "Randomized controlled pilot study of mindfulness-based stress reduction for persistently fatigued cancer survivors," *Psycho-Oncology* 24, no. 8 (August 2015): 885–93.

140. L. K. Sprod, I. D. Fernandez, M. C. Janelsins, et al., "Effects of yoga on cancer-related fatigue and global side-effect burden in older cancer survivors," *Journal of Geriatric Oncology* 6, no. 1 (January 2015): 8–14.

141. L. L. Zhang, S. Z. Wang, H. L. Chen, A. Z. Yuan, "Tai chi exercise for cancer-related fatigue in patients with lung cancer undergoing chemotherapy: a randomized controlled trial," *Journal of Pain and Symptom Management* 51, no. 3 (March 2016): 504–11.

142. K. Ackermann, V. L. Revell, O. Lao, et al., "Diurnal rhythms in blood cell populations and the effect of acute sleep deprivation in healthy young men," *Sleep* 35, no. 7 (July 2012): 933–40.

The Anticancer Living Guide to Better Sleep

1. R. A. Hendler, V. A. Ramchandani, J. Gilman, D. W. Hommer, "Stimulant and sedative effects of alcohol," *Current Topics in Behavioral Neurosciences* 13 (May 2013): 489–509.

2. Sleep Science, "Does your body temperature change while you sleep? Learn how your temperature guides you to and from dreamland each night.," www.sleep.org/articles/does-your-body-temperature-change-while-you-sleep.

Chapter Ten: Moving for Wellness

1. J. Lakerveld, A. Loyen, N. Schotman, et al., "Sitting too much: a hierarchy of socio-demographic correlates," *Preventive Medicine* 101 (August 2017): 77–83.

2. I. M. Lee, E. J. Shiroma, F. Lobelo, et al., "Effect of physical inactivity on major non-communicable diseases worldwide: an analysis of burden of disease and life expectancy," *The Lancet* 380, no. 9838 (July 2012): 219–29.

3. D. Kilari, E. Soto-Perez-de-Celis, S. G. Mohile, et al., "Designing exercise clinical trials for older adults with cancer: recommendations from 2015 Cancer and Aging Research Group NCI U13 Meeting," *Journal of Geriatric Oncology* 7, no. 4 (July 2016): 293–304.

4. R. J. Maddock, G. A. Casazza, D. H. Fernandez, M. I. Maddock, "Acute modulation of cortical glutamate and gaba content by physical activity," *Journal of Neuroscience* 36, no. 8 (February 2016): 2449–57.

5. K. L. Szuhany, M. Bugatti, M. W. Otto, "A meta-analytic review of the effects of exercise on brain-derived neurotrophic factor," *Journal of Psychiatric Research* 60 (October 2015): 56–64.

6. F. S. Routledge, T. S. Campbell, J. A. McFetridge-Durdle, S. L. Bacon, "Improvements in heart rate variability with exercise therapy," *Canadian Journal of Cardiology* 26, no. 6 (June-July 2010): 303–12.

7. S. Gujral, H. Aizenstein, C. F. Reynolds, M. A. Butters, K. I. Erickson, "Exercise effects on depression: possible neural mechanisms," *General Hospital Psychiatry* 49 (November 2017): 2–10.

8. R. J. Maddock, G. A. Casazza, M. H. Buonocore, C. Tanase, "Vigorous exercise increases brain lactate and glx (glutamate+glutamine): a dynamic 1h-mrs study," *Neuroimage* 57, no. 4 (August 2011): 1324–30.

9. UC Davis Health Newletter, "This is your brain on exercise," February 23, 2016, www.ucdmc.ucdavis.edu/publish/news/newsroom/10798.

10. A. Loudin, "Can exercise cure depression and anxiety?," *Washington Post*, May 2016, www.washingtonpost.com/national/health-science/can-exercise-cure-depression-and-anxiety/2016/05/09/2a938914-ed2f-11e5-bc08-3e03a5b41910_story.html?utm_term=.4a0b43ae9271.

11. T. Carter, I. Morres, J. Repper, P. Callaghan, "Exercise for adolescents with depression: valued aspects and perceived change," *Journal of Psychiatric and Mental Health Nursing* 23, no. 1 (February 2016): 37–44.

12. P. D. Loprinzi, B. J. Cardinal, "Association between objectively-measured physical activity and sleep, NHANES 2005–2006," *Mental Health and Physical Activity* 4, no. 2 (December 2011): 65–69.

13. Y. Yamanaka, K.-i. Honma, S. Hashimoto, et al., "Effects of physical exercise on human circadian rhythms," *Sleep and Biological Rhythms* 4, no. 3 (September 2006): 199–206.

14. Oregon State University News and Research Communications, "Study: physical activity impacts overall quality of sleep," November 22, 2011, www.oregonstate.edu /ua/ncs/archives/2011/nov/study-physical-activity-impacts-overall-quality-sleep.

15. U. Ladabaum, A. Mannalithara, P. A. Myer, G. Singh, "Obesity, abdominal obesity, physical activity, and caloric intake in U.S. adults: 1988 to 2010," *American Journal of Medicine* 127, no. 8 (August 2014): 717–27.

16. B. Hanlon, M. J. Larson, B. W. Bailey, J. D. LeCheminant, "Neural response to pictures of food after exercise in normal-weight and obese women," *Medicine and Science in Sports and Exercise* 44, no. 10 (October 2012): 1864–70.

17. J. Thompson Coon, K. Boddy, K. Stein, et al., "Does participating in physical activity in outdoor natural environments have a greater effect on physical and mental well-being than physical activity indoors? a systematic review," *Environmental Science & Technology* 45, no. 5 (March 2011): 1761–72.

18. V. F. Gladwell, D. K. Brown, C. Wood, G. R. Sandercock, J. L. Barton, "The great outdoors: how a green exercise environment can benefit all," *Extreme Physiology & Medicine* 2 (January 2013): 3.

19. P. C. Hallal, L. B. Andersen, F. C. Bull, et al., "Global physical activity levels: surveillance progress, pitfalls, and prospects," *The Lancet* 380, no. 9838 (July 2012): 247–57.

20. B. J. Park, Y. Tsunetsugu, T. Kasetani, T. Kagawa, Y. Miyazaki, "The physiological effects of shinrin-yoku (taking in the forest atmosphere or forest bathing): evidence

from field experiments in 24 forests across Japan," *Environmental Health and Preventive Medicine* 15, no. 1 (January 2010): 18–26.

21. B. C. Focht, "Brief walks in outdoor and laboratory environments: effects on affective responses, enjoyment, and intentions to walk for exercise," *Research Quarterly for Exercise and Sport* 80, no. 3 (September 2009): 611–20.

22. S. A. Tabish, "Is diabetes becoming the biggest epidemic of the twenty-first century?," *International Journal of Health Sciences* 1, no. 2 (July 2007): v–viii.

23. Centers for Disease Control and Prevention, "New CDC report: more than 100 million Americans have diabetes or prediabetes," July 18, 2017, www.cdc.gov/media/releases/2017/p0718-diabetes-report.html.

24. National Heart Lung and Blood Institute, "Coronary heart disease risk factors," 2016, www.nhlbi.nih.gov/health/health-topics/topics/hd/atrisk.

25. H. J. Baer, R. J. Glynn, F. B. Hu, et al., "Risk factors for mortality in the Nurses' Health Study: a competing risks analysis," *American Journal of Epidemiology* 173, no. 3 (February 2011): 319–29.

26. L. Soares-Miranda, D. S. Siscovick, B. M. Psaty, W. T. Longstreth, Jr., D. Mozaffarian, "Physical activity and risk of coronary heart disease and stroke in older adults: the cardiovascular health study," *Circulation* 133, no. 2 (January 2016): 147–55.

27. P. A. Sheridan, H. A. Paich, J. Handy, et al., "Obesity is associated with impaired immune response to influenza vaccination in humans," *International Journal of Obesity (2005)* 36, no. 8 (August 2012): 1072–77.

28. F. S. Luppino, L. M. de Wit, P. F. Bouvy, et al., "Overweight, obesity, and depression: a systematic review and meta-analysis of longitudinal studies," *Archives of General Psychiatry* 67, no. 3 (March 2010): 220–29.

29. S. A. Shapses, L. C. Pop, Y. Wang, "Obesity is a concern for bone health with aging," *Nutrition Research* 39 (March 2017): 1–13.

30. M. J. Ormsbee, C. M. Prado, J. Z. Ilich, et al., "Osteosarcopenic obesity: the role of bone, muscle, and fat on health," *Journal of Cachexia, Sarcopenia, and Muscle* 5, no. 3 (September 2014): 183–92.

31. D. J. Tomlinson, R. M. Erskine, C. I. Morse, K. Winwood, G. Onambele-Pearson, "The impact of obesity on skeletal muscle strength and structure through adolescence to old age," *Biogerontology* 17, no. 3 (June 2016): 467–83.

32. S. F. M. Chastin, E. Ferriolli, N. A. Stephens, K. C. H. Fearon, C. Greig, "Relationship between sedentary behaviour, physical activity, muscle quality and body composition in healthy older adults," *Age and Ageing* 41, no. 1 (January 2012): 111–14.

33. J. C. Nguyen, A. S. Killcross, T. A. Jenkins, "Obesity and cognitive decline: role of inflammation and vascular changes," *Frontiers in Neuroscience* 8 (December 2014): 375.

34. T. Tchkonia, D. E. Morbeck, T. von Zglinicki, et al., "Fat tissue, aging, and cellular senescence," *Aging Cell* 9, no. 5 (May 2010): 667–84.

35. E. I. Fishman, J. A. Steeves, V. Zipunnikov, et al., "Association between objectively measured physical activity and mortality in NHANES," *Medicine & Science in Sports & Exercise* 48, no. 7 (July 2016): 1303–11.

36. C. M. Friedenreich, Q. Wang, H. K. Neilson, et al., "Physical activity and survival after prostate cancer," *European Urology* 70, no. 4 (October 2016): 576–85.

37. M. D. Holmes, W. Y. Chen, D. Feskanich, C. H. Kroenke, G. A. Colditz, "Physical activity and survival after breast cancer diagnosis," *Journal of the American Medical Association* 293, no. 20 (May 2005): 2479–86.

38. J. Goh, E. A. Kirk, S. X. Lee, W. C. Ladiges, "Exercise, physical activity and breast cancer: the role of tumor-associated macrophages," *Exercise Immunology Review* 18 (August 2012): 158–76.

39. C. E. Champ, L. Francis, R. J. Klement, R. Dickerman, R. P. Smith, "Fortifying the treatment of prostate cancer with physical activity," *Prostate Cancer* 2016 (January 2016): 11.

40. L. M. Buffart, J. Kalter, M. G. Sweegers, et al., "Effects and moderators of exercise on quality of life and physical function in patients with cancer: an individual patient data meta-analysis of 34 RCTs," *Cancer Treatment Reviews* 52, no. Supplement C (January 2017): 91–104.

41. K. S. Courneya, D. C. McKenzie, J. R. Mackey, et al., "Effects of exercise dose and type during breast cancer chemotherapy: multicenter randomized trial," *Journal of the National Cancer Institute* 105, no. 23 (December 2013): 1821–32.

42. A. S. Betof, C. D. Lascola, D. Weitzel, et al., "Modulation of murine breast tumor vascularity, hypoxia and chemotherapeutic response by exercise," *Journal of the National Cancer Institute* 107, no. 5 (May 2015).

43. S. C. Moore, I. M. Lee, E. Weiderpass, et al., "Association of leisure-time physical activity with risk of 26 types of cancer in 1.44 million adults," *Journal of the American Medical Association Internal Medicine* 176, no. 6 (June 2016): 816–25.

44. National Cancer Institute, "Physical activity and cancer," January 27, 2017, www.cancer.gov/about-cancer/causes-prevention/risk/obesity/physical-activity-fact-sheet.

45. K. Y. Wolin, Y. Yan, G. A. Colditz, I. M. Lee, "Physical activity and colon cancer prevention: a meta-analysis," *British Journal of Cancer* 100, no. 4 (February 2009): 611–16.

46. American Institute for Cancer Research, "Getting up from your desk can put the 'breaks' on cancer," November 3, 2011, www.aicr.org/press/press-releases/getting-up-from-your-desk.html.

47. Y. Wu, D. Zhang, S. Kang, "Physical activity and risk of breast cancer: a meta-analysis of prospective studies," *Breast Cancer Research and Treatment* 137, no. 3 (February 2013): 869–82.

48. A. H. Eliassen, S. E. Hankinson, B. Rosner, M. D. Holmes, W. C. Willett, "Physical activity and risk of breast cancer among postmenopausal women," *Archives of Internal Medicine* 170, no. 19 (October 2010): 1758–64.

49. J. S. Hildebrand, S. M. Gapstur, P. T. Campbell, M. M. Gaudet, A. V. Patel, "Recreational physical activity and leisure-time sitting in relation to postmenopausal breast cancer risk," *Cancer Epidemiology, Biomarkers & Prevention* 22, no. 10 (October 2013): 1906–12.

50. A. Fournier, G. Dos Santos, G. Guillas, et al., "Recent recreational physical activity and breast cancer risk in postmenopausal women in the E3N cohort," *Cancer Epidemiology, Biomarkers & Prevention* 23, no. 9 (September 2014): 1893–1902.

51. D. Schmid, G. Behrens, M. Keimling, et al., "A systematic review and meta-analysis of physical activity and endometrial cancer risk," *European Journal of Epidemiology* 30, no. 5 (May 2015): 397–412.

52. M. Du, P. Kraft, A. H. Eliassen, et al., "Physical activity and risk of endometrial adenocarcinoma in the Nurses' Health Study," *International Journal of Cancer* 134, no. 11 (June 2014): 2707–16.

53. C. Friedenreich, A. Cust, P. H. Lahmann, et al., "Physical activity and risk of endometrial cancer: the European prospective investigation into cancer and nutrition," *International Journal of Cancer* 121, no. 2 (July 2007): 347–55.

54. K. S. Courneya, C. M. Friedenreich, R. D. Reid, et al., "Predictors of follow-up exercise behavior 6 months after a randomized trial of exercise training during breast cancer chemotherapy," *Breast Cancer Research and Treatment* 114, no. 1 (March 2009): 179–87.

55. K. S. Courneya, D. C. McKenzie, J. R. Mackey, et al., "Moderators of the effects of exercise training in breast cancer patients receiving chemotherapy: a randomized controlled trial," *Cancer* 112, no. 8 (April 2008): 1845–53.

56. R. Ballard-Barbash, C. M. Friedenreich, K. S. Courneya, et al., "Physical activity, biomarkers, and disease outcomes in cancer survivors: a systematic review," *Journal of the National Cancer Institute* 104, no. 11 (June 2012): 815–40.

57. K. M. Mustian, C. M. Alfano, C. Heckler, et al., "Comparison of pharmaceutical, psychological, and exercise treatments for cancer-related fatigue: a meta-analysis," *Journal of the American Medical Association Oncology* 3, no. 7 (July 2017): 961–68.

58. M. G. Sweegers, T. M. Altenburg, M. J. Chinapaw, et al., "Which exercise prescriptions improve quality of life and physical function in patients with cancer during and following treatment? A systematic review and meta-analysis of randomised controlled trials," *British Journal of Sports Medicine* (September 2017).

59. C. M. Friedenreich, H. K. Neilson, M. S. Farris, K. S. Courneya, "Physical activity and cancer outcomes: a precision medicine approach," *Clinical Cancer Research* 22, no. 19 (October 2016): 4766–75.

60. W. Demark-Wahnefried, E. A. Platz, J. A. Ligibel, et al., "The role of obesity in cancer survival and recurrence," *Cancer Epidemiology, Biomarkers & Prevention* 21, no. 8 (June 2012): 1244–59.

61. H. Arem, S. C. Moore, Y. Park, et al., "Physical activity and cancer-specific mortality in the NIH-AARP Diet and Health Study cohort," *International Journal of Cancer* 135, no. 2 (July 2014): 423–31.

62. S. E. Bonn, A. Sjolander, Y. T. Lagerros, et al., "Physical activity and survival among men diagnosed with prostate cancer," *Cancer Epidemiology, Biomarkers & Prevention* 24, no. 1 (January 2015): 57–64.

63. H. Arem, R. M. Pfeiffer, E. A. Engels, et al., "Pre- and postdiagnosis physical activity, television viewing, and mortality among patients with colorectal cancer in the National Institutes of Health-AARP Diet and Health Study," *Journal of Clinical Oncology* 33, no. 2 (January 2015): 180–88.

64. M. Fitzmaurice, "Exercising key to cancer battle, world expert tells Ulster University," December 7, 2015, www.belfastlive.co.uk/news/health/exercising-key-cancer-battle-world-10564610.

65. H. K. Sanoff, A. M. Deal, J. Krishnamurthy, et al., "Effect of cytotoxic chemotherapy on markers of molecular age in patients with breast cancer," *Journal of the National Cancer Institute* 106, no. 4 (April 2014): dju057.

66. L. W. Jones, L. A. Habel, E. Weltzien, et al., "Exercise and risk of cardiovascular events in women with nonmetastatic breast cancer," *Journal of Clinical Oncology* 34, no. 23 (August 2016): 2743–49.

67. L. W. Jones, D. R. Fels, M. West, et al., "Modulation of circulating angiogenic factors and tumor biology by aerobic training in breast cancer patients receiving neoadjuvant chemotherapy," *Cancer Prevention Research* 6, no. 9 (September 2013): 925–37.

68. W. E. Hornsby, P. S. Douglas, M. J. West, et al., "Safety and efficacy of aerobic training in operable breast cancer patients receiving neoadjuvant chemotherapy: a phase ii randomized trial," *Acta Oncologica* 53, no. 1 (January 2014): 65–74.

69. J. F. Meneses-Echavez, E. G. Jimenez, J. S. Rio-Valle, et al., "The insulin-like growth factor system is modulated by exercise in breast cancer survivors: a systematic review and meta-analysis," *BMC Cancer* 16, no. 1 (August 2016): 682.

70. J. F. Meneses-Echavez, J. E. Correa-Bautista, E. Gonzalez-Jimenez, et al., "The effect of exercise training on mediators of inflammation in breast cancer survivors: a systematic review with meta-analysis," *Cancer Epidemiology, Biomarkers & Prevention* 25, no. 7 (July 2016): 1009–17.

71. R. Ballard-Barbash, C. M. Friedenreich, K. S. Courneya, et al., "Physical activity, biomarkers, and disease outcomes in cancer survivors: a systematic review," *Journal of the National Cancer Institute* 104, no. 11 (June 2012): 815–40.

72. A. Ruiz-Casado, A. Martin-Ruiz, L. M. Perez, et al., "Exercise and the hallmarks of cancer," *Trends Cancer* 3, no. 6 (June 2017): 423–41.

73. G. J. Koelwyn, D. F. Quail, X. Zhang, R. M. White, L. W. Jones, "Exercise-dependent regulation of the tumour microenvironment," *Nature Reviews: Cancer* 17, no. 10 (September 2017): 620–32.

74. G. J. Koelwyn, E. Wennerberg, S. Demaria, L. W. Jones, "Exercise in regulation of inflammation-immune axis function in cancer initiation and progression," *Oncology* 29, no. 12 (December 2015): 908–20, 922.

75. O. K. Glass, B. A. Inman, G. Broadwater, et al., "Effect of aerobic training on the host systemic milieu in patients with solid tumours: an exploratory correlative study," *British Journal of Cancer* 112, no. 5 (March 2015): 825–31.

76. M. J. M. Magbanua, E. L. Richman, E. V. Sosa, et al., "Physical activity and prostate gene expression in men with low risk prostate cancer," *Cancer Causes & Control* 25, no. 4 (February 2014): 515–23.

77. M. E. Lindholm, F. Marabita, D. Gomez-Cabrero, et al., "An integrative analysis reveals coordinated reprogramming of the epigenome and the transcriptome in human skeletal muscle after training," *Epigenetics* 9, no. 12 (December 2014): 1557–69.

78. K. A. Ashcraft, R. M. Peace, A. S. Betof, M. W. Dewhirst, L. W. Jones, "Efficacy and mechanisms of aerobic exercise on cancer initiation, progression, and metastasis: a critical systematic review of in vivo preclinical data," *Cancer Research* 76, no. 14 (July 2016): 4032–50.

79. V. K. Verma, V. Singh, M. P. Singh, S. M. Singh, "Effect of physical exercise on tumor growth regulating factors of tumor microenvironment: Implications in exercise-dependent tumor growth retardation," *Immunopharmacology and Immunotoxicology* 31, no. 2 (June 2009): 274–82.

80. L. W. Jones, B. L. Viglianti, J. A. Tashjian, et al., "Effect of aerobic exercise on tumor physiology in an animal model of human breast cancer," *Journal of Applied Physiology* 108, no. 2 (February 2010): 343–48.

81. G. J. Koelwyn, D. F. Quail, X. Zhang, R. M. White, L. W. Jones, "Exercise-dependent regulation of the tumour microenvironment," *Nature Reviews: Cancer* 17, no. 10 (September 2017): 620–32.

82. Dialogue Blog from the Wilmot Cancer Institute, "Exercise and cancer research: Setting new standards, giving patients control," June 19, 2017, www.urmc.rochester.edu/cancer-institute/newsroom/dialogue-blog/june-2017/exercise-and-cancerresearch-settingnew-standard.aspx.

83. K. M. Mustian, L. K. Sprod, M. Janelsins, L. J. Peppone, S. Mohile, "Exercise recommendations for cancer-related fatigue, cognitive impairment, sleep problems, depression, pain, anxiety, and physical dysfunction: a review," *Oncolology Hematology Review* 8, no. 2 (January 2012): 81–88.

84. K. M. Mustian, J. A. Katula, H. Zhao, "A pilot study to assess the influence of tai chi chuan on functional capacity among breast cancer survivors," *Journal of Supportive Oncology* 4, no. 3 (March 2006): 139–45.

85. K. M. Mustian, O. G. Palesh, S. A. Flecksteiner, "Tai chi chuan for breast cancer survivors," *Medicine and Sport Science* 52 (May 2008): 209–17.

86. L. K. Sprod, I. D. Fernandez, M. C. Janelsins, et al., "Effects of yoga on cancer-related fatigue and global side-effect burden in older cancer survivors," *Journal of Geriatric Oncology* 6, no. 1 (January 2015): 8–14.

87. K. M. Mustian, L. K. Sprod, M. Janelsins, et al., "Multicenter, randomized controlled trial of yoga for sleep quality among cancer survivors," *Journal of Clinical Oncology* 31, no. 26 (September 2013): 3233–41.

88. B. Oh, P. N. Butow, B. A. Mullan, et al., "Effect of medical qigong on cognitive function, quality of life, and a biomarker of inflammation in cancer patients: a randomized controlled trial," *Supportive Care in Cancer* 20, no. 6 (June 2012): 1235–42.

89. B. Oh, P. Butow, B. Mullan, et al., "A critical review of the effects of medical qigong on quality of life, immune function, and survival in cancer patients," *Integrative Cancer Therapies* 11, no. 2 (June 2012): 101–10.

90. K. M. Mustian, L. Peppone, T. V. Darling, et al., "A 4-week home-based aerobic and resistance exercise program during radiation therapy: a pilot randomized clinical trial," *Journal of Supportive Oncology* 7, no. 5 (September–October 2009): 158–67.

91. National Comprehensive Cancer Network (NCCN), "Exercising during cancer treatment," 2017, www.nccn.org/patients/resources/life_with_cancer/exercise.aspx.

92. L. W. Jones, "Precision oncology framework for investigation of exercise as treatment for cancer," *Journal of Clinical Oncology* 33, no. 35 (December 2015): 4134–37.

93. D. Cohan, "Foundation for embodied medicine," 2017, www.embodiedmedicine.org

94. O. H. Zahrt, A. J. Crum, "Perceived physical activity and mortality: evidence from three nationally representative U.S. Samples," *Health Psychology* 36, no. 11 (November 2017): 1017–25.

95. D. Buettner, *The Blue Zones: 9 Lessons for Living Longer from the People Who've Lived the Longest* (Washington, D.C.: National Geographic, 2012).

96. American Cancer Society, "ACS guidelines on nutrition and physical activity for cancer prevention," February 5, 2016, www.cancer.org/healthy/eat-healthy-get -active/acs-guidelines-nutrition-physical-activity-cancer-prevention.html.

97. For a great book on this topic, see G. Reynolds, *The First 20 Minutes: Surprising Science Reveals How We Can Exercise Better, Train Smarter, Live Longer* (New York: Penguin, 2013).

98. J. B. Gillen, B. J. Martin, M. J. MacInnis, et al., "Twelve weeks of sprint interval training improves indices of cardiometabolic health similar to traditional endurance training despite a five-fold lower exercise volume and time commitment," *PloS One* 11, no. 4 (April 2016): e0154075.

99. D. M. Bhammar, S. S. Angadi, G. A. Gaesser, "Effects of fractionized and continuous exercise on 24-h ambulatory blood pressure," *Medicine and Science in Sports and Exercise* 44, no. 12 (December 2012): 2270–76.

100. B. M. F. M. Duvivier, N. C. Schaper, M. A. Bremers, et al., "Minimal intensity physical activity (standing and walking) of longer duration improves insulin action and plasma lipids more than shorter periods of moderate to vigorous exercise (cycling) in sedentary subjects when energy expenditure is comparable," *PloS One* 8, no. 2 (February 2013): e55542.

101. E. I. Fishman, J. A. Steeves, V. Zipunnikov, et al., "Association between objectively measured physical activity and mortality in nhanes," *Medicine and Science in Sports and Exercise* 48, no. 7 (July 2016): 1303–11.

102. L. Liu, Y. Shi, T. Li, et al., "Leisure time physical activity and cancer risk: evaluation of the WHO's recommendation based on 126 high-quality epidemiological studies," *British Journal of Sports Medicine* 50, no. 6 (March 2016): 372.

103. C. M. Phillips, C. B. Dillon, I. J. Perry, "Does replacing sedentary behaviour with light or moderate to vigorous physical activity modulate inflammatory status in adults?," *International Journal of Behavioral Nutrition and Physical Activity* 14 (October 2017): 138.

104. H. Arem, S. C. Moore, A. Patel, et al., "Leisure time physical activity and mortality: a detailed pooled analysis of the dose-response relationship," *Journal of the American Medical Association Internal Medicine* 175, no. 6 (June 2015): 959–67.

105. G. Canales, "Blue Cure," July 11, 2013, www.bluecure.org/gabe-canales.

Chapter Eleven: Food as Medicine

1. U.S. Department of Health and Human Services and U.S. Department of Agriculture," 2015–2020 dietary guidelines for Americans, 8th ed.," December 2015, www .health.gov/dietaryguidelines/2015/guidelines.

2. M. H. Carlsen, B. L. Halvorsen, K. Holte, et al., "The total antioxidant content of more than 3100 foods, beverages, spices, herbs and supplements used worldwide," *Nutrition Journal* 9 (January 2010): 3.

3. M. Greger, "Antioxidant content of 3,139 foods," www.nutritionfacts.org/video /antioxidant-content-of-3139-foods.

4. G. Diesing, "How a rooftop garden, local farming helped one hospital boost patient satisfaction," June 6, 2016, www.hhnmag.com/articles/7218-how-a-rooftop-garden -local-farming-helped-one-hospital-boost-patient-satisfaction.

5. D. M. Klurfeld, D. Kritchevsky, "The Western diet: an examination of its relationship with chronic disease," *Journal of the American College of Nutrition* 5, no. 5 (January 1986): 477–85.

6. A. Jemal, M. M. Center, C. DeSantis, E. M. Ward, "Global patterns of cancer incidence and mortality rates and trends," *Cancer Epidemiology, Biomarkers & Prevention* 19, no. 8 (August 2010): 1893–07.

7. L. Sharp, D. Donnelly, A. Hegarty, et al., "Risk of several cancers is higher in urban areas after adjusting for socioeconomic status. Results from a two-country population-based study of 18 common cancers," *Journal of Urban Health: Bulletin of the New York Academy of Medicine* 91, no. 3 (January 2014): 510–25.

8. L. A. Torre, R. L. Siegel, E. M. Ward, A. Jemal, "Global cancer incidence and mortality rates and trends—an update," *Cancer Epidemiology, Biomarkers & Prevention* 25, no. 1 (January 2016): 16–27.

9. S. J. D. O'Keefe, J. V. Li, L. Lahti, et al., "Fat, fiber and cancer risk in African Americans and rural Africans," *Nature Communications* 6 (April 2015): 6342.

10. Y. Fan, X. Jin, C. Man, Z. Gao, X. Wang, "Meta-analysis of the association between the inflammatory potential of diet and colorectal cancer risk," *Oncotarget* 8, no. 35 (August 2017): 59592–600.

11. Human Microbiome Project Consortium, "A framework for human microbiome research," *Nature* 486, no. 7402 (June 2012a): 215–21.

12. P. J. Turnbaugh, R. E. Ley, M. Hamady, et al., "The human microbiome project: exploring the microbial part of ourselves in a changing world," *Nature* 449, no. 7164 (October 2007): 804.

13. National Human Genome Research Institute, "The Human Genome Project," October 1, 2015, www.genome.gov/10001772/all-about-the-human-genome-project-hgp.

14. A. B. Hall, A. C. Tolonen, R. J. Xavier, "Human genetic variation and the gut microbiome in disease," *Nature Reviews: Genetics* 18, no. 11 (November 2017): 690–99.

15. A. B. Shreiner, J. Y. Kao, V. B. Young, "The gut microbiome in health and in disease," *Current Opinion in Gastroenterology* 31, no. 1 (January 2015): 69–75.

16. Institute of Medicine (US) Food Forum, "Influence of the Microbiome on the Metabolism of Diet and Dietary Components," in *The Human Microbiome, Diet, and Health: Workshop Summary* (Washington, D.C.: National Academies Press, 2013).

17. W. S. Garrett, "Cancer and the microbiota," *Science* 348, no. 6230 (April 2015): 80–86.

18. J. A. Segre, "MICROBIOME. Microbial growth dynamics and human disease," *Science* 349, no. 6252 (September 2015): 1058–59.

19. L. Zitvogel, M. Ayyoub, B. Routy, G. Kroemer, "Microbiome and anticancer immunosurveillance," *Cell* 165, no. 2 (April 2016): 276–87.

20. R. F. Schwabe, C. Jobin, "The microbiome and cancer," *Nature Reviews: Cancer* 13, no. 11 (October 2013): 800–12.

21. More details on the microbiome: In some cases the specific bacterial species are better understood and characterized. For example, in colon cancer patients the bacterial diversity was similar or slightly reduced in cancer patients compared to matched controls, and the composition of the microbiome was commonly driven by high prevalence and levels of fusobacterium and porphyromonas, as well as lower levels of ruminococcus in feces from colon cancer patients. However, because these and other studies are observational studies, the link between the microbiome as a causative factor remains unclear in human studies.

22. R. Francescone, V. Hou, S. I. Grivennikov, "Microbiome, inflammation and cancer," *Cancer Journal* 20, no. 3 (May–June 2014): 181–89.

23. S. V. Rajagopala, S. Vashee, L. M. Oldfield, et al., "The human microbiome and cancer," *Cancer Prevention Research* 10, no. 4 (April 2017): 226–34.

24. N. Shi, N. Li, X. Duan, H. Niu, "Interaction between the gut microbiome and mucosal immune system," *Military Medical Research* 4 (May 2017): 14.

25. Y. Belkaid, Timothy W. Hand, "Role of the microbiota in immunity and inflammation," *Cell* 157, no. 1 (March 2014): 121–41.

26. H. J. Wu, E. Wu, "The role of gut microbiota in immune homeostasis and autoimmunity," *Gut Microbes* 3, no. 1 (January–February 2012): 4–14.

27. V. Gopalakrishnan, C. N. Spencer, L. Nezi, et al., "Gut microbiome modulates response to anti-PD-1 immunotherapy in melanoma patients," *Science* (November 2017).

28. M. Glick-Bauer, M.-C. Yeh, "The health advantage of a vegan diet: exploring the gut microbiota connection," *Nutrients* 6, no. 11 (October 2014): 4822–38.

29. J. L. Sonnenburg, F. Backhed, "Diet-microbiota interactions as moderators of human metabolism," *Nature* 535, no. 7610 (July 2016): 56–64.

30. V. K. Ridaura, J. J. Faith, F. E. Rey, et al., "Gut microbiota from twins discordant for obesity modulate metabolism in mice," *Science* 341, no. 6150 (September 2013): 1241214.

31. D. Servan-Schreiber, *Anticancer: A New Way of Life* (New York: Viking, 2009).

32. Y. Barak, D. Fridman, "Impact of mediterranean diet on cancer: focused literature review," *Cancer Genomics & Proteomics* 14, no. 6 (November–December 2017): 403–8.

33. L. Schwingshackl, C. Schwedhelm, C. Galbete, G. Hoffmann, "Adherence to mediterranean diet and risk of cancer: an updated systematic review and meta-analysis," *Nutrients* 9, no. 10 (September 2017).

34. L. Schwingshackl, G. Hoffmann, "Does a Mediterranean-type diet reduce cancer risk?," *Current Nutrition Reports* 5 (September 2016): 9–17.

35. H. E. Bloomfield, E. Koeller, N. Greer, et al., "Effects on health outcomes of a Mediterranean diet with no restriction on fat intake: a systematic review and meta-analysis," *Annals of Internal Medicine* 165, no. 7 (October 2016): 491–500.

36. M. Dinu, G. Pagliai, A. Casini, F. Sofi, "Mediterranean diet and multiple health outcomes: an umbrella review of meta-analyses of observational studies and randomised trials," *European Journal of Clinical Nutrition* (May 2017).

37. Y. S. Aridi, J. L. Walker, O. R. L. Wright, "The association between the Mediterranean dietary pattern and cognitive health: a systematic review," *Nutrients* 9, no. 7 (June 2017).

38. M. Filomeno, C. Bosetti, E. Bidoli, et al., "Mediterranean diet and risk of endometrial cancer: a pooled analysis of three Italian case-control studies," *British Journal of Cancer* 112, no. 11 (May 2015): 1816–21.

39. P. A. van den Brandt, M. Schulpen, "Mediterranean diet adherence and risk of postmenopausal breast cancer: results of a cohort study and meta-analysis," *International Journal of Cancer* 140, no. 10 (May 2017): 2220–31.

40. National Cancer Institute, "Vitamin D and cancer prevention," October 21, 2013, www.cancer.gov/about-cancer/causes-prevention/risk/diet/vitamin-d-fact-sheet.
41. D. Aune, E. Giovannucci, P. Boffetta, et al., "Fruit and vegetable intake and the risk of cardiovascular disease, total cancer and all-cause mortality—a systematic review and dose-response meta-analysis of prospective studies," *International Journal of Epidemiology* 46, no. 3 (June 2017): 1029–56.
42. H. R. Harris, W. C. Willett, R. L. Vaidya, K. B. Michels, "An adolescent and early adulthood dietary pattern associated with inflammation and the incidence of breast cancer," *Cancer Research* 77, no. 5 (March 2017): 1179–87.
43. R. Estruch, E. Ros, J. Salas-Salvadó, et al., "Primary prevention of cardiovascular disease with a Mediterranean diet," *New England Journal of Medicine* 368, no. 14 (April 2013): 1279–90.
44. E. Toledo, F. B. Hu, R. Estruch, et al., "Effect of the Mediterranean diet on blood pressure in the PREDIMED trial: results from a randomized controlled trial," *BMC Medicine* 11 (September 2013): 207.
45. R. Estruch, "Anti-inflammatory effects of the Mediterranean diet: the experience of the PREDIMED study," *Proceedings of the Nutrition Society* 69, no. 3 (August 2010): 333 40.
46. J. Salas-Salvado, M. Bullo, N. Babio, et al., "Reduction in the incidence of type 2 diabetes with the Mediterranean diet: results of the PREDIMED-Reus nutrition intervention randomized trial," *Diabetes Care* 34, no. 1 (January 2011): 14–19.
47. N. Babio, E. Toledo, R. Estruch, et al., "Mediterranean diets and metabolic syndrome status in the PREDIMED randomized trial," *CMAJ : Canadian Medical Association Journal* 186, no. 17 (November 2014): E649–57.
48. E. Toledo, J. Salas-Salvado, C. Donat-Vargas, et al., "Mediterranean diet and invasive breast cancer risk among women at high cardiovascular risk in the PREDIMED trial: a randomized clinical trial," *Journal of the American Medical Association Internal Medicine* 175, no. 11 (November 2015): 1752–60.
49. More details on the Mediterranean diet: A placebo-controlled trial published in August 2017 of 10,061 patients with previous myocardial infarction and high C-reactive protein levels found that a drug that blocks inflammation, in this case blocking interleukin-1β—a part of our innate immune system—resulted in fewer cardiovascular events that was driven by reductions in CRP and not changes in lipid levels. Planned secondary analyses also found that cancer mortality was lower in the patients who were getting the anti-inflammatory drug, including reduced incidence of lung cancer and lung-cancer-related deaths. The provocative findings from this trial suggest that inflammation may be a common pathway linked to both cardiovascular disease and cancer. However, fatal infections or sepsis were significantly more common in the drug groups than in the placebo group, a side effect you will not have from eating a Mediterranean diet.
50. M. Yang, S. A. Kenfield, E. L. Van Blarigan, et al., "Dietary patterns after prostate cancer diagnosis in relation to disease-specific and total mortality," *Cancer Prevention Research* 8, no. 6 (June 2015): 545–51.
51. M. S. Donaldson, "Nutrition and cancer: a review of the evidence for an anti-cancer diet," *Nutrition Journal* 3, no. 1 (October 2004): 19.
52. D. Aune, N. Keum, E. Giovannucci, et al., "Whole grain consumption and risk of cardiovascular disease, cancer, and all cause and cause specific mortality: systematic review and dose-response meta-analysis of prospective studies," *British Medical Journal* 353 (June 2016): i2716.
53. G. Zong, A. Gao, F. B. Hu, Q. Sun, "Whole grain intake and mortality from all causes, cardiovascular disease, and cancer: a meta-analysis of prospective cohort studies," *Circulation* 133, no. 24 (June 2016): 2370–80.

54. More details on fiber: A meta-analysis published in 2016 that looked at fourteen long-term studies found that people who ate the most whole grains were 10 percent less likely to die of cancer. For every additional serving of whole grains, their cancer risk declined by an additional 5 percent (G. Zong, A. Gao, F. B. Hu, Q. Sun, "Whole grain intake and mortality from all causes, cardiovascular disease, and cancer: a meta-analysis of prospective cohort studies," *Circulation* 133, no. 24 [June 2016]: 2370–80).

The growing international concern about gluten sensitivity and intolerance has blossomed in the past ten years. Almost one in three American consumers now say they hope to cut back on the gluten in their diet. The market has responded to this perceived need with gluten-free food sales that topped $15 billion in 2016. Even products that never had gluten, like potato chips and popcorn, are now advertising their products as "gluten free." But what is the scientific evidence that gluten is the culprit behind concerns about digestive health?

My Florentine-based colleague Francesco Sofi, who works at the Careggie University Hospital in Florence, Italy, did not want to give up his wheat pasta, so he started researching the effects of ancient wheat compared to modern wheat. In one study, he found that organically grown khorasan wheat resulted in not only improved symptoms in those suffering from irritable bowel disease, but also a marked decrease in the inflammatory profile (F. Sofi, A. Whittaker, A. M. Gori, et al., "Effect of Triticum turgidum subsp. turanicum wheat on irritable bowel syndrome: a double-blinded randomised dietary intervention trial," *British Journal of Nutrition* 111, no. 11 [June 14, 2014]: 1992–99). Study participants who ate the ancient grain, which has kernels that contain more proteins, lipids, vitamins, minerals, and amino acids than modern wheat, had reductions in circulating levels of pro-inflammatory cytokines (including IL-6, IL-17, interferon-gama), monocyte chemotactic protein-1, and vascular endothelial growth factor, or VEGF. Inflammation and VEGF are both linked with key cancer hallmarks. In fact, inflammation itself has been labeled a cancer hallmark by some because it is increasingly clear that chronic inflammation increases cancer risk.

Francesco and his colleagues have conducted numerous trials comparing the effects of ancient versus modern wheat using randomized, controlled, blinded, cross-over design clinical trials. They have found benefits of ancient wheat and buckwheat for cardiovascular, diabetes, and inflammatory risk markers in both patient populations and healthy individuals (A. Whittaker, F. Sofi, M. L. Luisi, et al., "An organic khorasan wheat-based replacement diet improves risk profile of patients with acute coronary syndrome: a randomized crossover trial," *Nutrients* 7, no. 5 [May 11 2015]: 3401–15; A. Whittaker, M. Dinu, F. Cesari, et al., "A khorasan wheat-based replacement diet improves risk profile of patients with type 2 diabetes mellitus [T2DM]: a randomized crossover trial," *European Journal of Nutrition* 56, no. 3 [April 2017]: 1191–1200; A. Sereni, F. Cesari, A. M. Gori, et al., "Cardiovascular benefits from ancient grain bread consumption: findings from a double-blinded randomized crossover intervention trial," *International Journal of Food, Science, and Nutrition* 68, no. 1 [February 2017]: 97–103). Even comparing semi-whole-wheat ancient grains, which have a lower gluten content and increased bran and germ components, to semi-whole-wheat modern grains revealed substantially better biological profile for those eating the ancient grains. Ancient grains are naturally more nutritious and do not need the fortification that we see is necessary for modern wheat strains. So, for those who do not want to go totally gluten free but want to reduce the gluten content of your flour, try some of these ancient grains. For those going totally gluten free, you need to know that gluten-free grains are not always fortified with vitamins and iron and they often lack the fiber and phytochemicals of whole grains. It is therefore important to ensure you are getting these important nutrients through other parts of your diet.

55. A. M. Mileo, S. Miccadei, "Polyphenols as modulator of oxidative stress in cancer disease: new therapeutic strategies," *Oxidative Medicine and Cellular Longevity* 2016 (December 2016): 17.

56. M. H. Carlsen, B. L. Halvorsen, K. Holte, et al., "The total antioxidant content of more than 3100 foods, beverages, spices, herbs and supplements used worldwide," *Nutrition Journal* (January 2010): 3.

57. D. Boivin, S. Lamy, S. Lord-Dufour, et al., "Antiproliferative and antioxidant activities of common vegetables: a comparative study," *Food Chemistry* 112, no. 2 (January 2009): 374–80.

58. J. V. Higdon, B. Delage, D. E. Williams, R. H. Dashwood, "Cruciferous vegetables and human cancer risk: epidemiologic evidence and mechanistic basis," *Pharmacological Research* 55, no. 3 (January 2007): 224–36.

59. H. Wang, T. O. Khor, L. Shu, et al., "Plants against cancer: a review on natural phytochemicals in preventing and treating cancers and their druggability," *Anti-Cancer Agents in Medicinal Chemistry* 12, no. 10 (2012): 1281–1305.

60. T. M. Hardy, T. O. Tollefsbol, "Epigenetic diet: impact on the epigenome and cancer," *Epigenomics* 3, no. 4 (August 2011): 503 18.

61. G. Tse, G. D. Eslick, "Cruciferous vegetables and risk of colorectal neoplasms: a systematic review and meta-analysis," *Nutrition and Cancer* 66, no. 1 (December 2014): 128–39.

62. M. J. Clark, K. Robien, J. L. Slavin, "Effect of prebiotics on biomarkers of colorectal cancer in humans: a systematic review," *Nutrition Reviews* 70, no. 8 (August 2012): 436–43.

63. A. S. Tsao, D. Liu, J. Martin, et al., "Phase II randomized, placebo-controlled trial of green tea extract in patients with high-risk oral premalignant lesions," *Cancer Prevention Research* 2, no. 11 (November 2009): 931–41.

64. J. V. Heymach, T. J. Shackleford, H. T. Tran, et al., "Effect of low-fat diets on plasma levels of NF-kappaB-regulated inflammatory cytokines and angiogenic factors in men with prostate cancer," *Cancer Prevention Research* 4, no. 10 (October 2011): 1590–98.

65. J. Shi, L. Xiong, J. Li, et al., "A linear dose-response relationship between fasting plasma glucose and colorectal cancer risk: systematic review and meta-analysis," *Scientific Reports* 5 (December 2015): 17591.

66. T. J. Hartman, P. S. Albert, Z. Zhang, et al., "Consumption of a legume-enriched, low-glycemic index diet is associated with biomarkers of insulin resistance and inflammation among men at risk for colorectal cancer," *Journal of Nutrition* 140, no. 1 (January 2010): 60–67.

67. S. Aiko, I. Kumano, N. Yamanaka, et al., "Effects of an immuno-enhanced diet containing antioxidants in esophageal cancer surgery following neoadjuvant therapy," *Diseases of the Esophagus* 25, no. 2 (February 2012): 137–45.

68. S. S. Percival, J. P. Vanden Heuvel, C. J. Nieves, et al., "Bioavailability of herbs and spices in humans as determined by ex vivo inflammatory suppression and DNA strand breaks," *Journal of the American College of Nutrition* 31, no. 4 (August 2012): 28–94.

69. Z. Zhang, L. L. Atwell, P. E. Farris, E. Ho, J. Shannon, "Associations between cruciferous vegetable intake and selected biomarkers among women scheduled for breast biopsies," *Public Health Nutrition* 19, no. 7 (May 2016): 1288–95.

70. Y. Hu, G. H. McIntosh, R. K. Le Leu, et al., "Supplementation with Brazil nuts and green tea extract regulates targeted biomarkers related to colorectal cancer risk in humans," *British Journal of Nutrition* 116, no. 11 (December 2016): 1901–11.

71. C. S. Charron, H. D. Dawson, G. P. Albaugh, et al., "A single meal containing raw, crushed garlic influences expression of immunity- and cancer-related genes in whole blood of humans," *Journal of Nutrition* 145, no. 11 (November 2015): 2448–55.

72. M. Principi, A. Di Leo, M. Pricci, et al., "Phytoestrogens/insoluble fibers and colonic estrogen receptor β: randomized, double-blind, placebo-controlled study," *World Journal of Gastroenterology* 19, no. 27 (July 2013): 4325–33.

73. D. Trudel, D. P. Labbe, I. Bairati, et al., "Green tea for ovarian cancer prevention and treatment: a systematic review of the in vitro, in vivo and epidemiological studies," *Gynecologic Oncology* 126, no. 3 (September 2012): 491–98.

74. P. Chen, W. Zhang, X. Wang, et al., "Lycopene and risk of prostate cancer: a systematic review and meta-analysis," *Medicine* 94, no. 33 (August 2015): e1260.

75. E. C. Borresen, D. G. Brown, G. Harbison, et al., "A randomized controlled trial to increase navy bean or rice bran consumption in colorectal cancer survivors," *Nutrition and Cancer* 68, no. 8 (November–December 2016): 1269–80.

76. S. G. J. van Breda, E. van Agen, S. van Sanden, et al., "Vegetables affect the expression of genes involved in anticarcinogenic processes in the colonic mucosa of c57bl/6 female mice," *The Journal of Nutrition* 135, no. 8 (August 2005): 1879–88.

77. J. A. Meyerhardt, D. Niedzwiecki, D. Hollis, et al., "Association of dietary patterns with cancer recurrence and survival in patients with stage III colon cancer," *Journal of the American Medical Association* 298, no 7 (August 2007): 754–64.

78. D. Buettner, *The Blue Zones: 9 Lessons for Living Longer from the People Who've Lived the Longest* (Washington, D.C.: National Geographic, 2012).

79. Centers for Disease Control and Prevention, "Cancer and obesity," October 3, 2017, www.cdc.gov/vitalsigns/obesity-cancer/index.html.

80. G. M. Massetti, W. H. Dietz, L. C. Richardson, "Excessive weight gain, obesity, and cancer: opportunities for clinical intervention," *Journal of the American Medical Association* 318, no. 20 (November 2017): 1975–76.

81. American Institute for Cancer Research, "Obesity and cancer risk," 2017, www.aicr.org/reduce-your-cancer-risk/weight/reduce_weight_cancer_link.html.

82. National Cancer Institute, "Obesity and cancer," January 17, 2017, www.cancer.gov/about-cancer/causes-prevention/risk/obesity/obesity-fact-sheet.

83. K. Rtveladze, T. Marsh, L. Webber, et al., "Health and economic burden of obesity in Brazil," *PloS One* 8, no. 7 (July 2013): e68785.

84. F. Bray, I. Soerjomataram, "The changing global burden of cancer: transitions in human development and implications for cancer prevention and control," in *Cancer: Disease Control Priorities*, 3rd ed., eds. H. Gelband, P. Jha, and R. Sankaranrayanan, et al. (Washington, D.C.: The International Bank for Reconstruction and Development/The World Bank, 2015).

85. National Cancer Institute, "Study forecasts new breast cancer cases by 2030," April 23, 2015, www.cancer.gov/news-events/cancer-currents-blog/2015/breast-forecast.

86. American Institute for Cancer Research, "2017 AICR Cancer Risk Awareness Survey Report," 2017, www.vcloud.aicr.org/index.php/s/C6Q18hBpSQrukkC/download.

87. C. E. Kearns, L. A. Schmidt, S. A. Glantz, "Sugar industry and coronary heart disease research: a historical analysis of internal industry documents," *Journal of the American Medical Association Internal Medicine* 176, no. 11 (2016): 1680–85.

88. C. E. Kearns, D. Apollonio, S. A. Glantz, "Sugar industry sponsorship of germ-free rodent studies linking sucrose to hyperlipidemia and cancer: a historical analysis of internal documents," *PLoS Biology* 15, no. 11 (November 2017): e2003460.

89. Q. Yang, Z. Zhang, E. W. Gregg, et al., "Added sugar intake and cardiovascular diseases mortality among U.S. adults," *Journal of the American Medical Association Internal Medicine* 174, no. 4 (April 2014): 516–24.

90. C. Iadecola, "Sugar and Alzheimer's disease: a bittersweet truth," *Nature Neuroscience* 18, no. 4 (April 2015): 477–78.

91. J. M. Rippe, T. J. Angelopoulos, "Relationship between added sugars consumption and chronic disease risk factors: current understanding," *Nutrients* 8, no. 11 (November 2016): 697.

92. R. H. Lustig, L. A. Schmidt, C. D. Brindis, "Public health: the toxic truth about sugar," *Nature* 482, no. 7383 (February 2012): 27–29.

93. American Heart Association, "Added sugars add to your risk of dying from heart disease," September 16, 2016, www.heart.org/HEARTORG/HealthyLiving/Healthy Eating/Nutrition/Added-Sugars-Add-to-Your-Risk-of-Dying-from-Heart -Disease_UCM_460319_Article.jsp.

94. P. Gnagnarella, S. Gandini, C. La Vecchia, P. Maisonneuve, "Glycemic index, glycemic load, and cancer risk: a meta-analysis," *American Journal of Clinical Nutrition* 87, no. 6 (June 2008): 1793–1801.

95. I. Romieu, P. Ferrari, S. Rinaldi, et al., "Dietary glycemic index and glycemic load and breast cancer risk in the European Prospective Investigation into Cancer and Nutrition (EPIC)," *American Journal of Clinical Nutrition* 96, no. 2 (August 2012): 345–55.

96. Y. Choi, E. Giovannucci, J. E. Lee, "Glycaemic index and glycaemic load in relation to risk of diabetes-related cancers: a meta-analysis," *British Journal of Nutrition* 108, no. 11 (December 2012): 1934–47.

97. M. A. Fuchs, K. Sato, D. Niedzwiecki, et al., "Sugar-sweetened beverage intake and cancer recurrence and survival in CALGB 89803 (Alliance)," *PloS One* 9, no. 6 (June 2014): e99816.

98. J. M. Genkinger, R. Li, D. Spiegelman, et al., "Coffee, tea, and sugar-sweetened carbonated soft drink intake and pancreatic cancer risk: a pooled analysis of 14 cohort studies," *Cancer Epidemiology, Biomarkers & Prevention* 21, no. 2 (February 2012): 305–18.

99. N. Potischman, R. J. Coates, C. A. Swanson, et al., "Increased risk of early-stage breast cancer related to consumption of sweet foods among women less than age 45 in the United States," *Cancer Causes and Control* 13, no. 10 (December 2002): 937–46.

100. M. Lajous, M. C. Boutron-Ruault, A. Fabre, F. Clavel-Chapelon, I. Romieu, "Carbohydrate intake, glycemic index, glycemic load, and risk of postmenopausal breast cancer in a prospective study of French women," *American Journal of Clinical Nutrition* 87, no. 5 (May 2008): 1384–91.

101. G. C. Kabat, M. Y. Kim, H. D. Strickler, et al., "A longitudinal study of serum insulin and glucose levels in relation to colorectal cancer risk among postmenopausal women," *British Journal of Cancer* 106, no. 1 (January 2012): 227–32.

102. I. Drake, E. Sonestedt, B. Gullberg, et al., "Dietary intakes of carbohydrates in relation to prostate cancer risk: a prospective study in the Malmö diet and cancer cohort," *American Journal of Clinical Nutrition* 96, no. 6 (December 2012): 1409–18.

103. P. Hossain, B. Kawar, M. El Nahas, "Obesity and diabetes in the developing world— a growing challenge," *New England Journal of Medicine* 356, no. 3 (January 2007): 213–15.

104. World Health Organization, "Global report on diabetes," 2016, www.apps.who.int /iris/bitstream/10665/204871/1/9789241565257_eng.pdf?ua=1&utm_source= blog&utm_campaign=rc_blogpost.

105. J. Wojciechowska, W. Krajewski, M. Bolanowski, T. Krecicki, T. Zatonski, "Diabetes and cancer: a review of current knowledge," *Experimental and Clinical Endocrinology and Diabetes* 124, no. 5 (May 2016): 263–75.

106. More details on sugar: Research points to high sugar levels as the reason for the connection between diabetes and increased cancer risk. In 2013, scientists at the university Rey Juan Carlos in Madrid found that high sugar levels increase the

activity of a protein that has been connected to two key cancer hallmarks—cell immortality and cell proliferation. When responding to an uptick in sugars, cells in the intestine secrete a hormone that causes the pancreas to release insulin, which helps the body process sugar into energy or store it for future use. Dr. Garcia Jimenez and his colleagues studied this process at a molecular level. They discovered an unexpected side effect: An increase in ß-catenin (A. Chocarro-Calvo, J. M. Garcia-Martinez, S. Ardila-Gonzalez, A. De la Vieja, C. Garcia-Jimenez, "Glucose-induced beta-catenin acetylation enhances Wnt signaling in cancer," *Molecular Cell* 49, no. 3 [February 7, 2013]: 474–86). ß-catenin is a protein known to be a major factor in the development of different cancers. It can make normal cells immortal, an important early step in cancer progression. The accumulation of ß-catenin also leads to cell proliferation. This represents clear evidence of a molecular mechanism through which high blood-sugar levels could predispose the body to cancer, encouraging tumor creation and growth.

107. U.S. Department of Health and Human Services, "14th report on carcinogens," 2016, www.ntp.niehs.nih.gov/pubhealth/roc/index-1.html#toc1.

108. American Cancer Society, "Alcohol use and cancer," April 5, 2017, www.cancer.org/cancer/cancer-causes/diet-physical-activity/alcohol-use-and-cancer.html.

109. G. Testino, "The burden of cancer attributable to alcohol consumption," *Maedica* 6, no. 4 (October 2011): 313–20.

110. National Cancer Institute, "Alcohol and cancer risk," June 24, 2013, www.cancer.gov/about-cancer/causes-prevention/risk/alcohol/alcohol-fact-sheet.

111. H. K. Seitz, P. Becker, "Alcohol metabolism and cancer risk," www.pubs.niaaa.nih.gov/publications/arh301/38-47.htm.

112. P. Boffetta, M. Hashibe, C. La Vecchia, W. Zatonski, J. Rehm, "The burden of cancer attributable to alcohol drinking," *International Journal of Cancer* 119, no. 4 (August 2006): 884–87.

113. D. E. Nelson, D. W. Jarman, J. Rehm, et al., "Alcohol-attributable cancer deaths and years of potential life lost in the United States," *American Journal of Public Health* 103, no. 4 (April 2013): 641–48.

114. N. K. LoConte, A. M. Brewster, J. S. Kaur, J. K. Merrill, A. J. Alberg, "Alcohol and cancer: a statement of the American Society of Clinical Oncology," *Journal of Clinical Oncology* (November 2017): JCO2017761155.

115. Harvard Health Publishing, "Glycemic index and glycemic load for 100+ foods," August 27, 2015, www.health.harvard.edu/diseases-and-conditions/glycemic-index-and-glycemic-load-for-100-foods.

116. A. Chocarro-Calvo, J. M. Garcia-Martinez, S. Ardila-Gonzalez, A. De la Vieja, C. Garcia-Jimenez, "Glucose-induced beta-catenin acetylation enhances Wnt signaling in cancer," *Molecular Cell* 49, no. 3 (February 2013): 474–86.

117. C. Garcia-Jimenez, J. M. Garcia-Martinez, A. Chocarro-Calvo, A. De la Vieja, "A new link between diabetes and cancer: enhanced Wnt/beta-catenin signaling by high glucose," *Journal of Molecular Endocrinology* 52, no. 1 (February 2014): R51–66.

118. S. C. Melkonian, C. R. Daniel, Y. Ye, et al., "Glycemic index, glycemic load, and lung cancer risk in non-Hispanic whites," *Cancer Epidemiology Biomarkers & Prevention* 25, no. 3 (March 2016): 532–39.

119. Q. Yang, "Gain weight by 'going diet?' artificial sweeteners and the neurobiology of sugar cravings: Neuroscience 2010," *Yale Journal of Biology and Medicine* 83, no. 2 (June 2010): 101–8.

120. S. D. Anton, C. K. Martin, H. Han, et al., "Effects of stevia, aspartame, and sucrose on food intake, satiety, and postprandial glucose and insulin levels," *Appetite* 55, no. 1 (March 2010): 37–43.

121. S. E. Swithers, "Artificial sweeteners produce the counterintuitive effect of inducing metabolic derangements," *Trends in Endocrinology and Metabolism* 24, no. 9 (July 2013): 431–41.

122. L. S. Augustin, C. Galeone, L. Dal Maso, et al., "Glycemic index, glycemic load and risk of prostate cancer," *International Journal of Cancer* 112, no. 3 (November 2004): 446–50.

123. C. M. Nagle, F. Kolahdooz, T. I. Ibiebele, et al., "Carbohydrate intake, glycemic load, glycemic index, and risk of ovarian cancer," *Annals of Oncology* 22, no. 6 (June 2011): 1332–38.

124. V. Bouvard, D. Loomis, K. Z. Guyton, et al., "Carcinogenicity of consumption of red and processed meat," *The Lancet Oncology* 16, no. 16 (October 2015): 1599–1600.

125. M. A. Fini, A. Elias, R. J. Johnson, R. M. Wright, "Contribution of uric acid to cancer risk, recurrence, and mortality," *Clinical and Translational Medicine* 1 (August 2012): 1–16.

126. American Cancer Society, "World Health Organization says processed meat causes cancer," October 26, 2015, www.cancer.org/latest-news/world-health-organization -says-processed-meat-causes-cancer.html.

127. N. F. Aykan, "Red meat and colorectal cancer," *Oncology Reviews* 9, no. 1 (December 2015): 288.

128. J. M. Genkinger, A. Koushik, "Meat consumption and cancer risk," *PLoS Medicine* 4, no. 12 (December 2007): e345.

129. National Cancer Institute, "Chemicals in meat cooked at high temperatures and cancer risk," October 19, 2015, www.cancer.gov/about-cancer/causes-prevention /risk/diet/cooked-meats-fact-sheet.

130. R. L. Santarelli, F. Pierre, D. E. Corpet, "Processed meat and colorectal cancer: a review of epidemiologic and experimental evidence," *Nutrition and Cancer* 60, no. 2 (April 2008): 131–44.

131. American Cancer Society, "Acrylamide and cancer risk," March 10, 2016, www .cancer.org/cancer/cancer-causes/acrylamide.html.

132. More details on red meat: The cancer-causing substances released from cooking red meat include heterocyclic amines (HCA) and polycyclic aromatic hydrocarbons (PAH). These compounds are formed when meat is cooked at high temperatures or is charred. Unfortunately, they are also formed when meat is cooked at normal temperatures, including pan fried, broiled, or grilled. However, the longer meat is cooked, the higher the levels of HCA and PAH. These compounds are also present at high levels in grilled chicken. Both HCA and PAH have been classified as mutagens—substances that can initiate the cancer process (carcinogens)—and are known to cause DNA damage (a key cancer hallmark). Rodents fed a diet that included HCAs developed tumors in various organs, including the breast, colon, liver lung, and prostate. Rodents fed PAHs developed leukemia and tumors in their lungs and gastrointestinal tract. Red meat is also a high source of saturated fat, albeit at a higher level in some cuts than in others, and this can have an effect on cancer risk and can modulate hormonal function, relevant for cancers such as breast, endometrial, prostate, and ovarian.

Red meat also contains a chemical called heme—part of the red pigment in the blood, hemoglobin—a source of iron that is broken down in our gut to form a family of chemicals called n-nitroso compounds. N-nitroso compounds damage the cells that line the colon, forcing other cells to replicate more often in order to heal the damage. With excess cell replication comes an increased probability of cell mutations. If cell mutations are left unchecked, through changes in different cancer hallmarks, cancer will form and thrive. In addition, processed red meats contain chemicals that generate n-nitroso compounds, such as nitrite preservatives. When combined with HCA and PAH, these compounds create a perfect storm for cancers to form—HCA and PAH being mutagens and carcinogens combined with n-nitroso compounds cause cell damage and excess cell replication in the colon (all key cancer hallmarks).

133. C. A. Daley, A. Abbott, P. S. Doyle, G. A. Nader, S. Larson, "A review of fatty acid profiles and antioxidant content in grass-fed and grain-fed beef," *Nutrition Journal* 9 (March 2010): 10.

134. E. Patterson, R. Wall, G. F. Fitzgerald, R. P. Ross, C. Stanton, "Health implications of high dietary omega-6 polyunsaturated fatty acids," *Journal of Nutrition and Metabolism* 2012 (November 2012): 539426.

135. A. N. Samraj, O. M. T. Pearce, H. Läubli, et al., "A red-meat-derived glycan promotes inflammation and cancer progression," *Proceedings of the National Academy of Sciences of the United States of America* 112, no. 2 (December 2015): 542–47.

136. More details on meat: Researchers at the University of California, San Diego, may have discovered another key culprit linking red meat and cancer (also via inflammation) (A. N. Samraj, O. M. Pearce, H. Laubli, et al., "A red-meat-derived glycan promotes inflammation and cancer progression," *Proceeding of the National Academy of Sciences of the United States of America* 112, no. 2 [January 13, 2015]: 542–47). Pork, beef, and lamb contain a type of sugar that our bodies view as a foreign invader, which sparks an immune response and results in inflammation. In a 2014 study, the California scientists genetically engineered mice so they, like humans, did not naturally produce the sugar in question. The idea was that the mice would view the introduction of the sugar as a foreign substance and mount an inflammatory response. When those genetically altered mice were then fed the foreign sugar in red meats, they developed tumors. This could explain why consuming red meat does not cause disease in other carnivores that have the red-meat sugar in their system. For humans, red meat may not be perceived as a nutrient, but as an invasive compound.

137. M. S. Moss, *Salt Sugar Fat: How the Food Giants Hooked Us* (New York: Random House, 2014).

138. N. M. Avena, P. Rada, B. G. Hoebel, "Evidence for sugar addiction: behavioral and neurochemical effects of intermittent, excessive sugar intake," *Neuroscience and Biobehavioral Reviews* 32, no. 1 (May 2008): 20–39.

139. D. M. Blumenthal, M. S. Gold, "Neurobiology of food addiction," *Current Opinion in Clinical Nutrition and Metabolic Care* 13, no. 4 (July 2010): 359–65.

140. E. M. Schulte, N. M. Avena, A. N. Gearhardt, "Which foods may be addictive? The roles of processing, fat content, and glycemic load," *PloS One* 10, no. 2 (February 2015): e0117959.

141. More details on hunger hormones: Evidence suggests that not only are the brain reward circuits modified through exposure to these unhealthy foods that are high in salt, sugar, and fat, but they can also modulate key hormones that regulate our feelings of hunger and satiation—in other words, feeling full. The two key hormones important in this process of appetite stimulation are leptin and ghrelin. Leptin is made by fat cells and decreases our appetite. Ghrelin is released from the stomach and increases appetite through signals to the brain. Ghrelin also plays a role in body weight. Levels of leptin are lower when you're thin and higher when you're overweight. However, similar to people with diabetes having insulin resistance, many obese people have built up a resistance to the appetite-suppressing effects of leptin. As a result, the normal regulation of appetite through leptin is not registered and excess stores of fat are built up. People with leptin resistance are not getting appropriate feedback from these key regulatory hormones telling our bodies when to eat

and when we are full and should stop eating. High-fat meals have been shown to dysregulate the balance of these hormones. But researchers have shown that either a diet rich in "good" carbohydrates (like whole grains) or a diet high in protein suppresses ghrelin more effectively than a diet high in fat. Sleep deprivation, stress, and depression are also linked with dysregulation of ghrelin and leptin levels. This provides further evidence to avoid the dieting pitfalls and ensure you harness the correct Mix of Six for the ideal and sustainable changes you are seeking.

142. G. Holmboe-Ottesen, M. Wandel, "Changes in dietary habits after migration and consequences for health: a focus on South Asians in Europe," *Food & Nutrition Research* 56 (November 2012): 10.3402/fnr.v345i3400.18891.

143. B. K. Defo, "Demographic, epidemiological, and health transitions: are they relevant to population health patterns in Africa?," *Global Health Action* 7, no. 1 (May 2014): 10.3402/gha.v3407.22443.

144. T. J. Key, A. Schatzkin, W. C. Willett, et al., "Diet, nutrition and the prevention of cancer," *Public Health Nutrition* 7, no. 1A (February 2004): 187–200.

145. J. Upadhyay, O. Farr, N. Perakakis, W. Ghaly, C. Mantzoros, "Obesity as a disease," *Medical Clinics of North America* 102, no. 1 (January 2018): 13–33.

146. D. P. Rose, P. J. Gracheck, L. Vona-Davis, "The interactions of obesity, inflammation and insulin resistance in breast cancer," *Cancers* 7, no. 4 (October 2015): 2147 68.

147. K. Bowers, G. Liu, P. Wang, et al., "Birth weight, postnatal weight change, and risk for high blood pressure among Chinese children," *Pediatrics* 127, no. 5 (May 2011): e1272–79.

148. K. Strohacker, K. C. Carpenter, B. K. McFarlin, "Consequences of weight cycling: an increase in disease risk?," *International Journal of Exercise Science* 2, no. 3 (July 2009): 191–201.

149. J. W. Rich-Edwards, K. Kleinman, K. B. Michels, et al., "Longitudinal study of birth weight and adult body mass index in predicting risk of coronary heart disease and stroke in women," *British Medical Journal* 330, no. 7500 (May 2005): 1115.

150. V. J. Carey, E. E. Walters, G. A. Colditz, et al., "Body fat distribution and risk of non-insulin-dependent diabetes mellitus in women: The Nurses' Health Study," *American Journal of Epidemiology* 145, no. 7 (April 1997): 614–19.

151. Centers for Disease Control and Prevention, "National Diabetes Statistics Report," 2017, www.cdc.gov/diabetes/pdfs/data/statistics/national-diabetes-statistics-report.pdf.

152. Centers for Disease Control and Prevention, "The health effects of overweight and obesity," June 5, 2015, www.cdc.gov/healthyweight/effects/index.html.

153. World Health Organization, "Obesity and overweight fact sheet," October 2017, www.who.int/mediacentre/factsheets/fs311/en.

154. K. Neovius, M. Neovius, F. Rasmussen, "The combined effects of overweight and smoking in late adolescence on subsequent disability pension: a nationwide cohort study," *International Journal of Obesity (2005)* 34, no. 1 (January 2010): 75–82.

155. J. A. Ligibel, C. M. Alfano, K. S. Courneya, et al., "American Society of Clinical Oncology position statement on obesity and cancer," *Journal of Clinical Oncology* 32, no. 31 (November 2014): 3568–74.

156. E. J. Gallagher, D. LeRoith, "Epidemiology and molecular mechanisms tying obesity, diabetes, and the metabolic syndrome with cancer," *Diabetes Care* 36, no. Supplement 2 (July 2013): S233–39.

157. E. J. Gallagher, D. LeRoith, "Obesity and diabetes: the increased risk of cancer and cancer-related mortality," *Physiological Reviews* 95, no. 3 (June 2015): 72–48.

158. R. Divella, R. De Luca, I. Abbate, E. Naglieri, A. Daniele, "Obesity and cancer: the role of adipose tissue and adipo-cytokines-induced chronic inflammation," *Journal of Cancer* 7, no. 15 (November 2016): 2346–59.

159. B. D. Hopkins, M. D. Goncalves, L. C. Cantley, "Obesity and cancer mechanisms: cancer metabolism," *Journal of Clinical Oncology* 34, no. 35 (November 2016): 4277–83.

160. T. Deng, C. J. Lyon, S. Bergin, M. A. Caligiuri, W. A. Hsueh, "Obesity, inflammation, and cancer," *Annual Review of Pathology* 11 (May 2016): 421–49.

161. Q. Dai, Y.-T. Gao, X.-O. Shu, et al., "Oxidative stress, obesity, and breast cancer risk: results from the Shanghai women's health study," *Journal of Clinical Oncology* 27, no. 15 (May 2009): 2482–88.

162. L. Marseglia, S. Manti, G. D'Angelo, et al., "Oxidative stress in obesity: a critical component in human diseases," *International Journal of Molecular Sciences* 16, no. 1 (December 2014): 378–400.

163. J. Luo, R. T. Chlebowski, M. Hendryx, et al., "Intentional weight loss and endometrial cancer risk," *Journal of Clinical Oncology* 35, no. 11 (April 2017): 1189–93.

164. J. P. Pierce, L. Natarajan, B. J. Caan, et al., "Influence of a diet very high in vegetables, fruit, and fiber and low in fat on prognosis following treatment for breast cancer: the Women's Healthy Eating and Living (WHEL) randomized trial," *Journal of the American Medical Association* 298, no. 3 (July 2007): 289–98.

165. J. P. Pierce, "Diet and breast cancer prognosis: making sense of the WHEL and WINS trials," *Current Opinion in Obstetrics and Gynecology* 21, no. 1 (February 2009): 86–91.

166. More details on the WHEL Study: Another large randomized clinical trial, the Women's Healthy Eating and Living Study reported mixed results when placing breast cancer survivors on diets high in vegetables and fruits. Benefits were found only for women experiencing hot flashes at study entry. However, one limitation with this study was that the women in the control group were already eating the recommended five servings of fruits and vegetables a day. So everyone in the study was eating a healthy diet from the start. In addition, the principal investigator of the study, John Pierce, told me he and the other researchers were focusing on the wrong target in the WHEL study. At the time, they thought the active mechanism they should target in the women was to increase carotenoids, such as beta-carotene, and these would exert an effect through their antioxidant capacity. In hindsight he said they should have prescribed an anti-inflammatory diet. Adding to this limitation, in order to consume the needed fruits and vegetables in the WHEL study, women were provided with juicers. This could have inadvertently increased overall sugar consumption at the cost of the important fiber in these foods. Although carotenoid levels increased in the intervention compared to the control group, and high carotenoid levels were linked with reduced recurrence of disease, anti-inflammatory markers remained unchanged. Yet inflammation was also a predictor of survival. Targeting increases in carotenoid levels and reducing inflammation may together be the best approach.

167. C. A. Thomson, C. L. Rock, P. A. Thompson, et al., "Vegetable intake is associated with reduced breast cancer recurrence in tamoxifen users: a secondary analysis from the Women's Healthy Eating and Living Study," *Breast Cancer Research and Treatment* 125, no. 2 (January 2011): 519–27.

168. J. P. Pierce, M. L. Stefanick, S. W. Flatt, et al., "Greater survival after breast cancer in physically active women with high vegetable-fruit intake regardless of obesity," *Journal of Clinical Oncology* 25, no. 17 (June 2007): 2345–51.

169. C. A. Thomson, T. E. Crane, A. Miller, et al., "A randomized trial of diet and physical activity in women treated for stage II–IV ovarian cancer: rationale and design of the Lifestyle Intervention for Ovarian Cancer Enhanced Survival (LIVES): an NRG Oncology/Gynecologic Oncology Group (GOG-225) Study," *Contemporary Clinical Trials* 49 (July 2016): 181–89.

170. More details on diet and cancer: Thomson recently coauthored a study that looked at the link between "energy dense foods" and cancer. High DED (dietary energy

density) foods are those that demand a lot of metabolic resources to process but deliver low nutrition. She and her team found that there is a 10 percent increase in cancers typically associated with obesity—in postmenopausal women of normal weight. Low DED foods, on the other hand, deliver high-nutrient content with low calorie demands on the body. Thompson, herself a former cancer patient, relates that these finding are "novel and contrary to our hypothesis and this finding suggests that weight management alone may not protect against obesity-related cancer in women who favor a 'high-energy-density' diet." This may explain why there has been an uptake in the onset of certain cancers (such as breast, prostate, and colorectal) among younger people who may not be eating an anticancer diet.

171. C. A. Thomson, T. E. Crane, D. O. Garcia, et al., "Association between dietary energy density and obesity-associated cancer: results from the Women's Health Initiative," *Journal of the Academy of Nutrition and Dietetics* (August 2017).

172. G. D. Potter, D. J. Skene, J. Arendt, et al., "Circadian rhythm and sleep disruption: causes, metabolic consequences, and countermeasures," *Endocrine Reviews* 37, no. 6 (December 2016): 584–608.

173. S. Taheri, L. Lin, D. Austin, T. Young, E. Mignot, "Short sleep duration is associated with reduced leptin, elevated ghrelin, and increased body mass index," *PLoS Medicine* 1, no. 3 (December 2004): e62.

174. R. Leproult, E. Van Cauter, "Role of sleep and sleep loss in hormonal release and metabolism," *Endocrine Development* 17 (November 2010): 11–21.

175. F.-P. J. Martin, S. Rezzi, E. Peré-Trepat, et al., "Metabolic effects of dark chocolate consumption on energy, gut microbiota, and stress-related metabolism in free-living subjects," *Journal of Proteome Research* 8, no. 12 (December 2009): 5568–79.

176. J. K. Srivastava, E. Shankar, S. Gupta, "Chamomile: A herbal medicine of the past with bright future," *Molecular Medicine Reports* 3, no. 6 (November 2010): 895–901.

177. R. S. Thompson, R. Roller, A. Mika, et al., "Dietary prebiotics and bioactive milk fractions improve NREM sleep, enhance REM sleep rebound and attenuate the stress-induced decrease in diurnal temperature and gut microbial alpha diversity," *Frontiers in Behavioral Neuroscience* 10 (January 2017).

178. L. Sominsky, S. J. Spencer, "Eating behavior and stress: a pathway to obesity," *Frontiers in Psychology* 5 (May 2014): 434.

179. K. Aschbacher, S. Kornfeld, M. Picard, et al., "Chronic stress increases vulnerability to diet-related abdominal fat, oxidative stress, and metabolic risk," *Psychoneuroendocrinology* 46 (August 2014): 14–22.

180. J. A. Foster, L. Rinaman, J. F. Cryan, "Stress & the gut-brain axis: regulation by the microbiome," *Neurobiology of Stress* (March 2017).

181. M. Zhang, J. Huang, X. Xie, C. D. Holman, "Dietary intakes of mushrooms and green tea combine to reduce the risk of breast cancer in Chinese women," *International Journal of Cancer* 124, no. 6 (March 2009): 1404–08.

182. P. Ghadirian, S. Narod, E. Fafard, et al., "Breast cancer risk in relation to the joint effect of BRCA mutations and diet diversity," *Breast Cancer Research and Treatment* 117, no. 2 (September 2009): 417–22.

183. P. Maas, M. Barrdahl, A. D. Joshi, et al., "Breast cancer risk from modifiable and nonmodifiable risk factors among white women in the United States," *Journal of the American Medical Association Oncology* 2, no. 10 (October 2016): 1295–1302.

184. More details on diet-gene interaction: In a 2009 study of French-Canadian women who had BRCA mutations, researchers found significantly reduced risk of breast cancer in women who ate the greatest variety of vegetables (P. Ghadirian, S. Narod, E. Fafard, et al., "Breast cancer risk in relation to the joint effect of BRCA mutations and diet diversity," *Breast Cancer Research and Treatment* 117, no. 2 [September 2009]: 417–22). A 2013 study of Korean women with the BRCA mutation confirmed the

association between vegetable variety and lower risk and also found that soy consumption reduced breast cancer risk, regardless of whether women had the genetic mutation (K. P. Ko, S. W. Kim, S. H. Ma, et al., "Dietary intake and breast cancer among carriers and noncarriers of BRCA mutations in the Korean Hereditary Breast Cancer Study," *American Journal of Clinical Nutrition* 98, no. 6 [December 2013]: 1493–1501). Meanwhile, a cohort of men who were at a high risk of prostate cancer due to a genetic mutation (five times more likely than the general population) were able to neutralize their genetic risk by consuming fish on a regular basis (M. Hedelin, E. T. Chang, F. Wiklund, et al., "Association of frequent consumption of fatty fish with prostate cancer risk is modified by COX-2 polymorphism," *International Journal of Cancer* 120, no. 2 [January 15, 2007]: 398–405). More recently, a paper in the Journal of the American Medical Association examined the contribution of both nonmodifiable and modifiable risk factors for breast cancer. The nonmodifiable factors included gene-related mutations as assessed by a polygenic risk score (PRS) and other nonmodifiable risk factors including family history, age at first birth, parity, age at menarche, height, menopausal status, and age at menopause. The modifiable risk factors included body mass index, hormone therapy use, level of alcohol consumption, and smoking status. For women in the highest decile of risk owing to nonmodifiable factors, those who had low BMI, did not drink or smoke, and did not use hormone therapy had a breast cancer risk comparable to an average woman in the general population (Maas, M. Barrdahl, A. D. Joshi, et al., "Breast cancer risk from modifiable and nonmodifiable risk factors among white women in the United States," *Journal of the American Medical Association Oncology* 2, no. 10 [October 2016]: 1295–1302). This suggests that nonmodifiable risk factors such as cancer-specific gene mutations and other demographic factors can be modulated through lifestyle factors.

The Anticancer Living Guide to Nutrition

1. The Full Yield Inc., "The Full Yield," 2017, www.thefullyield.com.
2. Food and Agriculture Organization of the United Nations, "Food-based dietary guidelines—Japan," 2010, www.fao.org/nutrition/education/food-based-dietary-guidelines/regions/countries/japan/en.
3. G. Zong, A. Gao, F. B. Hu, Q. Sun, "Whole grain intake and mortality from all causes, cardiovascular disease, and cancer: a meta-analysis of prospective cohort studies," *Circulation* 133, no. 24 (June 2016): 2370–80.
4. P. Knekt, J. Kumpulainen, R. Jarvinen, et al., "Flavonoid intake and risk of chronic diseases," *American Journal of Clinical Nutrition* 76, no. 3 (September 2002): 560–68.
5. E. Moghaddam, J. A. Vogt, T. M. Wolever, "The effects of fat and protein on glycemic responses in nondiabetic humans vary with waist circumference, fasting plasma insulin, and dietary fiber intake," *Journal of Nutrition* 136, no. 10 (October 2006): 2506–11.
6. A. K. Kant, B. I. Graubard, "Eating out in America, 1987–2000: Trends and nutritional correlates," *Preventive Medicine* 38, no. 2 (February 2004): 243–49.
7. S. Vikraman, C. D. Fryar, C. L. Ogden, "Caloric intake from fast food among children and adolescents in the United States, 2011–2012. NCHS Data Brief No. 213," November 6, 2015, www.cdc.gov/nchs/products/databriefs/db213.htm.
8. C. Geisler, C. M. Prado, M. J. Müller, "Inadequacy of body weight-based recommendations for individual protein intake—lessons from body composition analysis," *Nutrients* 9, no. 1 (December 2017): 23.
9. P. Trumbo, S. Schlicker, A. A. Yates, M. Poos, "Dietary reference intakes for energy, carbohydrate, fiber, fat, fatty acids, cholesterol, protein and amino acids," *Journal of the American Dietetic Association* 102, no. 11 (November 2002): 1621–30.

10. S. Ahmed, N. H. Othman, "The anti-cancer effects of Tualang honey in modulating breast carcinogenesis: an experimental animal study," *BMC Complementary and Alternative Medicine* 17, no. 1 (April 2017): 208.

11. T. Yamamoto, K. Uemura, K. Moriyama, K. Mitamura, A. Taga, "Inhibitory effect of maple syrup on the cell growth and invasion of human colorectal cancer cells," *Oncology Reports* 33, no. 4 (April 2015): 1579–84.

12. R. J. Johnson, M. S. Segal, Y. Sautin, et al., "Potential role of sugar (fructose) in the epidemic of hypertension, obesity and the metabolic syndrome, diabetes, kidney disease, and cardiovascular disease," *American Journal of Clinical Nutrition* 86, no. 4 (October 2007): 899–906.

13. A. Bordoni, F. Danesi, D. Dardevet, et al., "Dairy products and inflammation: a review of the clinical evidence," *Critical Reviews in Food Science and Nutrition* 57, no. 12 (August 2017): 2497–2525.

14. Y. Song, J. E. Chavarro, Y. Cao, et al., "Whole milk intake is associated with prostate-cancer-specific mortality among U.S. male physicians," *Journal of Nutrition* 143, no. 2 (February 2013): 189–96.

15. K. L. Watson, L. Stalker, R. A. Jones, R. A. Moorehead, "High levels of dietary soy decrease mammary tumor latency and increase incidence in MTB-IGFIR transgenic mice," *BMC Cancer* 15, (February 2015): 37.

16. S. J. Nechuta, B. J. Caan, W. Y. Chen, et al., "Soy food intake after diagnosis of breast cancer and survival: an in-depth analysis of combined evidence from cohort studies of U.S. and Chinese women," *American Journal of Clinical Nutrition* 96, no. 1 (July 2012): 123–32.

17. A. Seow, W. T. Poh, M. Teh, et al., "Diet, reproductive factors and lung cancer risk among Chinese women in Singapore: evidence for a protective effect of soy in non-smokers," *International Journal of Cancer* 97, no. 3 (January 2002): 365–71.

18. K. Dechering, C. Boersma, S. Mosselman, "Estrogen receptors alpha and beta: two receptors of a kind?," *Current Medicinal Chemistry* 7, no. 5 (May 2000): 561–76.

19. S. Ali, R. C. Coombes, "Estrogen receptor alpha in human breast cancer: occurrence and significance," *Journal of Mammary Gland Biology and Neoplasia* 5, no. 3 (July 2000): 271–81.

20. D. M. Harris, E. Besselink, S. M. Henning, V. L. Go, D. Heber, "Phytoestrogens induce differential estrogen receptor alpha- or beta-mediated responses in transfected breast cancer cells," *Experimental Biology and Medicine* 230, no. 8 (September 2005): 558–68.

21. S. Ziaei, R. Halaby, "Dietary isoflavones and breast cancer risk," *Medicines* 4, no. 2 (April 2017): 18.

22. F. F. Zhang, D. E. Haslam, M. B. Terry, et al., "Dietary isoflavone intake and all-cause mortality in breast cancer survivors: the breast cancer family registry," *Cancer* 123, no. 11 (June 2017): 2070–79.

23. S. Simon, "How your diet may affect your risk of breast cancer," American Cancer Society, October 25, 2017, www.cancer.org/latest-news/how-your-diet-may-affect-your-risk-of-breast-cancer.html.

24. U.S. Department of Health and Human Services, "14th report on carcinogens," 2016, www.ntp.niehs.nih.gov/pubhealth/roc/index-1.html#toc1.

25. D. E. Nelson, D. W. Jarman, J. Rehm, et al., "Alcohol-attributable cancer deaths and years of potential life lost in the United States," *American Journal of Public Health* 103, no. 4 (April 2013): 641–48.

26. N. K. LoConte, A. M. Brewster, J. S. Kaur, J. K. Merrill, A. J. Alberg, "Alcohol and cancer: a statement of the American Society of Clinical Oncology," *Journal of Clinical Oncology* (November 2017): JCO2017761155.

27. A. Fullana, A. A. Carbonell-Barrachina, S. Sidhu, "Comparison of volatile aldehydes present in the cooking fumes of extra virgin olive, olive, and canola oils," *Journal of Agricultural and Food Chemistry* 52, no. 16 (August 2004): 5207–14.

28. B. M. Popkin, K. E. D'Anci, I. H. Rosenberg, "Water, hydration, and health," *Nutrition Reviews* 68, no. 8 (August 2010): 439–58.

29. E. T. Perrier, E. C. Johnson, A. L. McKenzie, L. A. Ellis, L. E. Armstrong, "Urine colour change as an indicator of change in daily water intake: a quantitative analysis," *European Journal of Nutrition* 55, no. 5 (August 2016): 1943–49.

30. National Cancer Institute, "Tea and cancer prevention," November 17, 2010, www .cancer.gov/about-cancer/causes-prevention/risk/diet/tea-fact-sheet.

31. About Herbs, "Green tea," August 16, 2017, www.mskcc.org/cancer-care/integrative -medicine/herbs/green-tea.

32. Men's Health, "Which bottled green tea packs the most nutritional punch?," October 5, 2010, www.menshealth.com/nutrition/best-green-tea.

33. S. Caini, S. Cattaruzza, B. Bendinelli, et al., "Coffee, tea and caffeine intake and the risk of non-melanoma skin cancer: a review of the literature and meta-analysis," *European Journal of Nutrition* 56, no. 1 (February 2017): 1–12.

34. D. Loomis, K. Z. Guyton, Y. Grosse, et al., "Carcinogenicity of drinking coffee, mate, and very hot beverages," *The Lancet Oncology* 17, no. 7 (July 2016): 877–78.

Chapter Twelve: The Environment and the Quest for Health

1. J. M. Shultz, S. Galea, "Mitigating the mental and physical health consequences of Hurricane Harvey," *Journal of the American Medical Association* 318, no. 15 (October 2017): 1437–38.

2. United States Environmental Protection Agency, "Universe of chemicals and general validation principles," 2012, www.epa.gov/sites/production/files/2015-07/docu ments/edsp_chemical_universe_and_general_validations_white_paper_11_12.pdf.

3. International Agency for Research on Cancer, "IARC monographs of the evaluation of carcinogenic risks to humans," World Health Organization, 2017, www.monographs .iarc.fr.

4. L. B. McKenzie, N. Ahir, U. Stolz, N. G. Nelson, "Household cleaning product-related injuries treated in U.S. emergency departments in 1990–2006," *Pediatrics* 126, no. 3 (September 2010): 509–16.

5. Q. Di, Y. Wang, A. Zanobetti, et al., "Air pollution and mortality in the Medicare population," *New England Journal of Medicine* 376, no. 26 (June 2017): 2513–22.

6. Y. Horii, K. Kannan, "Survey of organosilicone compounds, including cyclic and linear siloxanes, in personal care and household products," *Archives of Environmental Contamination and Toxicology* 55, no. 4 (November 2008): 701–10.

7. F. A. Caliman, M. Gavrilescu, "Pharmaceuticals, personal care products and endocrine disrupting agents in the environment—a review," *CLEAN–Soil, Air, Water* 37, no. 4–5 (April 2009): 277–303.

8. S. I. Korfali, R. Sabra, M. Jurdi, R. I. Taleb, "Assessment of toxic metals and phthalates in children's toys and clays," *Archives of Environmental Contamination and Toxicology* 65, no. 3 (October 2013): 368–81.

9. American Cancer Society, "Teflon and perfluorooctanoic acid (PFOA)," January 5, 2016, www.cancer.org/cancer/cancer-causes/teflon-and-perfluorooctanoic-acid-pfoa .html.

10. A. M. Hormann, F. S. Vom Saal, S. C. Nagel, et al., "Holding thermal receipt paper and eating food after using hand sanitizer results in high serum bioactive and urine total levels of bisphenol a (BPA)," *PloS One* 9, no. 10 (October 2014): e110509.

11. S. Babu, S. N. Uppu, B. Martin, O. A. Agu, R. M. Uppu, "Unusually high levels of bisphenol a (BPA) in thermal paper cash register receipts (CRS): development and

application of a robust LC-UV method to quantify BPA in CRS," *Toxicology Mechanisms and Methods* 25, no. 5 (May 2015): 410–16.

12. A. R. David, M. R. Zimmerman, "Cancer: an old disease, a new disease or something in between?," *Nature Reviews: Cancer* 10, no. 10 (October 2010): 728–33.

13. Centers for Disease Control and Prevention, "Cancer Clusters," December 18, 2013, www.cdc.gov/nceh/clusters.

14. J. R. Brown, J. L. Thornton, "Percivall Pott (1714-1788) and chimney sweepers' cancer of the scrotum," *British Journal of Industrial Medicine* 14, no. 1 (January 1957): 68–70.

15. W. Graebner, "Radium girls, corporate boys. [Review of: C. Clark, *Radium Girls: Women and Industrial Health Reform, 1910–1935* (Chapel Hill: University of North Carolina Press, 1997)]," *Reviews in American History* 26, no. 3 (September 1998): 587–92.

16. L. Kovács, D. Csupor, G. Lente, T. Gunda, "Catastrophes, poisons, chemicals," in *100 Chemical Myths*, eds. Lajos Kovács, Dezső Csupor, Gábor Lente, and Tamás Gunda (New York: Springer, 2014).

17. Integrated Risk Information System, "IRIS Bimonthly Public Science Meeting," October 2014, www.epa.gov/iris/iris-bimonthly-public-meeting-oct-2014.

18. Centers for Disease Control and Prevention, "World Trade Center Health Program—Program at a Glance," Centers for Disease Control and Prevention, 2016d.

19. Ibid., 2017e.

20. P. J. Lioy, C. P. Weisel, J. R. Millette, et al., "Characterization of the dust/smoke aerosol that settled east of the World Trade Center (WTC) in lower Manhattan after the collapse of the WTC 11 September 2001," *Environmental Health Perspectives* 110, no. 7 (July 2002): 703–14.

21. A. H. Mokdad, L. Dwyer-Lindgren, C. Fitzmaurice, et al., "Trends and patterns of disparities in cancer mortality among U.S. counties, 1980–2014," *Journal of the American Medical Association* 317, no. 4 (January 2017): 388–406.

22. M. Singer, "Down cancer alley: the lived experience of health and environmental suffering in Louisiana's chemical corridor," *Medical Anthropology Quarterly* 25, no. 2 (June 2011): 141–63.

23. L. Suarez, J. Martin, "Primary liver cancer mortality and incidence in Texas Mexican Americans, 1969–80," *American Journal of Public Health* 77, no. 5 (May 1987): 631–33.

24. A. Kirpich, E. Leary, "Superfund locations and potential associations with cancer incidence in Florida," *Statistics and Public Policy* 4, no. 1 (December 2017): 1–9.

25. Environmental Working Group, "About Us," 2017, www.ewg.org/about-us-#.Wnir2LynGUK./

26. A. Formuzis, "Chemical reform law falls short in protecting public health, environment," May 24, 2016, www.ewg.org/release/chemical-reform-law-falls-short-protecting-public-health-environment-.Wg3u0KIiVpu.

27. J. LaDou, B. Castleman, A. Frank, et al., "The case for a global ban on asbestos," *Environmental Health Perspectives* 118, no. 7 (July 2010): 897–901.

28. J. A. Swenberg, B. C. Moeller, K. Lu, et al., "Formaldehyde carcinogenicity research: 30 years and counting for mode of action, epidemiology, and cancer risk assessment," *Toxicologic Pathology* 41, no. 2 (February 2013): 181–89.

29. F. Suja, B. K. Pramanik, S. M. Zain, "Contamination, bioaccumulation and toxic effects of perfluorinated chemicals (PFCS) in the water environment: a review paper," *Water Science and Technology* 60, no. 6 (September 2009): 1533–44.

30. A. Blum, B. N. Ames, "Flame-retardant additives as possible cancer hazards," *Science* 195, no. 4273 (January 1977): 17–23.

31. K. Mulder, M. Knot, "PVC plastic: a history of systems development and entrenchment," *Technology in Society* 23, no. 2 (April 2001): 265–86.

32. Office of Environmental Health Hazard Assessment, "Bisphenol-A listed as known to the state of California to cause reproductive toxicity," May 11, 2015, www.oehha .ca.gov/proposition-65/crnr/bisphenol-listed-known-state-california-cause -reproductive-toxicity.

33. A. Miodovnik, S. M. Engel, C. Zhu, et al., "Endocrine disruptors and childhood social impairment," *Neurotoxicology* 32, no. 2 (March 2011): 261–67.

34. C. Casals-Casas, B. Desvergne, "Endocrine disruptors: from endocrine to metabolic disruption," *Annual Review of Physiology* 73 (November 2011): 135–62.

35. M. I. Cuomo, *A World Without Cancer: The Making of a New Cure and the Real Promise of Prevention* (New York: Rodale, 2012).

36. E. Swedenborg, J. Ruegg, S. Makela, I. Pongratz, "Endocrine disruptive chemicals: mechanisms of action and involvement in metabolic disorders," *Journal of Molecular Endocrinology* 43, no. 1 (July 2009): 1–10.

37. J. M. Gray, S. Rasanayagam, C. Engel, J. Rizzo, "State of the evidence 2017: an update on the connection between breast cancer and the environment," *Environmental Health* 16, no. 1 (September 2017): 94.

38. P. D. Darbre, P. W. Harvey, "Parabens can enable hallmarks and characteristics of cancer in human breast epithelial cells: a review of the literature with reference to new exposure data and regulatory status," *Journal of Applied Toxicology* 34, no. 9 (September 2014): 925–38.

39. D. E. Buttke, K. Sircar, C. Martin, "Exposures to endocrine-disrupting chemicals and age of menarche in adolescent girls in NHANES (2003–2008)," *Environmental Health Perspectives* 120, no. 11 (November 2012): 1613–18.

40. Environmental Protection Agency, "Endocrine disruption," November 22, 2017, www.epa.gov/endocrine-disruption.

41. R. H. Hill Jr., D. L. Ashley, S. L. Head, L. L. Needham, J. L. Pirkle, "p-Dichlorobenzene exposure among 1,000 adults in the United States," *Archives of Environmental Health* 50, no. 4 (July–August 1995): 277–80.

42. M. S. Wolff, S. L. Teitelbaum, K. McGovern, et al., "Environmental phenols and pubertal development in girls," *Environment International* 84 (November 2015): 174–80.

43. M. S. Wolff, S. L. Teitelbaum, G. Windham, et al., "Pilot study of urinary biomarkers of phytoestrogens, phthalates, and phenols in girls," *Environmental Health Perspectives* 115, no. 1 (January 2007): 116–21.

44. M. E. Herman-Giddens, J. Steffes, D. Harris, et al., "Secondary sexual characteristics in boys: data from the pediatric research in office settings network," *Pediatrics* 130, no. 5 (November 2012): e1058–68.

45. M. E. Herman-Giddens, L. Wang, G. Koch, "Secondary sexual characteristics in boys: estimates from the National Health and Nutrition Examination Survey III, 1988–1994," *Archives of Pediatrics and Adolescent Medicine* 155, no. 9 (September 2001): 1022–28.

46. Collaborative Group on Hormonal Factors in Breast Cancer, "Menarche, menopause, and breast cancer risk: individual participant meta-analysis, including 118,964 women with breast cancer from 117 epidemiological studies," *The Lancet Oncology* 13, no. 11 (November 2012): 1141–51.

47. F. R. Day, D. J. Thompson, H. Helgason, et al., "Genomic analyses identify hundreds of variants associated with age at menarche and support a role for puberty timing in cancer risk," *Nature Genetics* 49, no. 6 (June 2017): 834–41.

48. C. Bonilla, S. J. Lewis, R. M. Martin, et al., "Pubertal development and prostate cancer risk: Mendelian randomization study in a population-based cohort," *BMC Medicine* 14 (April 2016): 66.

49. E. Diamanti-Kandarakis, J. P. Bourguignon, L. C. Giudice, et al., "Endocrine-disrupting chemicals: an Endocrine Society scientific statement," *Endocrine Reviews* 30, no. 4 (June 2009): 293–342.

50. G. S. Prins, W. Y. Hu, G. B. Shi, et al., "Bisphenol A promotes human prostate stem-progenitor cell self-renewal and increases in vivo carcinogenesis in human prostate epithelium," *Endocrinology* 155, no. 3 (March 2014): 805–17.

51. Environmental Working Group, "Exposures add up survey results," 2017, www.ewg.org/skindeep/2004/06/15/exposures-add-up-survey-results/.Wg32G1UrJQJ.

52. Environmental Working Group, "Teen girls' body burden of hormone-altering cosmetics chemicals," September 24, 2008, www.ewg.org/research/teen-girls-body-burden-hormone-altering-cosmetics-chemicals.Wg33jlUrJQJ.

53. P. J. Lioy, R. Hauser, C. Gennings, et al., "Assessment of phthalates/phthalate alternatives in children's toys and childcare articles: review of the report including conclusions and recommendation of the Chronic Hazard Advisory Panel of the Consumer Product Safety Commission," *Journal of Exposure Science & Environmental Epidemiology* 25, no. 4 (July–August 2015): 343–53.

54. M. T. Dinwiddie, P. D. Terry, J. Chen, "Recent evidence regarding triclosan and cancer risk," *International Journal of Environmental Research and Public Health* 11, no. 2 (February 2014): 2209–17.

55. C. O'Neil, "Organic imports continue to rise alongside organic demand, research shows," October 25, 2017, www.ewg.org/agmag/2017/10/organic-imports-continue-rise-alongside-organic-demand-research-shows-.Wg36zKIiVps.

56. A. Bradman, L. Quiros-Alcala, R. Castorina, et al., "Effect of organic diet intervention on pesticide exposures in young children living in low-income urban and agricultural communities," *Environmental Health Perspectives* 123, no. 10 (October 2015): 1086–93.

57. CBS News, "60 Minutes found that Lumber Liquidators' Chinese-made laminate flooring contains amounts of toxic formaldehyde that may not meet health and safety standards," 2015, www.cbsnews.com/news/lumber-liquidators-linked-to-health-and-safety-violations.

58. H. Malcolm, "Subway: 'Yoga mat' chemical almost out of bread," April 11, 2014, www.usatoday.com/story/money/business/2014/04/11/subway-yoga-mat-chemical-almost-out-of-bread/7587787.

59. The Office of Environmental Health Hazard Assessment, "Notice of amendment of text Title 27, California Code of Regulations amendment of Section 25705 Specific Regulatory Levels: no significant risk levels 4-methylimidazole (4-MEI)," February 8, 2012, www.oehha.ca.gov/proposition-65/crnr/notice-amendment-text-title-27-california-code-regulations-amendment-section.

60. S. R. Lara, "Governor Brown signs Cleaning Product Right to Know Act to create first-in-nation label law for consumers," October 15, 2017, www.sd33.senate.ca.gov/news/2017-10-15-governor-brown-signs-cleaning-product-right-know-act-create-first-nation-label-law.

61. Governor Andrew M. Cuomo, "Governor Cuomo announces new regulations to require disclosure of chemicals in household cleaning products," April 25, 2017, www.governor.ny.gov/news/governor-cuomo-announces-new-regulations-require-disclosure-chemicals-household-cleaning.

62. SC Johnson Press Room, "SC Johnson introduces industry-first 100 percent fragrance transparency with new Glade® Fresh Citrus Blossoms Collection," February 11, 2016, www.scjohnson.com/en/press-room/press-releases/02-11-2016/sc-johnson-introduces-industry-first-100-percent-fragrance-transparency-with-new-glade-fresh-citrus-blossoms-collection.aspx.

63. Unilever, "What is Smartlabel™?," 2017, www.unileverusa.com/brands/smartlabel.
64. Procter & Gamble, "What are preservatives," 2017, www.us.pg.com/our-brands /product-safety/ingredient-safety/preservatives.
65. Campbell's, "Campbell to remove BPA from packaging by mid-2017," March 28, 2016, www.campbellsoupcompany.com/newsroom/press-releases/campbell-to-remove -bpa-from-packaging-by-mid-2017.
66. Getting to Know Cancer, "Assessing the carcinogenic potential of low dose exposures to chemical mixtures in the environment," 2017, www.gettingtoknowcancer .org/taskforce_environment.php.
67. Getting to Know Cancer, "The Halifax Project," September 20, 2016, www.getting toknowcancer.org/.
68. T. B. Hayes, V. Khoury, A. Narayan, et al., "Atrazine induces complete feminization and chemical castration in male African clawed frogs (Xenopus laevis)," *Proceedings of the National Academy of Sciences of the United States of America* 107, no. 10 (March 2010): 4612–17.
69. C. Cox, "Atrazine: toxicology," *Journal of Pesticide Reform* 21, no. 2 (Summer 2001a): 12–20.
70. A. Dorsey, "Toxicological profile for atrazine," Agency for Toxic Substances and Disease Registry, January 21, 2015, www.atsdr.cdc.gov/toxprofiles/tp.asp?id=338&tid=59.
71. K. Hu, Y. Tian, Y. Du, et al., "Atrazine promotes RM1 prostate cancer cell proliferation by activating STAT3 signaling," *International Journal of Oncology* 48, no. 5 (May 2016): 2166–74.
72. Anticancer Lifestyle Program, "Select comments from course participants," 2017, www.anticancerlifestyle.org/testimonials/page/4.
73. M. Hanna-Attisha, J. LaChance, R. C. Sadler, A. Champney Schnepp, "Elevated blood lead levels in children associated with the Flint drinking water crisis: a spatial analysis of risk and public health response," *American Journal of Public Health* 106, no. 2 (February 2016): 283–90.
74. Environmental Working Group, "Hidden carcinogen taints tap water, consumer products nationwide," September 6, 2017, www.ewg.org/release/hidden-carcinogen-taints-tap-water-consumer-products-nationwide-.Wign501TEdU.
75. J. E. Cooper, E. L. Kendig, S. M. Belcher, "Assessment of bisphenol A released from reusable plastic, aluminium and stainless steel water bottles," *Chemosphere* 85, no. 6 (October 2011): 943–47.
76. S. Eladak, T. Grisin, D. Moison, et al., "A new chapter in the bisphenol A story: bisphenol S and bisphenol F are not safe alternatives to this compound," *Fertility and Sterility* 103, no. 1 (January 2015): 11–21.
77. R. Vinas, C. S. Watson, "Bisphenol S disrupts estradiol-induced nongenomic signaling in a rat pituitary cell line: effects on cell functions," *Environmental Health Perspectives* 121, no. 3 (March 2013): 352–58.
78. A. Vaiserman, "Early-life exposure to endocrine disrupting chemicals and later-life health outcomes: an epigenetic bridge?," *Aging and Disease* 5, no. 6 (December 2014): 419–29.
79. L. Trasande, A. J. Spanier, S. Sathyanarayana, T. M. Attina, J. Blustein, "Urinary phthalates and increased insulin resistance in adolescents," *Pediatrics* 132, no. 3 (September 2013): e646–55.
80. P. Mirmira, C. Evans-Molina, "Bisphenol A, obesity, and type 2 diabetes mellitus: Genuine concern or unnecessary preoccupation?," *Translational Research: The Journal of Laboratory and Clinical Medicine* 164, no. 1 (July 2014): 13–21.
81. F. S. Vom Saal, S. C. Nagel, B. L. Coe, B. M. Angle, J. A. Taylor, "The estrogenic endocrine disrupting chemical bisphenol A (BPA) and obesity," *Molecular and Cellular Endocrinology* 354, no. 1–2 (May 2012): 74–84.

82. F. Grun, B. Blumberg, "Endocrine disrupters as obesogens," *Molecular and Cellular Endocrinology* 304, no. 1–2 (May 2009): 19–29.

83. H. A. Beydoun, M. A. Beydoun, H. A. Jeng, A. B. Zonderman, S. M. Eid, "Bisphenol-A and sleep adequacy among adults in the National Health and Nutrition Examination Surveys," *Sleep* 39, no. 2 (February 2016): 467–76.

84. S. A. Johnson, M. S. Painter, A. B. Javurek, et al., "Sex-dependent effects of developmental exposure to bisphenol A and ethinyl estradiol on metabolic parameters and voluntary physical activity," *Journal of Developmental Origins of Health and Disease* 6, no. 6 (December 2015): 539–52.

The Anticancer Living Guide to Detoxify Your Environment

1. M. Derudi, S. Gelosa, A. Sliepcevich, et al., "Emission of air pollutants from burning candles with different composition in indoor environments," *Environmental Science and Pollution Research International* 21, no. 6 (March 2014): 4320–30.

2. Centers for Disease Control and Prevention, "Occupational cancer," April 24, 2017, www.cdc.gov/niosh/topics/cancer/npotocca.html.

3. X. Zhang, S. K. Brar, S. Yan, R. D. Tyagi, R. Y. Surampalli, "Fate and transport of fragrance materials in principal environmental sinks," *Chemosphere* 93, no. 6 (October 2013): 857–69.

4. United States Environmental Protection Agency, "Volatile organic compounds' impact on indoor air quality," 2017, www.epa.gov/indoor-air-quality-iaq/volatile-organic-compounds-impact-indoor-air-quality.

5. R. A. Rudel, J. M. Ackerman, K. R. Attfield, J. G. Brody, "New exposure biomarkers as tools for breast cancer epidemiology, biomonitoring, and prevention: a systematic approach based on animal evidence," *Environmental Health Perspectives* 122, no. 9 (September 2014): 881–95.

6. Environmental Working Group, "EWG's healthy home tips: tip 7—filter your tap water," 2017, www.ewg.org/research/healthy-home-tips/tip-7-filter-your-tap-water-filter.

7. Environmental Working Group, "EWG's updated water filter buying guide," 2017, www.ewg.org/tapwater/water-filter-guide.php-.Wg4Ou1UrJQJ.

8. Environmental Working Group, "EWG's 2017 Shopper's Guide to Pesticides in Produce™," 2017, https://www.ewg.org/foodnews/dirty_dozen_list.php-.Wg4PI1UrJQI.

9. International Agency for Research on Cancer, "IARC classifies radiofrequency electromagnetic fields as possibly carcinogenic to humans," May 31, 2011, www.iarc.fr/en/media-centre/pr/2011/pdfs/pr208_E.pdf.

10. L. Kheifets, M. Repacholi, R. Saunders, E. van Deventer, "The sensitivity of children to electromagnetic fields," *Pediatrics* 116, no. 2 (August 2005): e303–13.

11. J. Schüz, "Exposure to electromagnetic fields and cancer: the epidemiological evidence," General Assembly and Scientific Symposium, 2011 XXXth URSI, 2011.

12. M. Gutierrez, "New records show how state reworked secret cell phone warnings," *San Francisco Chronicle*, May 19, 2017, www.sfchronicle.com/health/article/New-records-show-how-state-reworked-secret-cell-11160254.php.

13. California Department of Public Health, "Cell phones and health," California Department of Public Health, April 2014, www.sfchronicle.com/file/198/6/1986-Cell Phones 1-26-15.pdf.

14. N. R. Council, *Review of the Environmental Protection Agency's Draft IRIS Assessment of Tetrachloroethylene* (Washington, D.C.: National Academies Press, 2010).

15. E. Hartman, "The messy truth about dry cleaning," *Washington Post*, August 10, 2008, www.washingtonpost.com/wp-dyn/content/article/2008/08/07/AR2008080702759.html.

16. U.S. Environmental Protection Agency, "Reducing air pollution from dry cleaning operations," September 12, 2005, www.epa.gov/sites/production/files/2017-06/documents/drycleaners_comm_info.pdf.

17. U.S. Environmental Protection Agency, "Surfactant enhancement of liquid C02 for surface cleaning," May 13, 2003, www.cfpub.epa.gov/si/si_public_record_Report.cfm?dirEntryID=56445.

18. R. Gottlieb, L. Bechtel, J. Goodheart, P. Sinsheimer, C. Tranby, "Final report: evaluation and demonstration of wet cleaning alternatives to perchloroethylene-based garment care," 1997, www.cfpub.epa.gov/ncer_abstracts/index.cfm/fuseaction/display.highlight/abstract/945/report/F.

Concluding Thoughts

1. American Institute for Cancer Research, "Recommendations for cancer prevention," 2017, www.aicr.org/reduce-your-cancer-risk/recommendations-for-cancer-prevention.

2. B. Arun, T. Austin, G. V. Babiera, et al., "A comprehensive lifestyle randomized clinical trial: design and initial patient experience," *Integrative Cancer Therapies* 16, no. 1 (March 2017): 3–20.

Appendix A: The Cancer Hallmarks Explained

1. D. Hanahan, R. A. Weinberg, "The hallmarks of cancer," *Cell* 100, no. 1 (January 2000): 57–70.

2. D. Hanahan, R. A. Weinberg, "Hallmarks of cancer: the next generation," *Cell* 144, no. 5 (March 2011): 646–74.

Appendix B: Eating by Food Groups—A New Pattern

1. H. L. Nicastro, S. A. Ross, J. A. Milner, "Garlic and onions: their cancer prevention properties," *Cancer Prevention Research* 8, no. 3 (March 2015): 181–89.

2. D. Boivin, S. Lamy, S. Lord-Dufour, et al., "Antiproliferative and antioxidant activities of common vegetables: a comparative study," *Food Chemistry* 112, no. 2 (January 2009): 374–80.

3. A. Sengupta, S. Ghosh, S. Bhattacharjee, "Allium vegetables in cancer prevention: an overview," *Asian Pacific Journal of Cancer Prevention* 5, no. 3 (July–September 2004): 237–45.

4. A. W. Hsing, A. P. Chokkalingam, Y. T. Gao, et al., "Allium vegetables and risk of prostate cancer: a population-based study," *Journal of the National Cancer Institute* 94, no. 21 (November 2002): 1648–51.

5. C. A. Thomson, C. L. Rock, B. J. Caan, et al., "Increase in cruciferous vegetable intake in women previously treated for breast cancer participating in a dietary intervention trial," *Nutrition and Cancer* 57, no. 1 (May 2007): 11–19.

6. C. A. Thomson, E. Ho, M. B. Strom, "Chemopreventive properties of 3,3'-diindolylmethane in breast cancer: evidence from experimental and human studies," *Nutrition Reviews* 74, no. 7 (July 2016): 432–43.

7. M. Lenzi, C. Fimognari, P. Hrelia, "Sulforaphane as a promising molecule for fighting cancer," *Cancer Treatment and Research* 159 (October 2014): 207–23.

8. K. L. Kaspar, J. S. Park, C. R. Brown, et al., "Pigmented potato consumption alters oxidative stress and inflammatory damage in men," *Journal of Nutrition* 141, no. 1 (January 2011): 108–11.

9. S. Lim, J. Xu, J. Kim, et al., "Role of anthocyanin-enriched purple-fleshed sweet potato p40 in colorectal cancer prevention," *Molecular Nutrition & Food Research* 57, no. 11 (November 2013): 1908–17.

10. G. Block, B. Patterson, A. Subar, "Fruit, vegetables, and cancer prevention: a review of the epidemiological evidence," *Nutrition and Cancer* 18, no. 1 (January 1992): 1–29.

11. M. Zhang, J. Huang, X. Xie, C. D. Holman, "Dietary intakes of mushrooms and green tea combine to reduce the risk of breast cancer in Chinese women," *International Journal of Cancer* 124, no. 6 (March 2009): 1404–8.

12. E. N. Alonso, M. J. Ferronato, N. A. Gandini, et al., "Antitumoral effects of D-Fraction from grifola frondosa (maitake) mushroom in breast cancer," *Nutrition and Cancer* 69, no. 1 (January 2017): 29–43.

13. M. E. Balandaykin, I. V. Zmitrovich, "Review on chaga medicinal mushroom, inonotus obliquus (higher basidiomycetes): realm of medicinal applications and approaches on estimating its resource potential," *International Journal of Medicinal Mushrooms* 17, no. 2 (March 2015): 95–104.

14. American Institute for Cancer Research, "Berries," American Institute for Cancer Research, 2017, www.aicr.org/foods-that-fight-cancer/foodsthatfightcancer_berries .html.

15. G. D. Stoner, L.-S. Wang, N. Zikri, et al., "Cancer prevention with freeze-dried berries and berry components," *Seminars in Cancer Biology* 17, no. 5 (May 2007): 403–10.

16. A. Basu, M. Rhone, T. J. Lyons, "Berries: emerging impact on cardiovascular health," *Nutrition Reviews* 68, no. 3 (March 2010): 168–77.

17. H. N. Luu, W. J. Blot, Y. B. Xiang, et al., "Prospective evaluation of the association of nut/peanut consumption with total and cause-specific mortality," *Journal of the American Medical Association: Internal Medicine* 175, no. 5 (May 2015): 755–66.

18. X. Su, R. M. Tamimi, L. C. Collins, et al., "Intake of fiber and nuts during adolescence and incidence of proliferative benign breast disease," *Cancer Causes and Control* 21, no. 7 (July 2010): 1033–46.

19. C. Sanchez-Gonzalez, C. J. Ciudad, V. Noe, M. Izquierdo-Pulido, "Health benefits of walnut polyphenols: an exploration beyond their lipid profile," *Critical Reviews in Food Science and Nutrition* 57, no. 16 (November 2017): 3373–83.

20. L. R. Jimenez, W. A. Hall, M. S. Rodriquez, et al., "Quantifying residues from postharvest propylene oxide fumigation of almonds and walnuts," *Journal of AOAC International* 98, no. 5 (September–October 2015): 1423–27.

21. M. D. Danyluk, T. M. Jones, S. J. Abd, et al., "Prevalence and amounts of salmonella found on raw California almonds," *Journal of Food Protection* 70, no. 4 (April 2007): 820–27.

22. L. U. Thompson, J. M. Chen, T. Li, K. Strasser-Weippl, P. E. Goss, "Dietary flaxseed alters tumor biological markers in postmenopausal breast cancer," *Clinical Cancer Research* 11, no. 10 (May 2005): 3828–35.

23. A. K. Wiggins, J. K. Mason, L. U. Thompson, "Beneficial influence of diets enriched with flaxseed and flaxseed oil on cancer," in *Cancer Chemoprevention and Treatment by Diet Therapy*, ed. William C. S. Cho (Dordrecht, The Netherlands: Springer, 2013), 55–89.

24. J. K. Mason, L. U. Thompson, "Flaxseed and its lignan and oil components: can they play a role in reducing the risk of and improving the treatment of breast cancer?," *Applied Physiology, Nutrition, and Metabolism. Physiologie Appliquée, Nutrition et Métabolisme* 39, no. 6 (June 2014): 663–78.

25. T. Huang, M. Xu, A. Lee, S. Cho, L. Qi, "Consumption of whole grains and cereal fiber and total and cause-specific mortality: prospective analysis of 367,442 individuals," *BMC Medicine* 13 (March 2015): 59.

26. R. C. Masters, A. D. Liese, S. M. Haffner, L. E. Wagenknecht, A. J. Hanley, "Whole and refined grain intakes are related to inflammatory protein concentrations in human plasma," *Journal of Nutrition* 140, no. 3 (March 2010): 587–94.

27. M. Lefevre, S. Jonnalagadda, "Effect of whole grains on markers of subclinical inflammation," *Nutrition Reviews* 70, no. 7 (July 2012): 387–96.

28. A. M. Troen, "Folate and vitamin B12: function and importance in cognitive development," *Nestle Nutrition Institute Workshop Series* 70 (January 2012): 161–71.

29. American Institute for Cancer Research, "Legumes," American Institute for Cancer Research, 2017, www.aicr.org/foods-that-fight-cancer/foodsthatfightcancer_berries .html.

30. H. Wang, M. S. Geier, G. S. Howarth, "Prebiotics: a potential treatment strategy for the chemotherapy-damaged gut?," *Critical Reviews in Food Science and Nutrition* 56, no. 6 (August 2016): 946–56.

31. B. Petschow, J. Dore, P. Hibberd, et al., "Probiotics, prebiotics, and the host microbiome: the science of translation," *Annals of the New York Academy of Sciences* 1306 (December 2013): 1–17.

32. S. J. Bultman, "The microbiome and its potential as a cancer preventive intervention," *Seminars in Oncology* 43, no. 1 (September 2016): 97–106.

33. A. Riviere, M. Selak, D. Lantin, F. Leroy, L. De Vuyst, "Bifidobacteria and butyrate-producing colon bacteria: importance and strategies for their stimulation in the human gut," *Frontiers in Microbiology* 7 (July 2016): 979.

34. H. M. Chen, Y. N. Yu, J. L. Wang, et al., "Decreased dietary fiber intake and structural alteration of gut microbiota in patients with advanced colorectal adenoma," *The American Journal of Clinical Nutrition* 97, no. 5 (May 2013): 1044–52.

35. M. G. Gareau, P. M. Sherman, W. A. Walker, "Probiotics and the gut microbiota in intestinal health and disease," *Nature Reviews Gastroenterology & Hepatology* 7, no. 9 (September 2010): 503–14.

36. Human Microbiome Project Consortium, "Structure, function and diversity of the healthy human microbiome," *Nature* 486, no. 7402 (June 2012b): 207–14.

37. S. J. Hewlings, D. S. Kalman, "Curcumin: a review of its effects on human health," *Foods* 6, no. 10 (October 2017).

38. G. P. Lim, T. Chu, F. Yang, et al., "The curry spice curcumin reduces oxidative damage and amyloid pathology in an Alzheimer transgenic mouse," *Journal of Neuroscience* 21, no. 21 (November 2001): 8370–77.

39. R. Wilken, M. S. Veena, M. B. Wang, E. S. Srivatsan, "Curcumin: a review of anti-cancer properties and therapeutic activity in head and neck squamous cell carcinoma," *Molecular Cancer* 10 (February 2011): 12.

40. S. S. Percival, J. P. Vanden Heuvel, C. J. Nieves, et al., "Bioavailability of herbs and spices in humans as determined by ex vivo inflammatory suppression and DNA strand breaks," *Journal of the American College of Nutrition* 31, no. 4 (August 2012): 288–94.

41. K. Griffiths, B. B. Aggarwal, R. B. Singh, et al., "Food antioxidants and their anti-inflammatory properties: a potential role in cardiovascular diseases and cancer prevention," *Diseases* 4, no. 3 (August 2016).

Appendix C: Environmental Toxin Hit List

1. T. B. Hayes, V. Khoury, A. Narayan, et al., "Atrazine induces complete feminization and chemical castration in male African clawed frogs (Xenopus laevis)," *Proceedings of the National Academy of Sciences of the United States of America* 107, no. 10 (March 2010): 4612–17.

2. C. Cox, "Herbicide Factsheet Atrazine: Toxicology," *Journal of Pesticide Reform* 21, no. 2 (Summer 2001b).

3. M. C. Alavanja, C. Samanic, M. Dosemeci, et al., "Use of agricultural pesticides and prostate cancer risk in the Agricultural Health Study cohort," *American Journal of Epidemiology* 157, no. 9 (May 2003): 800–14.

4. K. Hu, Y. Tian, Y. Du, et al., "Atrazine promotes RM1 prostate cancer cell proliferation by activating STAT3 signaling," *International Journal of Oncology* 48, no. 5 (May 2016): 2166–74.

5. J. R. Rochester, "Bisphenol A and human health: a review of the literature," *Reproductive Toxicology* 42 (December 2013): 132–55.

6. S. Eladak, T. Grisin, D. Moison, et al., "A new chapter in the bisphenol A story: bisphenol S and bisphenol F are not safe alternatives to this compound," *Fertility and Sterility* 103, no. 1 (January 2015): 11–21.

7. F. Salazar-Garcia, E. Gallardo-Diaz, P. Ceron-Mireles, D. Loomis, V. H. Borja-Aburto, "Reproductive effects of occupational DDT exposure among male malaria control workers," *Environmental Health Perspectives* 112, no. 5 (April 2004): 542–47.

8. N. Shivapurkar, K. L. Hoover, L. A. Poirier, "Effect of methionine and choline on liver tumor promotion by phenobarbital and DDT in diethylnitrosamine-initiated rats," *Carcinogenesis* 7, no. 4 (April 1986): 547–50.

9. M. Kogevinas, "Human health effects of dioxins: cancer, reproductive and endocrine system effects," *Human Reproduction Update* 7, no. 3 (May–June 2001): 331–39.

10. S. N. Bhupathiraju, F. Grodstein, M. J. Stampfer, et al., "Exogenous hormone use: oral contraceptives, postmenopausal hormone therapy, and health outcomes in the Nurses' Health Study," *American Journal of Public Health* 106, no. 9 (September 2016): 1631–37.

11. M. E. Samson, S. A. Adams, C. M. Mulatya, et al., "Types of oral contraceptives and breast cancer survival among women enrolled in Medicaid: a competing-risk model," *Maturitas* 95 (January 2017): 42–49.

12. U.S. Food and Drug Administration, "Fragrances in cosmetics," November 25, 2017, www.fda.gov/Cosmetics/ProductsIngredients/Ingredients/ucm388821.htm.

13. F. A. Caliman, M. Gavrilescu, "Pharmaceuticals, personal care products and endocrine disrupting agents in the environment—a review," *CLEAN–Soil, Air, Water* 37, no. 4–5 (April 2009): 277–303.

14. Environmental Working Group, "Not so sexy: hidden chemicals in perfume and cologne," May 12, 2010, www.ewg.org/research/not-so-sexy-.Wh3IDFVKsdV.

15. B. Eskenazi, A. Bradman, R. Castorina, "Exposures of children to organophosphate pesticides and their potential adverse health effects," *Environmental Health Perspectives* 107, Supplement 3 (June 1999): 409–19.

16. P. D. Darbre, P. W. Harvey, "Parabens can enable hallmarks and characteristics of cancer in human breast epithelial cells: a review of the literature with reference to new exposure data and regulatory status," *Journal of Applied Toxicology* 34, no. 9 (September 2014): 925–38.

17. A. M. Leung, E. N. Pearce, L. E. Braverman, "Perchlorate, iodine and the thyroid," *Best Practice & Research: Clinical Endocrinology & Metabolism* 24, no. 1 (February 2010): 133–41.

18. K. M. Rappazzo, E. Coffman, E. P. Hines, "Exposure to perfluorinated alkyl substances and health outcomes in children: a systematic review of the epidemiologic literature," *International Journal of Environmental Research and Public Health* 14, no. 7 (June 2017): 691.

19. C. Lau, "Perfluorinated compounds: an overview," in *Toxicological Effects of Perfluoroalkyl and Polyfluoroalkyl Substances*, ed. Jamie C. DeWitt (Cham, Switzerland: Humana Press, 2015), 1–21.

20. J. D. Meeker, K. K. Ferguson, "Urinary phthalate metabolites are associated with decreased serum testosterone in men, women, and children from NHANES 2011–2012," *Journal of Clinical Endocrinology and Metabolism* 99, no. 11 (November 2014): 4346–52.

21. W. J. Cowell, S. A. Lederman, A. Sjödin, et al., "Prenatal exposure to polybrominated diphenyl ethers and child attention problems at 3–7 years," *Neurotoxicology and Teratology* 52 (Pt B) (November–December 2015): 143–50.

22. V. Linares, M. Belles, J. L. Domingo, "Human exposure to PBDE and critical evaluation of health hazards," *Archives of Toxicology* 89, no. 3 (March 2015): 335–56.

23. K. A. Jarema, D. L. Hunter, R. M. Shaffer, M. Behl, S. Padilla, "Acute and developmental behavioral effects of flame retardants and related chemicals in zebrafish," *Neurotoxicology and Teratology* 52 (Pt B) (November–December 2015): 194–209.

24. L. G. Costa, G. Giordano, "Developmental neurotoxicity of polybrominated diphenyl ether (PBDE) flame retardants," *Neurotoxicology* 28, no. 6 (November 2007): 1047–67.

25. M.F. Yueh, K. Taniguchi, S. Chen, et al., "The commonly used antimicrobial additive triclosan is a liver tumor promoter," *Proceedings of the National Academy of Sciences of the United States of America* 111, no. 48 (November 2014): 17200–17205.

26. National Toxicology Program, "Report on carcinogens, fourteenth edition," U.S. Department of Health and Human Services, Public Health Service, 2016b.

27. Health and Food Safety Scientific Committee, "Opinion concerning banning of dialkanolamines which are still in the inventory adopted by the plenary session of the SCCNFP on 17 February 1999," February 17, 1999, www.ec.europa.eu/health /scientific_committees/consumer_safety/opinions/sccnfp_opinions_97_04/sccp _out64_en.htm.

28. J. B. Knaak, H. W. Leung, W. T. Stott, J. Busch, J. Bilsky, "Toxicology of mono-, di-, and triethanolamine," *Reviews of Environmental Contamination and Toxicology* 149 (January 1997): 1–86.

29. The Agency for Toxic Substances and Disease Registry (ATSDR), "Toxic substances portal—ethylene oxide," July 1999, www.atsdr.cdc.gov/toxfaqs/tf.asp?id=733&tid=133.

30. M. M. Peters, T. W. Jones, T. J. Monks, S. S. Lau, "Cytotoxicity and cell proliferation induced by the nephrocarcinogen hydroquinone and its nephrotoxic metabolite 2,3,5-(tris-glutathion-S-yl)hydroquinone," *Carcinogenesis* 18, no. 12 (December 1997): 2393–401.

31. G. Bjorklund, M. Dadar, J. Mutter, J. Aaseth, "The toxicology of mercury: current research and emerging trends," *Environmental Research* 159 (November 2017): 545–54.

32. P. Boffetta, E. Merler, H. Vainio, "Carcinogenicity of mercury and mercury compounds," *Scandinavian Journal of Work, Environment and Health* 19, no. 1 (February 1993): 1–7.

33. IARC Working Group on the Evaluation of Carcinogenic Risk to Humans, ed., "Mineral oils, untreated or mildly treated," in *Chemical Agents and Related Occupations* (Lyon, France: WHO International Agency for Research on Cancer, 2014).

34. S. Maipas, P. Nicolopoulou-Stamati, "Sun lotion chemicals as endocrine disruptors," *Hormones* 14, no. 1 (January–March 2015): 32–46.

35. S. Heikkinen, J. Pitkaniemi, T. Sarkeala, N. Malila, M. Koskenvuo, "Does hair dye use increase the risk of breast cancer? A population-based case-control study of Finnish women," *PLoS One* 10, no. 8 (August 2015): e0135190.

36. The Agency for Toxic Substances and Disease Registry (ATSDR), "Toxic substances portal—ethylene oxide," July 1999, www.atsdr.cdc.gov/toxfaqs/tf.asp?id=733&tid= 133.

37. The Agency for Toxic Substances and Disease Registry (ATSDR), "Toxic substances portal1—dioxane," September 2007, www.atsdr.cdc.gov/toxfaqs/tf.asp?id=954& tid=199.

38. H.J. Jang, C. Y. Shin, K.-B. Kim, "Safety evaluation of polyethylene glycol (PEG) compounds for cosmetic use," *Toxicological Research* 31, no. 2 (June 2015): 105–36.

39. L. Montenegro, D. Paolino, G. Puglisi, "Effects of silicone emulsifiers on in vitro skin permeation of sunscreens from cosmetic emulsions," *Journal of Cosmetic Science* 55, no. 6 (November–December 2004): 509–18.

40. C. A. Bondi, J. L. Marks, L. B. Wroblewski, et al., "Human and environmental toxicity of sodium lauryl sulfate (SLS): evidence for safe use in household cleaning products," *Environmental Health Insights* 9 (November 2015): 27–32.

41. R. Penninkilampi, G. D. Eslick, "Perineal talc use and ovarian cancer: a systematic review and meta-analysis," *Epidemiology* (August 2017).

42. C. M. Filley, W. Halliday, B. K. Kleinschmidt-DeMasters, "The effects of toluene on the central nervous system," *Journal of Neuropathology and Experimental Neurology* 63, no. 1 (January 2004): 1–12.

INDEX

Page numbers in italics refer to charts and tables.

Abrams, Donald, 91–92
acceptance of cancer, 10, 18
activating invasion and metastases hallmark
    of cancer, 53, 54, 304
  sleep and, 167
  social support and, 99
acute stress, 138
acute stress disorder (ASD), 124
adverse childhood experiences (ACE), 62,
    141–43
aerobic glycolysis, 304–5
agave nectar, 256
air pollution, 267
alcohol, 258
  as carcinogen, 43, 234, 258
  in combination with tobacco use, 44–45
aldehydes, 258
alliums, 309
altruistic behavior, 85–86
Alzheimer's disease, 176, 200
American Cancer Society, 24
American Institute for Cancer Research, 24
Ancoli-Israel, Sonia, 183–84, 185
Andersen, Barbara, 73
angiogenesis, 53, 55, 302, 303–4
  diet and, 228
  social support and, 99
angiogenesis inhibitors, 56
anoikis, 47, 304
Anticancer Lifestyle Program, 7, 36,
    112–13, 276
anticancer living. See lifestyle
Anticancer (Schreiber), 11, 69, 226, 287
anticancer team, building
  support areas, 116–17
  weak spots, building up your, 117–18
Antoni, Mike, 145–46

apoptosis, cancer's ability to avoid, 53, 302
apoptosis inducers, 56
apples, 252
arsenic, 317
asbestos, 268–69
asparagus, 254
atrazine, 275–76, 315
avocado oil, 259
Awakening the Spine: Yoga for Health,
    Vitality and Energy (Scaravelli), 153
azodicarbonamide, 274

beans, 252, 257–58
beets, 254
behavioral therapy programs
  beneficial genetic expression profile
    changes resulting from, 140
  cognitive behavioral therapy (CBT), 152,
    180, 181, 189
behavior change, overcoming barriers to,
    319–30
  focusing on what can be achieved, 319–20
  high-risk events and triggers, dealing with,
    321–24
  houseguests, challenges posed by, 322–23
  lapses/relapses, dealing with, 323, 324
  plan for dealing with high-risk events or
    lapses/relapses, 324
  reframing your thoughts, 319, 320–21
  travel, challenges posed by, 322–23,
    325–28
bell curve for cancer prevention and control,
    14–16, 15
Benson, Herbert, 130
benzodiazepines, 179–80
berries, 252, 312
beta-amyloid, 176

Biden, Joe, 293
biological therapies, 58
bisphenol A (BPA), 269, 271, 272, 275, 276–77, 278, 315
bisphenol S (BPS), 277
Blackburn, Elizabeth, 64, 136, 147
blaming yourself for getting cancer, 6–7
blueberries, 252
Blue Cure Foundation, 213, 296
Blue Zones, 90, 229–30
body, reducing toxins put in or on your, 283–86
body clock, 162, 163
body weight
    cancer and, 238–44
    conditions negatively impacted by, 241–42
    obesity (*See* obesity)
Bolt, Usain, 170
bone health, 200
brain cleansing, and sleep, 175–76
BRCA-1 and BRCA-2 genes, 39–40
breakfast, 251–52
breast cancer
    body weight and, 241
    BRCA-1 and BRCA-2 genes and risk of, 39–40
    cancer prevention guidelines, risk and mortality reduction from following, 24, *25*
    cognitive behavioral stress management (CBSM) program, study on impact of, 145–46
    connectedness and survival rates, study on, 88–89
    early detection of, 6, 49
    early stage low-grade cancers, treatment decision for, 6, 49
    exercise and, 202–3, 208
    lifestyle intervention, study on impact of, 73–74, *74*
    Mediterranean diet and, 226, 228
    Rafte's experience and founding of support group for metastatic breast cancer, 83–85, 86, 296
    rates of, in U.S., 14
    sleep deprivation and, 177
    soy and, 257–58
    treatment decisions for low-risk disease, 49
    Women's Healthy Eating and Living (WHEL) Study on effect of vegetable intake on, 244–46, *245*
broccoli, 254
Brockovich, Erin, 266
Brown, Jerry, 274
Brucett M., breast cancer survivor, 133–34, 179

brussels sprouts, 254
Buettner, Dan, 212
Burke Harris, Nadine, 142–43

caffeine, 247
California Cleaning Product Right to Know Act, 274
Campbell Soup Company, 274–75
Canales, Gabe, 40–42, 112, 213–14, 296
cancer
    acceptance of diagnosis, 10, 18
    aging and, 5
    blaming yourself for, 6–7
    body weight and, 238–44
    causes of, 38–45
    cells (*See* cancer cells)
    death rates, 5
    diet and, 43, 223–24, 231, 232, 233–36
    early detection, 6, 47–48, 49
    as evolutionary response to modern life, 65–67
    funding for research, 9–10
    hallmarks of (*See* hallmarks of cancer model)
    healing versus curing, 29–31
    history of, 48–52
    hopelessness and despair, impact of, 34
    industrialization and, 265–66
    innovations in diagnosing and fighting, 4
    isolation felt by patients and, 35–36
    lifestyle and (*See* lifestyle)
    living with, 3–4
    microbiome and, 56, 225
    proactive healing, examples of (*See* proactive healing, examples of)
    psychological impact of diagnosis, 18
    rates of, 5, 14
    red and processed meats and, 236–37
    sleep deprivation and, 177–78
    soy and, 257–58
    standard of care, 18–23
    statistics on, dangers posed by, 10–12
    sugar consumption and, 233–34
    survival rates, 6
    tobacco consumption and, 8–10
    treatment (*See* cancer treatment)
    war metaphors in talking about, impact of, 31–32
    in younger people, 5–6
Cancer Alley, in Louisiana, 267
cancer cells, 46–58, 307
    cell mutations, initial bodily responses to, 46–47
    gestational period of, 47
    metastasis, 47–48
    treatment of (*See* cancer treatment)

cancer clusters, 266–68
Cancer Connection, 114
Cancer Genome Atlas project, 57
Cancer Moonshot, 293
cancer prevention
    bell curve for cancer prevention and
        control, 14–16, 15
    funding for research, 9–10
    guidelines for, risk and mortality reduction
        associated with following, 24, 25
    lifestyle and (See lifestyle)
    tobacco consumption and, 9
cancer proliferation loop, 134–35
cancer-related fatigue (CRF), 182–85, 205
cancer stem cells, 307
cancer treatment, 4–5
    biological therapies, 58
    chemotherapy, 43, 51–52, 207
    exercise as element of, 204–7
    gene behavior and, 52–55
    gene therapies, 58
    history of, 48–52
    immunotherapies, 52, 57–58, 225, 305
    palliative care, 50
    radiation, 51–52
    surgical treatment, 50–52
    targeted cancer therapies, 52, 55–57
    vaccines targeting cancer-causing viruses,
        57, 58
canola oil, 258, 259
car cleaning products, 287
Cardinal, Brad, 198
cardiovascular disease. See heart/
    cardiovascular disease
caregivers, and stress, 123, 136–37
CaringBridge, 103
carrots, 254
Carskadon, Mary, 171
Carter, Jennifer, 197
catechins, 261
cauliflower, 254
causes of cancer, 38–45
    chemical agents as, 42–44
    genetics and, 38–39
CBSM. See cognitive behavioral stress
    management (CBSM)
CBT. See cognitive behavioral
    therapy (CBT)
CDC-Kaiser ACE study, 141–42
cell phone use, 287
cell suicide. See apoptosis, cancer's ability to
    avoid
centenarians, 90
Chaoul, Alejandro, 159
checkpoint inhibitors, 305
chemical agents, 42–44

chemicals/chemical toxins. See environment/
    environmental toxins
chemotherapy, 43, 51–52, 207
children
    adverse childhood experiences (ACE),
        impact of, 62, 141–43
    anticancer living and, 77, 95
    reaction to parent's cancer diagnosis,
        96–97
    sharing new cancer diagnosis with, 96
    sleep deprivation, effects of, 170–71
chives, 309
chromosomal instability, 135–36
chronic stress, 61–63, 70, 134–39
    bodies response to, 122–23, 137–39
    cancer proliferation loop and, 134–35
    telomere shortening and, 135–36, 147–48
    See also stress
Church Health, 110–11
cigarettes. See tobacco consumption
circadian arousal system, 164
circadian rhythm, 162, 163, 164–65
CO_2 cleaning, 288
coal tar, 317
coconut oil, 258
coffee, 261
cognitive behavioral stress management
    (CBSM), 145–46
cognitive behavioral therapy (CBT)
    sleep quality improvement and, 180,
        181, 189
    stress reduction and, 152
Cohan, Deborah, 210–11
Colditz, Graham, 7
Cole, Steve, 45, 61–63, 67, 99, 100, 105, 106,
    112, 140, 152
colon/colorectal cancer
    body weight and, 241
    cancer prevention guidelines, risk and
        mortality reduction from following,
        24, 25
    exercise and, 203
    sleep deprivation and, 177–78
    in younger population, 5–6
colonization, 304
Commonweal, 101–2
community support, 117
compassion-based meditation, 131, 157–58
Comprehensive Lifestyle Study (CompLife),
    32–33, 35, 87, 113–14, 222–23, 291
connectedness. See love and social support
Cook, Ken, 268
cooking temperature, 258–59
cookware, 286
core values, 118–20
corn oil, 258

cortisol, 137–38, 164, 181
Courneya, Kerry, 204–5, 206
CRF. *See* cancer-related fatigue (CRF)
cruciferous vegetables, 228–29, 245–46,
　254, 309
Crum, Alia, 211
Cuomo, Andrew, 274
Cuomo, Margaret I., 269–70, 297
curing versus healing, 29–31
cytokines, 135

dairy, 256–57
dancing, 210–11
David, Rosalie, 265
Davidson, Richard, 130
DDT (di-cholor-diphenyl-trichloroethane), 315
DEA, 317
*The Deepest Well: Healing the Long-Term
　Effects of Childhood Adversity* (Burke
　Harris), 142–43
Dekker, Thomas, 163
dementia, 176, 200
DePinho, Ron, 231
depression
　emotional trauma of cancer and, 124
　gene expression and, 61
　gratitude and, 145
　sedentary lifestyle and, 200
　sleep deprivation and, 173
　volunteer work and reduced rates of, 85
despair, 34
detoxifying your environment, guide to,
　280–90
　body, reducing toxins put in or on your,
　　283–86
　car cleaning products, 287
　cell phone use, 287
　cleanup and elimination of potentially
　　hazardous products, 281–82
　dry cleaning, 287–88
　establishing anticancer environment, 280
　home, removing chemicals from, 281–82
　larger environment, limiting exposure to
　　toxins in, 286–88
　precautionary principle and, 280
　summary, 289–90
　water, filtering, 282
diabetes
　body weight and, 240
　chemical toxins and, 278
　diet and, 226
　sedentary lifestyle and, 199
　sleep deprivation and, 172, 173, 177
　sugar consumption and, 233–34
diaphragmatic breathing, 152, 154–55
dichlorobenzene, 271

diet, 24–25, 70, 221–61
　in Blue Zones, 229–30
　body weight cancer connection, 238–40
　as cause of cancer, 43, 223–24, 231, 232,
　　233–37
　exercise and, *246*, 246–47
　food groups, eating by, 309–14
　fruit, 227, 228, 232, 251–53, 311
　glycemic load, reducing, 235–36
　guide to nutrition (*See* nutrition, guide to)
　healing powers of, 221–22
　healthy choices and, 237–38
　highly processed foods, addictive nature
　　of, 238
　Mediterranean diet, 226–29
　microbiome and, 224–25
　plant-based diet, adopting, 226–29
　for prostate cancer, 17
　purpose of food, 222
　red and processed meats, 232, 236–37
　stress, impact of, 147–49
　sugar, 233–34, 255
　sugar substitutes, 235, 256
　supplements in, 227, 259
　synergy with other lifestyle factors,
　　247–48
　traveling, while, 327–28
　vegetables (*See* vegetables)
Dietary Guidelines, 222
diethylstilbestrol (DES) exposure, epigenetic
　effects of, 64–65
dinner, 252–53
dioxin, 315
doctors and health-care providers
　selection of, 93–94
　social support networks, role in helping
　　patients engage with, 94–95
Dorothy P., breast cancer survivor, 101, 112,
　221–22
dry cleaning, 287–88
ductal carcinoma in situ, 49
DuPont Chemical Company, 42

early detection of cancers, 6, 47–48, 49
early onset puberty, 271
Elaine W., breast cancer survivor, 19–21
electromagnetic fields, 287
Emmons, Robert, 145
emotional social support, 35–36
emotional stress, of cancer diagnosis,
　123–24
emotional support, 117
emotions of mortality, 124–27
empathy, 97, 144
endocrine disrupting chemicals (EDCs),
　270–73, 315–17

endometrial cancer
   body weight and, 241, 243
   cancer prevention guidelines, risk and
      mortality reduction from following, 24
   exercise and, 203–4
   Mediterranean diet and, 226
endothelial cells, 307
energy metabolism, cancer's reprogramming
   of, 53, 304–5
Environmental Working Group (EWG), 268
environment/environmental toxins, 24–25,
   43–44, 70–71, 263–90
   cancer clusters, 266–68
   detoxifying your environment, guide to
      (See subhead: detoxifying your
      environment, guide to)
   endocrine disruption and, 270–73, 315–17
   Halifax Project and, 275
   industrialization, and cancer prevalence,
      265–66
   ingredient labeling by manufacturers,
      274–75
   known carcinogenic chemicals still in use,
      268–69
   products containing, 264–65, 283–86
   public awareness of, 273
   synergy with other lifestyle factors,
      278–79
   traveling, encountered while, 328
   understanding scope of problem and
      limiting exposure to, 275–78
Epel, Elissa, 61, 64, 128–29, 136, 147, 303
epigenetics, 59–68
   of childhood experiences, 62
   defined, 59
   diethylstilbestrol (DES) exposure,
      epigenetic effects of, 64–65
   endocrine-disrupting compounds, effects
      of, 272
   evolutionary aspects of epigenetic
      experiences, 63–65
   external factors, 60
   Holocaust survivor descendants, stress
      profiles of, 63–64
   Human Epigenome Project (HEP), 63
   lifestyle and, 60–63, 67–68
   metastases as evolutionary adaptation,
      65–67
   reversibility of epigenetic influence, 64–65
   social genomics and, 60–63
epigenome, 60
epinephrine, 137–38
estrogen production, and body weight, 242
ethanolamine compounds (DEA/TEA/
   MEA), 317
ethinyl estradiol, 315–16

ethoxylated surfactants and 1,4-dioxane, 317
eudaimonic well-being, 104–5, 106, 118–20
   core values, discovering, 118–20
   supporting others, 120
European Epigenome Project, 63
exercise, 23–24, 24–25, 70, 196–220
   amount of, 212–13
   best types for fighting cancer, 208–9
   biological effects of, 207–8
   cancer risk and, 203–4
   cancer treatment protocol, adding exercise
      to, 204–7
   chemical toxins and, 278–79
   chemotherapy and, 207
   comparing yourself to others, effect of,
      211–12
   daily routine, incorporating movement
      into, 200–2
   dancing, 210–11
   defined, 197
   determining what works best for you,
      209–10
   diet and, 246, 246–47
   guide to developing exercise routine (See
      exercise routine, guide to developing)
   obesity and, 198, 241
   sedentary lifestyle, health problems
      associated with, 199–200
   sleep and, 184–85, 190, 198
   stress reduction and, 197–98
   synergy with other lifestyle factors, 197–99
   traveling, while, 326–27
exercise routine, guide to developing, 215–19
   active lifestyle, adopting, 218
   daily movement, monitoring, 215–16
   exercise bursts, 217–18
   fitness routine, developing, 217
   sitting time, breaking up, 216
   travel, staying active during, 218–19
   walking instead of sitting, 216–17

faith communities, 107–11
fasting, 328
fatigue, 23, 123, 140, 142, 153, 180, 181,
   184, 205. See also cancer-related
   fatigue (CRF)
Federer, Roger, 170
Feinberg, Andrew, 63
fibroblasts, 307
fight-or-flight response and, 122
filter systems, for water, 260, 282
fire retardants, 269
Fishman, Ezra, 202
flavonoids, 252, 261
Fleishman, Stewart, 105–6, 107
Flint, Michigan water crisis, 276

Florida Superfund sites, 268
focused-attention meditation, 131, 155–56
Folkman, Judah, 54–55
food addictions, 238
food groups, eating by, 251, 309–14
food packaging, 286
food storage, 286
forced optimism, 128
forest environments, health benefits of
    walking in, 199
formaldehyde, 269, 274, 317
Foundation for Embodied Medicine, 211
4-methylimidazole, 274
fragrance, 265, 274, 277–78, 316
Frankl, Viktor, 104
Fredrickson, Barbara, 85–86, 112
free radicals, 168
fruit, 227, 228, 232, 251–53, 311

gardening, 209
garlic, 309
gene expression, 52
    epigenetics, 59–68
    eudaimonic well-being and, 104–5, 106
    meditation and, 132
    social genomics, 60–63
    social ties and genetic expression,
        connection between, 104–5
    stress and, 139–40
gene regulation, 52
gene therapies, 58
genetics, 39–40
    externally triggered gene malfunctions, 39
    gene behavior, 52–55
    gene therapies, 58
    inherited genetic mutations, 39–40
genome instability and mutation, 54, 305, 306
Gibala, Martin, 212
Glaser, Janice Keicolt, 138–39
Glaser, Ron, 138–39
glucose, 304, 305
glycemic index, 235–36
glycolysis, 304–5
glymphatic system, 176
Gould, Stephen Jay, 11
grass-fed animals, 256–57
gratitude, 144–45
Gray, Janet, 65, 271–72
green onions, 309
green tea, 261
group support, 100–101
growth suppressor evasion, 53, 105, 242, 301–2

Halifax Project, 275
Hall, Martica (Tica), 178–79

hallmarks of cancer model, 53–54, 301–7
    activating invasion and metastases (See
        activating invasion and metastases
        hallmark of cancer)
    angiogenesis, inducing (See angiogenesis)
    apoptosis, cancer's ability to avoid, 53, 302
    enabling characteristics, 53–54, 305–6
    energy metabolism, reprogramming of, 53, 304–5
    genome instability and mutation, 54, 305, 306
    growth suppressors, evading, 53, 105, 242, 301–2
    immune function (See immune function)
    inflammation (See inflammation)
    proliferative signaling (See proliferative
        signaling)
    replicative immortality, 53, 167, 302–3
    tumor microenvironment, 307
Hanahan, Douglas, 53–54, 301
Harvard Study of Adult Development, 103–4
Hashmat E., breast cancer survivor, 72–73
head and neck cancer, 24
healing
    curing versus, 29–31
    proactive healing, examples of (See
        proactive healing, examples of)
Healing Circles, 102
healing communities, 101–3
heart/cardiovascular disease
    diet and, 226, 227, 228
    lifestyle change, effect of, 74–75
    Roseto effect and, 89
    sedentary lifestyle and, 199–200
    sleep deprivation and, 172, 177
hedonic well-being, 104–5, 106
herbs, 313–14
highly processed foods, addictive nature
    of, 238
Hinckley, California tainted water case, 266
Hippocrates, 48
Hirshberg, Meg, 7, 36, 112–13, 276, 295–96
Holocaust survivors' descendants, stress
    hormone profile of, 64
Holt-Lunstad, Julianne, 98
home, removing chemicals from, 281–82
homeostatic sleep process, 165
honey, 256
hopefulness, 129
hopelessness, 34
hormone interference, and body weight, 242
hormone therapies, 56
houseguests, challenges posed by, 322–23
household chores, 209–10
Human Epigenome Project (HEP), 63
human growth hormone (HGH), 167

human papilloma virus (HPV) vaccine, 57, 58
hydroquinone, 317

Idealist, 120
immune function
   body weight and, 242
   cancer cells ability to avoid immune
      destruction, 53, 54, 99, 305
   exercise and, 207
   meditation and, 130–31
   microbiome and, 225
   sleep and, 167, 168, 185
   social support and, 98–99, 105
   stress and, 122–23, 138–39, 146
immunotherapies, 52, 57–58, 225, 305
inflammation
   body weight and, 242
   cancer growth and, 53, 54, 305, 306
   cytokines and, 135
   dairy and, 256–57
   exercise and, 207
   microbiome and, 225
   negative mind-set and, 139, 143
   sleep and, 167, 168, 175
   social support and, 98–99, 104–5, 106
   stress and, 122–23, 135, 146, 147
informational support, 117
inherited genetic mutations, 39–40
instrumental social support, 35
insulin resistance, 199
   body weight and, 242
   microbiome and, 225
integrative oncology, 9
interleukin-6 (IL-6) levels, and social
      support, 99
Irwin, Michael, 174–75, 180–81, 185
isolation, health effects of, 35–36, 98
Issa, Jean-Pierre, 63

James, LeBron, 169–70
Jana L., breast cancer survivor, 109, 112
Jones, Lee, 207
joy, 149–50

Kabat-Zinn, Jon, 130–31
kale, 254
Katz, Aaron, 41
Katz, David, 7, 230
Kennedy, John F., 8
kindness towards others, impact on genes of,
      104–5
Kushi, Lawrence (Larry), 271

labels on food, reading, 255
lapses, 323, 324
Lazar, Sara, 131–32

lead, 317
Lee C., breast cancer survivor, 32–33
leeks, 309
Lerner, Michael, 30, 101–2, 128
lifestyle, 3, 4, 291–99
   awareness of anticancer lifestyle,
      spreading, 297
   bell curve for cancer prevention and
      control, 14–16, 15
   cancer incidence and death rates
      potentially prevented by, 7–8
   cancer prevention guidelines, risk and
      mortality reduction from following,
      24, 25
   children and, 77
   diet (See diet)
   environment (See environment)
   epigenetics and, 60–63, 67–68
   exercise (See exercise)
   hallmark processes of cancer addressed
      by, 54
   interrelationship between lifestyle factors,
      71–72
   key principles of, 76
   living for health, 293–99
   love and social support (See love and social
      support)
   post-treatment healing and, 26–27
   proactive healing, examples of (See
      proactive healing, examples of)
   sleep (See sleep)
   social genomics, 60–63
   social support (See love and social support)
   standard of care and, 18–23
   stress (See stress)
   synergistic healing and (See synergy/
      synergistic healing)
   taking care of oneself first, 294–95
   tobacco consumption and, 9
light therapy, 183–84, 189
Lindsay, Diana, 27–29, 102, 129, 149–50
liver cancer, and body weight, 241
loneliness, health effects of, 35–36, 98
love and social support, 24–25, 69,
      83–121, 294
   altruistic behavior, health benefits of, 85–86
   anticancer team, building, 116–18
   Blue Zones and, 90
   cancer progression and, 98–100
   cancer's power to unite social networks,
      86–88
   Church Health and, 110–11
   community support, 90
   doctors and health care providers, role of,
      94–95
   emotional social support, 35–36

love and social support (*cont.*)
    empathy and, 97
    eudaimonic well-being, 104–5, 106, 118–20
    faith communities and, 107–11
    as foundation for lifestyle changes, 83, 294
    genetic expression and, 104–5
    giving support, health benefits of,
        85–86, 120
    group support, power of, 100–101
    guide for, 116–20
    healing communities, 101–3
    instrumental social support, 35
    isolation, effects of, 35–36, 98
    kindness towards others, impact on genes
        of, 104–5
    loneliness and isolation, effects of,
        35–36, 98
    loved ones, discussing cancer diagnosis
        with, 95–96
    Mailman's experience and, 91–94
    married partners, support of, 97–98
    medical team, selection of, 93
    pets and, 105–7
    positive mind-set and, 143–44
    purposeful living and, 103–5
    Rafte's experience and, 83–85, 86, 296
    Roseto effect and, 89
    staying connected, importance of, 88–89
    stress levels and, 98–100
    summary, 121
    synergistic effect of, 112–15
    traveling and, 325–26
    withdrawal of patient from, 96–97
loved ones, discussing cancer diagnosis with,
    95–96
loving-kindness meditation, 131, 157–58
Lowe, Leroy, 275
Lumber Liquidators, 274
lung cancer, 9
Lutgendorf, Susan, 35, 99, 100, 104–5, 112
Lyubomirsky, Sonja, 105

Maddock, Richard, 197
Mailman, Josh, 91–94, 101, 296
Man's Search for Meaning (Frankl), 104
maple syrup, 256
Markel, Howard, 48
married partners, support of, 97–98
MEA, 317
"The Median Isn't the Message" (Gould), 11
medical team, selection of, 93
meditation
    beneficial genetic expression profile
        changes resulting from, 140
    benefits of, 132–34
    compassion-based meditation, 131, 157–58

diaphragmatic breathing, 154–55
    focused-attention meditation, 131, 155–56
    guide to developing daily practice, 154–58
    immune system function and, 130–31
    mindfulness-based stress reduction
        (MBSR), 130–32
    mindfulness meditation, 131, 156
    sleep quality improvement and, 181
    stress hormone levels and, 123
    stress reduction and, 152
    Tibetan monks control of physiological
        processes through, 130
    traveling, while, 326
meditation moments, 159
Mediterranean diet, 226–29
melatonin, 165, 181
mental health
    exercise and, 197–98
    sedentary lifestyle and, 200
    sleep and, 173
mercury, 317–18
metastases, 47–48, 53, 65–67, 134. *See also*
        activating invasion and metastases
        hallmark of cancer
Michelene H., breast cancer survivor,
        113–15, 143
Michels, Karin, 227
microbiome, 56, 224–25
mind-body practices
    beneficial genetic expression profile
        changes resulting from, 140, 181
    cognitive behavioral therapy (CBT), 152,
        180, 181, 189
    deep diaphragmatic breathing, 152
    goals of, 151
    guide to, 151–60
    meditation (*See* meditation)
    mindfulness-based stress reduction
        (MBSR), 130–32, 185
    nature, being in, 153
    qigong, 140, 153
    stress and, 129–34
    tai chi (*See* tai chi)
    traveling, while, 326
    yoga (*See* yoga)
mindfulness-based stress reduction (MBSR),
        130–32, 185
mindfulness meditation, 131, 156
mineral oil, 318
Molly M., glioblastoma multiforme survivor,
        12–14, 108–9, 127, 144, 152, 295
monoclonal antibody therapies, 56
Morris, Scott, 110–11
mortality, emotions of, 124–27
motivational support, 117
movement. *See* exercise

multiple myeloma, and body weight, 241
muscle health, 200
Mustian, Karen, 208
mutation. *See* genome instability and
    mutation

napping, 190
National Cancer Act, 51
National Drinking Water Database, 260
nature, 153, 199
necrosis, 301
Nedergaard, Maiken, 175–76
negative mind-set, 139, 143
Nella A., hormone positive cancer survivor,
    243–44, 298–99
neurotransmitters, 197
newly diagnosed patients, sharing of cancer
    diagnosis with loved ones, 95–96
n of 1 (Sabin), 79
norepinephrine, 134–35, 137–38
    social support and levels of, 99
*Not the Last Goodbye: Reflections on Life,
    Death, Healing and Cancer* (Servan-
    Schreiber), 129
nutrition, guide to, 249–62
    alcohol, 258
    beverage choices, 259–61
    breakfast, 251–52
    cancer treatment, protein intake when
        undergoing, 255–56
    coffee, 261
    cooking temperature, 258–59
    dairy, 256–57
    dinner, 252–53
    eating out and, 255
    evaluating current diet, 249–51
    food groups, eating by, 251, 309–14
    green tea, 261
    health-sustaining versus health-depleting
        foods, ratio of, 249–50, *250*
    labels, reading, 254–55
    preplanning meals, 252
    redesigning your plate, 251–53
    shopping healthier, 254
    soy, 257–58
    sugar, avoiding, 255
    sugar substitutes, 256
    summary, 262
    supplements, 259
    water, 259–61
nuts, 229, 252, 311

oats, 252
obesity, 43, 232
    cancer and, 238–44
    chemical toxins and, 278

conditions negatively impacted by, 241–42
lack of exercise and, 198, 241
sleep and, 172, 173
stress and, 147
O'Keefe, Stephen, 223, 224
Okinawa Centenarian Study, 90
olive oil, 258–59
omega-6 and omega 3 fatty acids, in red
    meat, 236–37, 256–57
oncologists, selection of, 93
onion, 309
online resources
    for healing communities, 102–3
    National Drinking Water Database, 260
    volunteering opportunities, 120
organic farming, 274
organic foods, 286
organophosphates, 316
Ornish, Dean, 17, 74–76
outdoors. *See* nature
ovarian cancer
    BRCA-1 and BRCA-2 genes and risk of,
        39–40
    cancer prevention guidelines, risk and
        mortality reduction from following, 24
    social support and cancer hallmark levels
        in patients with, 99
oversleeping, 174–75
oxidative stress, and body weight, 242
oxybenzone, 318

palliative care, 50
pancreatic cancer, and body weight, 241
parabens, 273, 316
paraphenylenediamine (PPD), 318
PBDEs (polybrominated diethyl ethers), 316
PCBs (polychlorinated biphenyls), 318
peak performance, and sleep, 169–70
pears, 252
perchlorate, 316
PERC (percholoethylene
    tetrachloroethylene), 287–88
perfluorinated chemicals (PFCs), 269, 316
pets, 105–7
Phelps, Michael, 169
phthalates, 269, 273, 316
phthalate syndrome, 273
physical activity
    defined, 197
    exercise (*See* exercise)
Pink Ribbons Project, 84, 86
Pink Ribbons Volunteer desk, 84–85
plant-based diet, 226–29
plant-based proteins, 312
polyphenols, 261
polyethylene glycol (PEG), 318

positive mind-set, 128–29, 319
　cultivating, 143–44
　forced optimism versus, 128
　sleep and, 173
post-traumatic stress disorder (PTSD), 124
practical support, 116
prebiotics, 313
precancerous states, 49
precautionary principle, 277–78, 280
precision medicine, 4, 209
prehabilitation, 169
prevention. *See* cancer prevention
proactive healing, examples of
　Brucett M., breast cancer survivor,
　　133–34, 179
　Diana Lindsay, rectal and lung cancer
　　survivor, 27–29, 102, 129, 149–50
　Dorothy P., breast cancer survivor, 101,
　　112, 221–22
　Elaine W., breast cancer survivor, 19–21
　Gabe Canales, prostate cancer survivor,
　　40–42, 112, 213–14, 296
　Glenn Sabin, chronic lymphocytic
　　leukemia survivor, 76–80, 129, 206, 277
　Hashmat E., breast cancer survivor, 72–73
　Jana L., breast cancer survivor, 109, 112
　Josh Mailman, neuroendocrine cancer
　　survivor, 91–94, 101, 296
　Lee C., breast cancer survivor, 32–33
　Michelene H., breast cancer survivor,
　　113–15, 143
　Molly M., glioblastoma multiforme
　　survivor, 12–14, 108–9, 127, 144, 152, 295
　Nella A., hormone positive cancer
　　survivor, 243–44, 298–99
　Susan Rafte, metastatic breast cancer
　　survivor, 83–85, 86, 296
　Verna G., endometrial cancer survivor, 240
probiotics, 313
Proctor & Gamble, 274
proliferative signaling, 53, 54, 301
　body weight and, 242
　exercise and, 207
　obesity and, 242
　sleep and, 167
　social support and, 99, 105
prostate cancer, 17
　dairy consumption and, 256–57
　diet and, 228
　early detection of, 6, 49
　early stage low-grade cancers, treatment
　　decision for, 6, 49
　exercise and, 202–3, 208
　lifestyle change, study on effect of, 74–76
psychological impact of diagnosis, 18
purposeful living, 103–5, 295–97

qigong, 140, 153

radiation
　as carcinogen, 43
　as treatment, 51–52
radio-frequency radiation, 287
Rafte, Jane, 84
Rafte, Susan, 83–85, 86, 296
raspberries, 252
reality, embracing, 127, 295
red and processed meats, 232, 236–37
red cabbage, 254
reflective writing, 160
relapses, 323, 324
REM (rapid eye movement) sleep, 168
replicative immortality, 53, 167, 302–3
rest and recovery. *See* sleep
root vegetables, 310
Roseto effect, 89

Sabin, Glenn, 76–80, 129, 206, 277
Sanoff, Hanna, 207
Saslow, Debbie, 57
Scaravelli, Vanda, 153
SC Johnson, 274
sedentary lifestyle, 165–66
　being overweight combined with, effects
　　of, 241
　cancer incidence and, 43
　cancer survivors' reduction of, 205–6
　health problems associated with, 199–200
seeds, 229, 312
senescence, 302–3
Servan-Schreiber, David, 8, 10–12, 22, 31, 69,
　120, 129, 226, 275–76, 287, 291
shallots, 309
shinrin-yoku (forest-bathing), 199
shopping for food, 254
showerheads, adding filters to, 282
signal transduction inhibitors, 56
silicone cleaning, 288
silicone-derived emollients, 318
sitting, 196, 216. *See also* sedentary lifestyle
60 Minutes (TV show), 274
sleep, 24–25, 70, 162–95
　benefits of, 173
　body, effect on, 177
　body clock and, 162, 163
　brain cleansing during, 175–76
　cancer-related fatigue (CRF) and, 182–85
　cancer risk and prognosis and, 177–78
　chemical toxins and, 278
　circadian rhythm and, 162, 163, 164–65
　cognitive behavioral therapy-insomnia
　　(CBT-I) and, 180, 181, 189
　cycles, 167

dreaming phases of (REM sleep), 168
economic cost of lack of, 172
electricity and technology, impacts on our
    biological clock of, 165–66
guide to sleeping better (*See* sleep
    solutions, guide to)
healing powers of, 166–69
light therapy and, 183–84, 189
listening to your body, importance of,
    184–86
meditation and, 181
methods for improving, 180–82
napping and, 190
negative biological consequences of lack
    of, 162–63, 170–73
optimum amount of, 173–74, *174*
oversleeping, effects of, 174–75
peak performance and, 169–70
physical activity and, 184–85, 190, 198
routine for, 190
sleeping pills and, 179–80
stress and, 171–72, 178–79
tai chi and, 180–81
telomere shortening and lack of, 168–69
traveling, while, 326
yoga and, 182
sleeping pills, 179–80
sleep medicine, 172
sleep solutions, guide to, 187–95
bedroom and, 189
daytime activities that will improve sleep,
    189–90
evaluating sleep health, 187–88
feeling sleepy and, 192–93
health-care professional, determining
    whether to consult, 189
sleeping patterns and challenges,
    identifying, 188–89
smell and, 190
sound solutions and, 191–92
summary of, 194–95
taste barriers to, 192
using your senses to optimize sleep,
    190–93
visual stimuli and, 191
Smith, Casey, 170
social genomics, 60–63
social jet lag, 173
social support. *See* love and social support
sodium lauryl sulfate, 318
Sood, Anil, 99, 100, 112, 134–35, 240
soy/soybeans, 257–58
spices, 313–14
Spiegel, David, 100
spinach, 247, 254
steel-cut oats, 252

stress, 24–25, 69–70, 122–61, 294
acute stress, 138
bodies response to, 122–23, 137–39
cancer diagnosis, emotional stress of,
    123–24
cancer proliferation loop and, 134–35
cancer risk and progression, effect on,
    122–23, 134–36
caregivers and, 136–37
childhood abuse and neglect and, 141–43
chronic stress, 61–63, 70, 122–23, 134–39
defined, 122
dietary benefits canceled out by, 147–49
emotions of mortality, 124–27
exercise and, 197–98
fight-or-flight response and, 122
forced optimism and, 128
gene expression and, 61, 139–40
gratitude, cultivating, 144–45
guide to stress reduction (*See* stress
    reduction guide)
healthy lifestyle, impact of, 147–48, *148*
hopefulness and, 129
immune system, effect on, 122–23,
    138–39
joy and, 149–50
long-term stressors, impact of, 140
management programs, impact of,
    145–46
mind-body practices and, 129–34
positive attitude and, 128–29, 143–44
reality, embracing, 127
as saboteur of healthy intentions, 146–49
sleep deprivation and, 171–72, 178–79
social support and levels of, 98–100
telomere shortening and, 135–36, 147–48
stress reduction guide, 151–61
goals of, 151
meditation moments, 159
meditation practice, developing, 154–58
mind-body practices, types of (*See*
    mind-body practices)
reflective writing, 160
summary of steps to de-stress, 161
stroke, 172, 200, 227, 228
Subway, 274
sugar, 233–34, 255
sugar substitutes, 235, 256
sunflower oil, 258
supplements, 227
support groups, 100–101
surgical treatment, 50–52
synergy/synergistic healing, 24–26, 73–80
defined, 24
diet and, 247–48
environment and, 278–79

synergy/synergistic healing (*cont.*)
    exercise and, 197–99
    love and social support and, 112–15
    system K4, 288

tai chi, 61
    beneficial genetic expression profile
        changes resulting from, 140, 181
    cancer-related fatigue (CRF) and, 185
    sleep quality improvement and, 180–81
    stress reduction and, 153
talc, 318
targeted cancer therapies, 52, 55–57
tea, 261
telomerase, 136, 303
telomere attrition, 136
Telomere Effect, The (Epel), 128–29, 303
telomeres, 303
    sleep deprivation and, 168–69
    stress and, 135–36, 147–48
Terry, Luther L., 8
therapy dogs, 105–7
Thomson, Cynthia, 244–45, 246–47
Tibetan monks, 130
tobacco consumption, 8–10
    benefits of quitting smoking, 44
    as carcinogen, 43
    in combination with alcohol use, 44–45
toluene, 318
Totten, Zoe Finch, 249
Townsend, Jeffrey, 66
Toxic Substances Control Act of 1976, 268
toxins. *See* environment/environmental
    toxins
traveling, staying healthy while, 322–23,
    325–28
    diet and, 327–28
    environment and, 328
    exercise and, 218–19, 326–27
    mind-body practice and, 326
    planning ahead, 325
    sleep and, 326
    social support and, 325–26
triclosan, 271, 273, 317
True Health Initiative, 7
tumorigenesis, 305–6
tumor microenvironment, 307
2,5-dichlorophenol, 271

Unilever, 274
United Nations online volunteering
    options, 120

vaccines targeting cancer-causing viruses,
    57, 58
vagal tone, and altruistic behavior, 85–86

vaporized nicotine (vaping), 9
vascular endothelial growth factor (VEGF)
    levels, and social support, 99
vasculogenesis, 303
vegetables, 227, 228–29, 232
    alliums, 309
    cruciferous vegetables, 228–29, 245–46,
        254, 309
    daily cooking, tips for, 253–54
    food groups, eating by, 309–10
    redesigning meals to include, 251–53
    root vegetables, 310
Verna G., endometrial cancer
    survivor, 240
vinyl chloride, 269
viral infections, 43
Volunteer Match, 120
volunteer work, 85–86, 120

Waldinger, Robert, 104
walking, 209–10
walnut oil, 258
Warburg, Otto, 304
Wargo, Jennifer, 225
water, 259–61, 282
Watson, Cheryl, 277
weight gain, 177
Weinberg, Robert, 53–54, 301
wet cleaning, 288
whole grains, 229, 252, 312
Willett, Walter, 240–41
Williams, Venus, 170
withdrawal of patient, 96–97
Women's Healthy Eating and Living (WHEL)
    Study, 244–46, *245*
A World Without Cancer: The Making of a
    New Cure and the Promise of Prevention
    (Cuomo), 269–70
World Trade Center attack of
    September 11, 2001, cancers
    associated with, 266–67
Wu, Xifeng, 235

Yehuda, Rachel, 64
yoga, 61, 132, 133
    beneficial genetic expression profile
        changes resulting from, 140
    cancer-related fatigue (CRF) and, 185
    sleep quality improvement and, 182
    stress hormone levels and, 123
    stress reduction and, 153
    traveling, while, 326
yogurt, 252

Zahrt, Octavia, 211
Zimmerman, Michael, 265